Perceptions of

Phobia *and* Phobics

The Quest for Control

The sketches on the title page and on page 64 are by Sipke Huismans, Dutch graphic artist.

(These sketches represent the phenomenon of "it", the spatial-emotional dimensions of the mother-child relations underlying depersonalization and derealization)

Perceptions of
Phobia *and* Phobics
The Quest for Control

BEULAH McNAB
Senior Lecturer of the former Department of Personality and Clinical Psychology, University of Amsterdam, The Netherlands

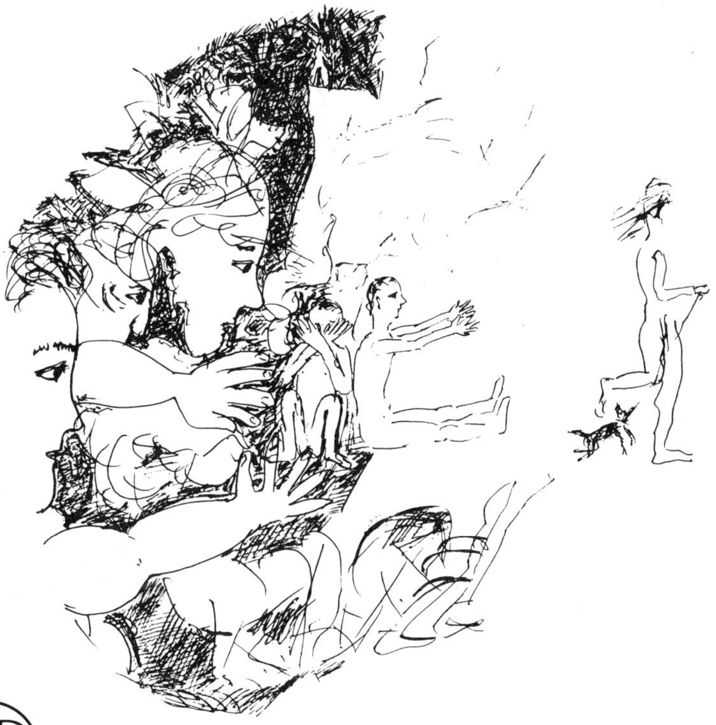

ACADEMIC PRESS
Harcourt Brace & Company, Publishers
London San Diego New York Boston Sydney Tokyo Toronto

This book is printed on acid-free paper.

Academic Press Limited
24–28 Oval Road
London NW1 7DX

United States edition published by
Academic Press Inc.
San Diego, CA 92101

A catalogue record for this book is available from the British Library

ISBN 0-12-485960-7

Typeset by Mathematical Composition Setters Ltd, Salisbury, Wiltshire
Printed and bound in Great Britain by The University Printing House, Cambridge.

Contents

Credits

Grateful acknowledgement is made to the following authors and publishers for permission to quote from their works:

Chapter I, pages 3–6: I.M. Marks. *Living with Fear. Understanding and Coping with Anxiety*, pages 79, 80, 81, 98 and 99. Copyright 1978 by McGraw-Hill, Incorporated, New York. Reprinted with permission of the author and publisher.

Chapter II, pages 14–17: R.L. Gregory. "The Confounded Eye". In: R.L. Gregory & E.H. Gombrich. *Illusions in Nature and Art*, chapter 2, pages 50, 56–57, 76–78 and 94. Copyright 1973 by Gerald Duckworth and Company, Ltd., London; R.L. Gregory. *Concepts and Mechanisms of Perception*, pages xviii–v, xx, 50, 199, 348, 354, 374, 590, 592–3, 596, 597 and 599. Copyright 1974 by Gerald Duckworth and Company, Ltd., London. Excerpts from both works reprinted with permission of the author and publisher.

Pages 17–25 and 31–32: J.J. Gibson. *The Ecological Approach to Visual Perception*, pages xiii, 8, 9, 12, 16, 32, 49, 52, 56, 75, 79, 107, 116, 117, 118, 122, 128, 135, 137, 139, 178, 194, 195, 197, 205, 219, 223, 245, 247 and 250. Copyright 1979 (originally) by Houghton Mifflin Company, Boston, Massachusetts, now by Lawrence Erlbaum Associates, Inc., Hillsdale, New Jersey. Reprinted with permission of the late author's wife, E.J. Gibson, and the publisher, Lawrence Erlbaum Associates, Inc.

Pages 21, 24 and 25: J.J. Gibson. *The Senses Considered as Perceptual Systems*, pages 280, 303–304. Copyright 1966 by James J. Gibson. Reprinted with permission of the late author's wife, E.J. Gibson, and the publisher, Houghton Mifflin Company, Boston, Massachusetts.

Pages 25–27: J.A. Fodor and Z.W. Pylyshyn. "How direct is visual perception? Some reflections on Gibson's 'Ecological Approach'," pages 141, 147, 148 and 152. In: *Cognition*, vol. 9, pp. 139–196. Copyright 1981 by Elsevier Science Publishers B.V. Amsterdam. Reprinted with permission of the publisher.

Pages 28, 33 and 34: in R. Shaw & J. Bransford (eds.). *Perceiving, Acting and Knowing. Towards an Ecological Psychology*. W.M. Mace. "James J. Gibson's strategy for perceiving", page 44; K.H. Pribram. "Some comments on the nature of the perceived universe", page 94; M.T. Turvey. "Preliminaries to a Theory of Action with reference to Vision", pages 214 and 257. Copyright 1977 by Lawrence Erlbaum Associates, Inc., Hillsdale, New Jersey. Reprinted with permission of the publisher.

Page 34: D. Marr. *Vision. A computational investigation into the human representation and processing of visual information*, page 30. Copyright 1982 by W.H. Freeman and Company, San Francisco and New York. Reprinted with permission of the publisher.

Pags 35–36: K.H. Pribram. *Brain and Perception. Holonomy and Structure in Figural Processing*, pages 14–16. Copyright 1991 by Lawrence Erlbaum Associates, Inc., New Jersey. Reprinted with permission of the publisher.

Acknowledgements

First and foremost to my promotor, Nico Frijda, Professor of Psychological Functions at the University of Amsterdam who, on the death of his friend, Johan Barendregt, took over where he had left off, guiding this work to completion and making the process memorable by his literary good sense, astringent wit and kind heart. And, by all these services to his late friend, thereby allowing me to benefit from his enduring care. My debt to him is profound.

In memory of the late Bob Nieuwenhuyse and Ron Ramsay, professors of psychology at the same university: my gratitude to the former for a pleasurable collaboration on the height-distance ratio [H/D] experiments (in Chapter V); to the latter for enlightening comments while reading Part One a few months before his death. To two other professors at this university many thanks: Erie Fournier (now emeritus), who encouraged me to speculate on the implications of my investigations for her field of child psychology; and Jan Elshout, for his brief and splendid comment on the work.

My gratitude extends also to Pieter Boeke, Emeritus Professor of Clinical Psychology (University of Groningen), and to Henk Barendregt, Professor of Mathematical Logic (University of Nijmegen) and eldest son of Johan Barendregt, for their memorable rôles as opponents of the work at my inauguration into the scientific community.

Without the interest, enthusiasm, support and criticism of a number of colleagues at the University of Amsterdam this work would have been less inspired: Wim Brinkman, psychologist, behavioural therapist, and psychoanalyst; Boudewijn Chabot, psychiatrist and psychotherapist; Peter van Haasen, child diagnostician and clinical psychologist; Jaap van Heerden, psychologist, methodologist and philosopher; and especially Igor van Krogten, clinical psychologist, personality theorist and adept of Proust and Musil, and Floris Pelgrim (University of Leiden), clinical psychologist and psychotherapist, who not only critically and patiently read the whole text but also shared with me his professional and intimate knowledge of the nature of phobic experiences.

To all the patients who remain unnamed but from whom I have learned much; and to those students who carried out the greater part of the investigations cheerfully, a special thanks.

To the supporting cast in the wings, who know themselves without being named, my gratitude for gifts of help and healing, great and small.

To Sipke Huismans, Dutch graphic artist and director of the AKI [*Akademie voor Beeldende Kunst*] in Enschede, who visualized the phenomenon of "it", the spatial-emotional dimensions of the mother-child relations underlying depersonalization and derealization, for his conception, understanding and care, a special mention.

My thanks too to my editor, Andrew Carrick, Kate Brewin, and Sutapas Bhattacharya, and to Academic Press and its staff for their generous help and painstaking efforts in preparing the manuscript for publication, which have been inestimable.

Last but certainly not least, a profound debt of gratitude is due to the Greats in psychology, Ernest Hilgard, Karl Pribram, Hans Eysenck and Adriaan de Groot. I am also indebted to James Pennebaker (*The Psychology of Physical Symptoms*, 1982) and to Thomas Lombardo (*The Reciprocity of Perceiver and Environment*, 1987). By their warm reception of the work and critical appreciation of my attempts to build bridges across disciplines and integrate seemingly unrelated facts, they allowed it to pass from the dark into the light, a tribute to Johan Barendregt.

Preface

The work in this book forms one small part of an innovative, perhaps even revolutionary project that was initiated and built up by Johan Barendregt, who held the Chair of Personality and Clinical Psychology at the University of Amsterdam from 1962–1982. Before taking up this post, as a postgraduate he was a member of J.J. Groen's multidisciplinary team doing research on medical, psychiatric and psychological problems, the *Psychosomatische Werkgroep* in the Academic Hospital, Wilhelmina Gasthuis in Amsterdam. This team was subsidized by the Rockefeller Foundation.

In his capacity as a member of this team, Barendregt worked for a short period at the Maudsley Hospital in London with Hans Eysenck, studying his techniques. On his return to Amsterdam he completed his dissertation (1954) on psychosomatic specificity in patients suffering from asthma-bronchialis [promotor: Adriaan de Groot]. Together with his first promovendus, G.J. Wilde, he would later develop the ABV (*Amsterdamse Biografische Vragenlijst*), which is still used as a clinical diagnostic instrument.

Becoming increasingly sceptical about the then prevailing psychological doctrines and the reductionistic, often piecemeal and intuitive-individualistic approaches in the investigation of complex psychological behaviours; and desirous of building a solid scientific foundation on which the study of the psychological personality and clinical psychology could be based, on assuming the Chair of Personality and Clinical Psychology, he conceived a plan that would later take form in what became known as the Amsterdam *Phobia-project, from different perspectives.*

In this school he gathered around him about thirty, mainly young researchers and a few experienced clinicians, and attempted to train us to become a multidisciplinary team in our approach to personality and clinical problems. Each one of the group was allotted a specific field in which to become competent – emotion and motivation, learning, cognition, perception, social interaction and interpersonal aspects, neurophysiology, neuropsychology, developmental psychology, psychodiagnostics, and therapeutic applications. He hoped that, by allowing us room to become experts in our own field, while participating in frequent discussions to disseminate one's ideas and fructify one another's, we would together arrive at a profound scientific understanding of a given clinical syndrome or personality problem.

He built up a tripartite institute – research, diagnostics and therapy – and used it also as a training-base for generations of graduate students. Each new clinical graduate who was a product of this school would be skilled not only in diagnostics and therapeutic applications but also in competent research procedures. To avoid this project developing into a tower of Babel, he chose to concentrate all efforts on one specific syndrome, one which he then thought might be relatively simple to tackle and which would quickly yield to this concerted effort, namely, phobia. In so doing, he aimed to achieve a proper scientific understanding of phobia, so that therapeutic intervention could more appropriately take into account the different characteristics of aetiological importance in different individuals. His line of reasoning was as follows:

Phobic and normal groups differ significantly on many variables. Although individual phobics deviate from the normal range, they do so on different variables. These differences in deviations from the normal range on different variables may indicate that phobics differ in characteristics that may be of aetiological importance even when their symptoms are relatively homogeneous. Therapists from different schools rely on different concepts to study and alter behaviour. These concepts differ in their appropriateness to account for different aetiological factors. Thus phobics might profit more from therapy whose central concept agrees best with and therefore can account better for their individual characteristics of aetiological importance (Barendregt, 1975).

But the project was doomed to fail; and its demise was hastened by the untimely death of its innovator. Why was this promise not fulfilled? Is no human endeavour in principle realizable in its pristine beauty? Or is it because a group of people, in which all compete for the highest honour or for a try at the brass ring, will inevitably tend to undermine one another's efforts rather than cooperate to achieve together the desired goal? Is it because the innovator himself was a man of strongly opposed tendencies, each warring within himself to gain ascendancy over the others? A chess-player of stature, he described his approach to life and to science in the following terms: "One is always the opposer, the contradictor, the underminer. I am always playing chess: if you claim something, I will refute it. There was a time in psychology when one came nearest to the truth by contravention." (Barendregt, 1982). One of his early collaborators, a psychiatrist of repute, summed up his scientific persona succinctly. "Hermeneutic among the methodologists, methodologist among the hermeneutic." (A. van Dantzig, 1989, in an interview with the author).

He was a nominalist in his philosophical orientation, and a pessimist about human nature. Extremely shrewd of mind, creative and inventive in his own work, a pace-maker in psychology, he was also an iconoclast, a scourge of the sacred cows of others. A thwarter par excellence he would, with flair and erudition, destroy the arguments of friend and foe alike, and take obvious delight in doing so. He was also a man unafraid to show to the discerning his softer side. Sometimes he would come to the laboratory in the early morning with shining eyes, fresh from a dewy perambulation around his garden, where as he would tell me he had counted before breakfast at least twelve new flowers that had opened their faces to the sun for the first time that year, and give me the Latin names of each and a little treatise on their care.

Yet at another moment, and even on the same day, he would gleefully dampen my enthusiasm for some new discovery in psychology by sombrely reflecting on the state of the art in psychology today, warning that my efforts too would come to nothing. In still another moment, frustrated by the slow pace at which my work progressed, he would stick his head around the door of my room, and say: "If you'd read less and think more, we'd progress faster", leaving me to cope with my mental disarray at this remark.

This book describes my own little odyssey within the greater whole. My field of competence is perception, and my secondary love the psychodynamics of being. This is a story of a voyage of discovery; but, like some creative processes, it begins at sea.

Almost all the experimental work had been done before I arrived at a less confused understanding of the nature of the information available to perceptual systems, of perceptual process, and of perceptual control. As I shall try to make clear, not all of this confusion is due to hardheadedness on my part, but may reflect the state of knowledge on these subjects in psychology today. Only after I had reluctantly let go of the axioms of the representational approach for long enough to explore other models (for example, the ecological one), did light enter the tunnel and the way out become clearer. As I moved backward to the beginning but forward in time, I glimpsed possible ways in which these approaches might be reconciled. Whether these insights contribute anything real to our knowledge of perceptual aspects of phobia, or are merely chimeras of an overheated or hallucinating brain, only time will tell.

The relative neglect of perceptual systems other than the visual one in this study may turn out to be a serious error. However, it is my hope that the more inclusive view on perceptual control opted for here may partially compensate for this omission. Since the basic principles described for vision may apply equally well to other perceptual systems and their functions, the reader will find the problem of generalization to these a relatively simple one.

What may one hope to find in this book? In science, as in life, one likes to be prepared for what is to come. Only in detective stories would this spoil all the fun. This is a detective story of sorts, wherein clue upon clue is piled as the story progresses (some of them misleading too) until the picture becomes clearer and possible solutions present themselves. But there are some in science who dislike detective stories, and who will not even read a work that does not first spell out what one may expect to find within. If you, the reader, are a lover of detective stories, move straight to Chapter I. If you are a no-nonsense scientist, though, with little inclination for suspense, then read on.

Chapter I is the only chapter in the book specifically concerned with theoretical definitions in theories of phobia (although Chapter III is an in-depth discussion on the merits and shortcomings of the psychodynamic approach). One will look in vain for comparisons between contemporary theories of phobia in this work, and in this the title of the book may be a little misleading. In tracing the historical roots in phobia in Chapter I, I argue for a multi-dimensional approach in understanding phobia. For even if our inferences are merely based on what patients over the centuries have told us about their experiences, it is clear that phobia must be multiply determined and can only fully be understood from different perspectives.

Chapter II contains a more general treatment of contemporary theories of perception, organized around three important questions which still are not definitively answered:

1. the nature of the information available to perceptual systems;
2. the nature of perceptual process; and
3. the nature of perceptual control.

The problems involved demonstrate the limitations of the theoretical assumptions and empirical findings of contemporary perception theorists. So as not to swamp the reader with a dissection of all the fruit on the many-splendoured tree of perception, these problems are discussed by focusing on the controversy still raging today between theorists who support the representational standpoint and those who support the ecological one. Briefly, the representational standpoint views perception as an inferential activity that is mediated by internal representations (models) of an essentially unknowable world. In this view, perception entails a construction of reality and is thus indirect. The ecological standpoint views perception as essentially a non-inferential activity, perceptual systems being geared to a direct pickup of information from an in principle knowable and highly structured world. The perceiver discovers, rather than constructs, persisting and changing relations in the information available in the surrounding stimulation. Both schools of thought view perception as a cognitive function, as the first source of knowledge about the environment. In assessing the pros and cons of these theories and the experimental efforts to substantiate these, I make a plausible argument for the need to reconcile both standpoints.

In Chapter III I discuss the theoretical approaches to neurosis and phobia of three contemporary clinicians (Freud, Matte-Blanco, and Barendregt) who can be classified as psychodynamic in orientation. In doing so, I show the weaknesses and strengths of Freud's ideas, which are to some extent compensated and made falsifiable by the work and thought of Matte-Blanco and of Barendregt. From a perceptual point of view, all three clinicians belong to the representational school of thought. All three also try to provide answers to the three fundamental questions of perception delineated earlier; but for obvious reasons (being clinicians) are mostly concerned with the third question, that of control. However, as I briefly describe their dilemma, one comes to see that, having provided plausible answers to the nature of process and control, they remain nonplussed by the nature of the information available to perceptual systems in neurosis and psychosis.

At this point I backtrack to the content of Chapter II in which, to my mind, some answers to their dilemma are provided. Drawing the theoretical and empirical work from general perceptual theory and that from clinical theory and practice together, I show how many puzzles can be resolved. This forms the content of Chapter IV, that is, the answer to the question which perplexed the clinicians – the nature of the information available to perceptual systems that initiates and maintains the phobia or neurosis. This is not achieved, though, without raising new and intriguing questions (for example, those relating to perceptual process and the dynamics of control in normal and phobic behaviours). With this problem addressed, Part One [Theoretical Issues] is concluded.

Part Two [An Empirical Inquiry] begins in Chapter V with my own experimental work on perception, which was designed to solve the question of the information actually available to phobic patients (and to normal people) in situations that have been clinically described as phobogenic. I contrast my findings with those of others in the literature representing the different schools of thought, and show that the representational approach may not be as adequate as has been supposed to explain the findings. The results of this inquiry into the nature of the information available to perceptual systems might rightly lead one to conclude that, in the area of affective psychophysics, one can go above and beyond Berlyne.

In Chapter VI, concerned with the strategies of perceptual control that emerge from the data in the previous chapter, it becomes clear that in perceptual process, the assumptions of the representationists regarding mechanisms of constancy seem to provide a more adequate explanation of the findings than, at present, the assumptions of the ecologists.

In Chapters VII to IX, which describe my own findings regarding the nature of perceptual control in normals and phobics, we see that these data cannot be understood properly without Gibson's contributions to the study of perception in his ecological approach. Nor, I might add, without taking into consideration what psychodynamic theorists and clinicians tell us about the nature of neurosis and phobia.

In Chapter X [General Discussion], I show that the apparently circuitous route, through perceptual theory and clinical theory, through empirical work in both fields, has been a very fruitful one. Not only can we describe with much more certainty than before the effective variables operating in normal and phobic perception in daily situations (which yield such strong feelings of anxiety and avoidance); but this peregrination shows more clearly than ever which problems still remain to be addressed (for example, the mechanisms of constancy, conflict, and control). Also, the relative weaknesses and strengths of the different theoretical approaches are discussed in this context. As in earlier chapters (especially Chapter VI), I briefly review certain behaviours which yield symptom formation and displacement of symptoms, in showing how these are directly linked to perceptual and cognitive issues. In this context, reasons are proposed why certain therapeutic methods might be more, and others less effective in treating these behaviours.

These findings indicate that simplistic theories of phobia and neurosis, and partial understanding of the nature of perception which adherence to one or other school of thought necessarily implicates, prevent us from obtaining a clear, rounded picture of the phenomenon under discussion; this, notwithstanding the fact that limits are imposed on our understanding of pathological behaviour by viewing it only from the perspective of perception.

In memory of my father, James Henry McNab,
who nurtured my love for both the sciences and the arts;
and Johan Barendregt, Professor of Psychology
at the University of Amsterdam (1962–1982),
who further educated me in both domains
by his critical, inquiring mind,
caustic wit and gentle art of
making enemies

PART ONE

THEORETICAL ISSUES

No, no, go not to Lethe, neither twist
  Wolf's-bane, tight-rooted, for its poisonous wine;
Nor suffer thy pale forehead to be kiss'd
  By nightshade, ruby grapes of Proserpine;
Make not your rosary of yew-berries,
  Nor let the beetle nor the death-moth be
    Your mournful Psyche, nor the downy owl
A partner in your sorrow's mysteries;
  For shade to shade will come too drowsily,
    And drown the wakeful anguish of the soul.

John Keats, 1820, *Ode on Melancholy*

I

Introduction

Statement of the Problem

In the context of this study, perception is defined as an epistemic act, that is, as the first source of knowledge of organisms (human or animal) in a given habitat. Perception in this sense implies an interaction between conscious, though not necessarily self-conscious, organisms and their environment, whereby relevant information may be abstracted and acted upon to facilitate successful adaptation to prevailing conditions. For the human being, the natural environment includes physical, phenomenal and socio-cultural structures, which in principle are available in a given habitat.

In this context I shall use the term *perceptual control* in a dual capacity, to refer on the one hand to the constraints imposed on perceptual systems by the nature of environmental stimulation and, on the other, to the regulating, guiding and steering perceptual actions resulting from information thus acquired.

Within this frame of reference I shall try to establish the grounds for the hypothesis that in the perception of phobic persons, and probably in that of others with allied clinical complaints, certain configurations of objects, structures and/or events that define environmental relations are systematically distorted. This distortion involves substantial over- and under-estimation of parameters of environmental conditions. This, in turn, may give rise to experiences of being overpowered and/or alienated by the environment, as well as to experiences of instability in or fluctuation of (parts of) the surround. The frequency and intensity of these experiences are such that severe disorientation may occur. If this disorientation persists, it will soon be accompanied by other experiences of derealization and depersonalization. In this view, the phobic phenomenon, at least in part, can be understood in terms of problems of perceptual control, as symptomatic of inadequate attempts to come to grips with reality.

In many psychological theories of phobia the environment is given only cursory attention, amounting to little more than to represent it as the inappropriate substitute for unresolved psychic conflict. Though environmental structure may assume such function in neurosis, it deserves more attention than this, seeing that aspects of its structure play a rôle in phobia which are not randomly selected, nor random in their effects. On the contrary, they form an integral component of the phobic phenomenon.

Throughout the ages sufferers from phobia have intuitively recognized the importance of environmental conditions to their complaints, and have been impressed by their impelling effects. The pull of these has often been so great that, even when through therapeutic intervention they have been enlightened about the real source of their troubles, these patients have been unable to ignore the environmental contribution.

Clinical theorists, on the other hand, impressed by the strength and tenacity of the phobic reaction, have tended to play down the environmental aspect and sought to explain it in terms of repressed traumatic experiences, or of intractable habits. However, though environmental effects are of greater significance to the complaint than many clinicians suspect, these comprise only one of the components of rather complex interactions between person and environment. Insofar as psychological theories of phobia have been reluctant to give due weight to its multiple determinants, these have gone astray. The tendency of many theorists to lose sight of other important factors while concentrating on the ones they advocate may have contributed not a little to the present confusion in definition of phobia. For example, and depending on the viewpoint of the theorist, phobia is defined by:

> The ramification of the fears that occur in anxiety neurosis (the latter being produced by anything) which withholds somatic sexual tension from the psychical and interferes with its elaboration within the psychical field (Freud's earliest formulation, 1892); a projection in that (phobias) replace an internal, instinctual danger by an external, perceptual one (his later formulation, 1936, p. 40).

In the latter formulation, Freud qualified this definition by the statement that the instinctual danger, fear of castration, is a pressing problem only because its expression would involve an external danger, the danger of loss of love or separation, or even moral or social anxiety ("Gewissensangst"). "Thus what happens in a phobia in the last resort is merely that one external danger is replaced by another" (p. 40).

> A persistent, excessive fear attached to an object or a situation that, objectively, is not a significant source of danger (Frazier & Carr, p. 906, in Freedman & Kaplan,1967).
> A conditioned fear response to what was originally a neutral stimulus, or by second-order conditioning (Wolpe, p. 182, in Spielberger, 1966).
> The avoidance of a rôle-relevant situation because, as the patient says, in this situation he or she is too emotional, mostly too anxious (Barendregt's ostensive definition, 1972, p. 107); an unpleasant experience, whose cause is wholly or partially wrongly situated by the patient. By adhering to this error, the situation is avoided (his essential definition, 1974, p. 295).

Nor has the *embarras de richesse* of symptoms accompanying the phobic reaction made classification tasks any easier. In fact, such is the state of affairs that many authorities (cf. Freedman & Kaplan, 1967) would prefer to view phobias rather as symptoms that are superimposed on, or extensions of, other, more basic personality configurations or reactions than as distinct syndromes.

That such a state of affairs hardly entails an advance on ancient conceptualizations, and from a certain standpoint may even be said to represent retrogression, I shall illustrate by a brief digression to the historical roots. Yet the main reason for this digression is to highlight the parallels in the phenomenon, by comparing contemporary descriptions of phobia with ancient ones. For though the determinants of phobia may be multiple, its protean manifestations could be mere illusion; illusion that masks fundamental consistency in its structure.

In Search of the Origins of Phobia: Descriptions and Definitions Through the Ages

The phobic phenomenon has occurred in all ages and probably in all cultures, and its symptoms and pluriformity of appearance have been noted and documented in myth, literature and clinical description from ancient times up to the present. Formerly subsumed under Melancholia, Neurasthenia and Anxiety Hysteria, it disappeared for a while from view but flourished nevertheless. As a distinct syndrome it reappeared once again in the mid-19th century in a publication by Westphal (1871).

The insights of the ancients rivalled our own, as their observations and descriptions of the phenomenon show. These agree so well with ours that, but for the quaint language, they could have been lifted from contemporary dossiers. Nor were their explanations of the complaint any less bizarre.

The term *phobia* is said to derive from the Greek word *Phobos*. In Greek mythology *Phobos* (Fright) was one of the sons or squires of *Ares*, god of war. Together with his brother *Deimos* (Fear), and supported by the companions *Eris* (Strife), insatiable in her fury, *Enyo*, she who destroys cities, and the *Keres*, sombre divinities eager to drink the black blood of the dying, he accompanied *Ares* on the battlefield, sowing disease and striking terror and fright in all beings who crossed their paths (Guirand, 1963).

The ancient Greeks tended to describe classes of phenomena outside their control and prediction by mythical representation, thereby achieving some understanding of the forces of nature (in both her human and physical aspects) in terms of gods who not only rule the visible world, but also the fortune and the hearts of men, as Bowra (1957) notes. Indeed, their powers of observation were formidable. The qualities attributed to *Phobos* and his retinue describe without doubt, and in apt detail, the traits and states of this pathological condition.

To the ancient Greeks and Romans, and to those of earlier and later civilizations, the morbid fears currently described in contemporary dossiers were well-known phenomena. Fear of arcadian places, of heights, walking alone far from home, fear of the dark, and the like, are expressed in the following excerpts. Even hints are given that some of these fears may have had sexual overtones. Arcadian places were often associated with the cult of *Pan* (later incorporated in the retinue of *Dionysus* or *Bacchus*). In the fertility rites of those times matrons and maids, in large companies, would spend whole nights on the bare hills in dances which simulated ecstasy, and in an intoxication partly alcoholic, partly mystical. According to Bertrand Russell (1949; 1974), husbands found the practice annoying, but did not dare to oppose religion. But the proverbial Arcadia, which townsmen imagined to be idyllic, was really full of barbaric horrors; and not less so in (pre-)medieval times:

> At every rustle of breeze he quakes, he starts at every sound (*Omnes se terrent auras, sonus excitat omnis – Virgil*, 70–19 B.C.)
>
> One is afraid of the fall of the cruets, another will not drink, as fancying himself a brick, and fearing he should be dissolved by the liquid (*Aretaeus of Cappodocia*, circa A.D. 30–90).
>
> Some there are who dared not to be alone in the dark for fear of hobgoblins and devils; he suspects every thing he hears or sees to be a devil, or enchanted, and imagineth a

thousand chimeras and visions which in his thinking he certainly sees, bugbears, talks with black men, ghosts, goblins (*Galen*, circa A.D. 130–200).

Another dares not to go over a bridge, come near a pool, rock or steep hill, for fear he be tempted to hang, drown or precipitate himself (*Ibn Sina/Avicenna*, circa A.D. 980–1037).

And 'tis strange what women and children will conceive unto themselves, if they go over a churchyard in the night, lie alone or be alone in a dark room, how they sweat and tremble on a sudden (Many, but not all quotations from ancient writings derive from Robert Burton, 1621/1972.)

Compare such descriptions with excerpts taken from contemporary dossiers of phobics (Marks, 1978):

I would give anything to be helped with my phobia because I'm afraid of losing my job. If there is a storm while I'm on a bus, for instance, I scream and feel sick and have an upset stomach afterwards. People think I'm crazy. I can't stop myself when a storm is on, but I'm just as frightened and hysterical when I'm with people during a storm.

A fear of open spaces has been at times very pronounced. Many a time I have slunk in alleys instead of keeping on the broad streets, and have often walked long distances, a mile or more, to avoid crossing some pasture or open square. I cannot bear to look across any wide expanse of water, feeling almost impelled to jump in out of sheer desperation.

I was taken suddenly with "spells" while I was attending a funeral of a relative. After a boy in the village was murdered, I almost feared to be alone, was afraid to go to the barn in the daytime, and suffered when put to bed at night. During the months which followed, I experienced the first symptoms of agoraphobia. One evening while coasting with other boys in the neighbourhood, I experienced an uncomfortable feeling each time I returned to the top of the hill. Since then I dread high things, to ascend anything high; an immense building or a high rocky bluff fills me with dread.

On the street I feel I am walking on shifting ground which is always falling or rising like a deck of a pitching and rolling ship.

On the street my legs feel like they are made of jelly and like I'm walking on cotton wool.

As it is today, these fears were found to occur more often in women than in men. Men in ancient times confessed more often to fear of assemblies and public places. As far back as the days of Homer, *agon* denoted an assembly, a meeting-place of the people usually for the discussion of public affairs, games or contests. Contests might be athletic, or a poetic competition, or a mental one between dramatists. Any such contest was known as an *agonia*. Another word for the *agon* was the *agora* (or public place where *agonias* took place). The term *agonia*, which later came to mean mental anguish specifically, originally referred to any testing of one's skills in one or other rôle. Today we call those who fear such tests of their skills in assemblies or public places *social phobics*, and those who fear open places *agoraphobics*. Hardly progress.

Hippocrates of Cos, a contemporary of Socrates (469–399 B.C.), described these agoraphobics as:

Men who feared that which need not be feared (...), who dared not come in company for fear he should be misused, disgraced, overshoot himself in gesture or speech, or be sick; he thinks every man observes him, aims at him, derides him, owes him malice.

> Another through bashfulness, suspicion, and timorousness will not be seen abroad, loves darkness as life, and cannot endure the light, or to sit in lightsome places, his hat in his eyes, he will neither see nor be seen by his good will (*Lib. de insania et melancholia*).

Fear overwhelmed many men who were to speak or show themselves in public assemblies or before great personages. Tully confessed that he still trembled at the beginning of his speech; and Demosthenes too before Phillipus.

> It confounds the voice so much afraid of his auditory, when he was to make a speech to the rest of the gods, that he could not utter a ready word, but was compelled to use Mercury's help in prompting (*Lucian, circa A.D. 120, Jupiter Tragoedus*).
>
> Many lamentable effects this fear causeth in man, as to be red, pale, tremble, sweat; it makes sudden cold and heat to come over all the body, palpitation of the heart, syncope. It hinders most honourable attempts and makes the heart ache, sad, heavy. They that live in fear are never merry, resolute, secure, but in continued pain. No greater misery, no rack, no torture like unto it; ever suspicious, anxious, solicitous, they are childishly drooping without reason, without judgment (*Plutarch, circa A.D. 45–120*).
>
> They fear where there is no ground for fear, they are alarmed at trifles (*Gordonius*). Although not all alike, some fear with an extraordinary and mighty fear (*Altomarus*). Some fear all alike, some certain men, and cannot endure their companies, are sick of them, or if they be from home. Some suspect treason, still others are afraid of their nearest and dearest friends (*Melanelius; Galen; Ruffus; Aëtius; in Burton*, 1621).

Hippocrates, who decried the attribution of these and other diseases to supernatural powers, indicates how various forms were blamed on different gods:

> If he utter a piercing and loud cry, they liken him to a horse and blame Poseidon (...). If he foam at the mouth and kick, Ares has the blame. When at night occur fears and terrors, delirium, jumpings from the bed and rushings out of doors, they say Hecate is attacking or that heroes are assaulting.

Excellent descriptions of what is nowadays called *social phobia*, complete with hyperventilation. Whereas in earlier times this occurred mostly in men, now that women are allowed into the modern *agoras* they, too, suffer from these fears; though to a lesser degree than men. Of more interest is the fact that the relating of these fears to (fear of) inadequacy or deficiency in the performance of one's rôle, whether in a physical or mental domain, is not new but of ancient origin (cf. Barendregt's definition of phobia, 1972; and recently, Van Zuuren, 1982).

Marks (1978) notes as characteristic of social phobics "the awareness of being observed and the inability to perform as long as anybody is watching". A glance from someone else will precipitate a panic. As one person said: "When I go out to eat in strange places I cannot eat, my throat feels a quarter of an inch wide, and I sweat". The fear is usually worse in smart, crowded restaurants, and less in the safety of the home.

> For fear of shaking, blushing, sweating, or looking ridiculous some affected persons will not sit facing another passenger in a bus or train, nor walk past a waiting line of people. They are terrified of attracting attention by behaving awkwardly or fainting. Some will avoid talking to superiors, and stage fright will prevent them from appearing in front of an audience. Social phobics are often afraid even to write in public (e.g., sign a check at a bank), or even handle money in front of others. For fear of shaking, a secretary may

> become unable to take dictation, a teacher may stop writing on a black-board in front of a class, an assembly line worker finds it impossible to perform routine acts necessary for assembling a product in a factory.
>
> One of these phobic patients described his inability to cope in these situations as follows: "Times more than I recall I have gone into restaurants or dining rooms, ordered a meal and left it untouched (...). Times more than I recall I have bought tickets to theatres, concerts, fairs or whatnot, merely to give them away when the critical moment arrived and I realised the impossibility of my facing the throng with composure".

Avicenna noted that sufferers often found some reduction of the complaints were to be had from alcoholic beverages, or even biscuits. Today we speak of "anxiety reducers".

> If he be in a silent auditory, or at a sermon, he is afraid he shall speak aloud unawares, something indecent, unfit to be said. If he be locked in a close room, he is afraid of being stifled for want of air, and still carries biscuits, aquavitae, or some strong waters about him, for fear of deliquiums, or being sick; or if he be in a throng, middle of a church, multitude, where he may not well get out, though he sit at ease, he is so misaffected. He will freely promise, undertake any business beforehand, but when it comes to be performed, he dare not adventure, but fears an infinite number of dangers, disasters.

More recently one reads in Marks:

> The first noticeable symptoms which manifested themselves were extreme nervous irritability, sleeplessness, loss of appetite, palpitation, spasmodic breathing, dilation of the eyes and nostrils, convulsive movements of the muscles, difficulty in articulation, etcetera, were the more prominent features. A sense of impending danger seemed to descend, spoiling every pleasure, thwarting every ambition (...). I became morbidly sensitive about being brought into close contact with any large number of people. Finding myself in the midst of a large gathering would inspire a feeling of terror on my part. This could be relieved in but one way – by getting away from the spot as soon as possible. Acting on this impulse I have left churches, theatres, even funerals, simply because of an utter inability to control myself to stay.

Some suffered from more than one kind of phobia too; and symptom substitution was not unknown. Nor was the tendency of sufferers to complain at length absent in those olden days (compare this with "*klaaggedrag*" [complaining behaviour] noted by Van Haasen, 1972, and by Schaper, 1974).

> Pacify them for one, they are instantly troubled by some other fear; always afraid of something which they foolishly imagine or conceive to themselves, which never peradventure was, never can be, never likely to be; troubled in mind upon every small occasion, unquiet, still, complaining, grieving, vexing, suspecting, grudging, discontent. Or if their minds be more quiet for the present, and they are free from foreign fears, outward accidents, yet their bodies are out of tune, they suspect some part or other to be amiss; now their head aches, heart, stomach, spleen is misaffected, they shall surely have this or that disease. Yet for all this, in other things they are wise, staid, discreet, and do nothing unbecoming their dignity, person, or place, this foolish, ridiculous and childish fear excepted (*Rhazes ad Almanzor*, A.D. 864–925).

Marks and others (e.g., Van Zuuren, 1982) comment too on the lack of self-assertion in social phobics, though they may otherwise be well-adjusted. Conforming too in their attitudes, "doing nothing unbecoming to their dignity, person, or place".

Aretaeus of Cappodocia was of the opinion that persons who are mad see as others do but do not form a correct judgment on what they have seen. (The word *madness* was used loosely by the ancients, as it is today, to characterize widely varying phenomena; from queer or unreasonable behaviour, to neuroses or psychoses, as Rosen, 1968, notes.) Aretaeus' insight is the more astonishing when one pauses to consider that he reached this conclusion about 1900 years before a modern-day clinician arrived at a similar conception (see Barendregt's formulation, 1974).

Fear of the *agora*, of open and enclosed spaces, were not the only fears suffered in ancient times either. Fear of events to come, fear of death, loss of life or goods, of being burned alive, or of execution, fear of disease, and of water were just as common.

> Some are afraid to be burned, or that the ground will sink under them or swallow them up quick, or that the king will call them in question for some fact they never did, and they will surely be executed (*Rhazes ad Almanzor*). Many fear death so much that, in a contrary humor, they make away with themselves (*Galen*). They are afraid of some loss, danger, that they will surely lose their lives, goods, and all they have, but why they know not (*Trincavellius*). Themiston, the physician, fell into an hydrophobia, by seeing one sick of that disease (*Dioscorides, 1st century A.D.*).

Nor was anxiety the main negative emotion evidenced. Then, as now, some phobics felt not anxious but angry; not cast-down or depressed but aggressive (cf. Barendregt, 1972, 1973; Marks, 1978).

> Fear and sorrow are no common symptoms (to all melancholy). Upon serious consideration, I find some are not so at all. Some indeed are sad, and not fearful; some fearful and not sad; some neither fearful nor sad; some both. Some are filled with anger, distrust, suspicion (*Diocles, circa 384–322 B.C.*).

And so one might go on *ad infinitum*; and wonder with Rhazes whether this disease did not proceed especially from the devil, and from him alone, for its symptoms are infinite.

Implications

From a historical point of view, then, very little seems to have changed in the phobic phenomenon, in spite of the many classification disguises it has worn. Though once-lost insights, through empirical inquiry, have been recovered today, this is at the cost of some etymological confusion. *Agoraphobia* is a case in point. From the ancient and medieval reports it is apparent that a relation was observed between fear of public performance in the *agora*, and rôle-deficiency or inadequacy, in men. Fear of open, arcadian spaces, and long, lonely pathways was also connected to a longing for, but apprehensiveness of, sexual excitement, especially in women and young girls.

The confusion sets in with the reappearance of agoraphobia as a clinical syndrome in modern times. Westphal (1871, 1872) published reports on three male patients with fears of open or public places, which he described as the impossibility of walking through certain streets or squares, or of doing so only with resultant dread or anxiety.

This condition he labelled *Agoraphobia*. Westphal's description suggests both a fear of performance in the *agora* and a fear of open spaces or streets.

More recently (Wurmser & McDaniel, 1978) we are told that though a frequent misusage of the word agoraphobia interprets it as being a fear of open spaces, this misusage should not be laid at the door of Westphal, who actually picked the term to illustrate its more specific meaning, namely, a fear of public places of assembly. However this may be, the fact is that at the time of his publications this may not have been so clear, since Freud (1917), though he carefully pointed out that a fear of open spaces, of lengthy roads or streets is linked to repressed sexual excitement, adopted the classification of *agoraphobia* for these cases. Sometimes he referred to this syndrome as *topophobia*. The making synonymous of *topophobia* with *agoraphobia* is reflected in its modern classification under *situation phobia* (see Marks, 1978 and Van Zuuren, 1982).

Contemporarily (Barendregt, 1972, 1973; Marks, 1978; Van Zuuren, 1976, 1982), the fear of social or professional situations in which one's skills can be, and frequently are, put to the test has been explicitly linked to rôle-deficiency or inadequacy, and described as essentially distinct from a fear of open spaces. Since its proper designation had traditionally been usurped, a new term was introduced. But thus to perpetuate the etymological confusion is to place one's hard-won insights open to the non-negligible risk of being once again lost in future times.

Of more relevance to this study are other implications of this comparison of ancient with modern descriptions of phobia. The comparison helps to bring out its essential universality and stability over time. Possibly this may mean that the phenomenon derives from certain, perhaps not even now well-understood, interactions between relatively permanent structures common to all environments in all ages, their perceptual transformations, and inadequate forms of perceptual control more often found in persons with certain types of personality configurations. Some of the issues involved, which are derived from the descriptions of phobia in the above, are enumerated below.

Differential Effects of Environmental Objects, Structures, Events

Throughout one can see that certain environmental objects, structures or events are more often the focus of attention in phobias than others. For example, open spaces, enclosed spaces, heights, dark and depleted spatial conditions, crowds (in social or professional assemblies), death and disease (loss of life but also rotting bodies), uncertainty of events yet to come. To state that in phobic syndromes objects, structures, and events in the environment exert differential effects, some being more and others less significant, is almost to state the obvious. But, given their relative neglect in theories of phobia, in this context perhaps not superfluous.

Relative Instability of Environmental Structure and Objects, and of the Phobic Person's Own Movement

Compared to non-sufferers, not only do certain characteristics of the environment seem more unstable (e.g., sharp fluctuations in intensity and quality of objects, uncontrollable expansion and contraction of spatiotemporal relations), but also the person's movement in space often seems outside his or her own control. These observations suggest differences between sufferers and non-sufferers in perceived stability of structure and of oneself in relation to this, thus in perceptual control over self and environment. This, in turn, suggests that there may be systematic differences in the way that phobic persons, compared to normal persons, interact perceptually with their environment.

Individual Differences Among Sufferers, not only in the Degree to which Certain Objects, Structures or Events Affect Them, but also in the Range that is Effective

Such differences indicate that developmental influences, socio-cultural differences and learning play important rôles in the perceptual or conceptual categories of these people.

Disturbances in Physiological Function and Instability of Emotions

In almost all cases, there is overwhelming evidence of disturbed activity in physiological and emotional systems, manifesting in overt symptoms, such as hyperventilation, blushing, etc., but also in heightened emotional states, distressing bodily experiences, and labile emotional control.

Differences in Susceptibility Related to Differences in Personality Configuration

Most observers, ancient and modern, remark on the personality configurations of these sufferers. In general these people are shy, unassuming, unassertive, insecure, conforming, inhibited and often suspicious. The characteristic common to these differing personality configurations might be described as a self-denying or self-rejecting attitude. The importance of familial and developmental conditions in acquiring such attitudes towards oneself is incontrovertible.

Although these enumerated aspects may not describe all the issues involved in phobia, they may well be the main ones, and can serve as starting-points for empirical investigation. In this study, and as a working hypothesis, I shall entertain this assumption in postulating that, when the above-mentioned interactions between person and environment are found, phobia will result. When the interactions between person and environment are not (or are less) pronounced, other forms of anxiety neurosis, or even psychosis, will probably be the case.

Anticipating some of the issues to be explored in the next three chapters, this statement may be understood as follows: if the orderly perception of certain environmental relations (e.g., ratios of stimulation) is crucial to maintaining stability in and constancy of environmental structures, and if the self provides the primary frame of reference in this perceptual activity, then severe disturbances or distortions in the (experience of) self will inevitably lead to instability and inconstancy in the perception of the environmental surround, and of the self-in-surround.

In normal vision and hearing, sensory representations of direction and distance vary widely as a function of change in observer posture, locomotion and head- and eye-movements, although perceived location of object and source remains relatively unchanged. (Such effects are called *egocentric constancies*.) Stability and constancy in the environment are known to be functions of orderly and gradated change in observer position, posture, and so on. But in phobic behaviour, and in the behaviour of depersonalized people, one frequently observes tendencies to freezing postures, rigid attitudes, stereotypic, erratic and uncontrolled movements. It is clear that under such conditions perception of environmental relations can hardly be optimal, and may even be minimal.

Even more striking in these patients is their inclination to a constant, almost obsessive self-observation, with concomitant disregard for other objects and structures in the environment. This inordinate self-observation is, in itself, an indication of serious dysfunction in self- and egosystems. Psychodynamically-oriented developmental psychologists have long noted that systematic relations exist between early disturbances in ego-integrative processes and the development of neurotic and/or psychotic syndromes in later years. Contemporary theorists (e.g., Kernberg, 1966; Mahler, 1968b; Masterson & Rinsley, 1980) argue that the amount, intensity and kind of stimulation in the mother-infant interactions determine later responses to environment and self. For instance, and especially in infancy, overstimulation is equated by the infant with unpleasure and pain, and is therefore to some extent traumatogenic, whereas moderate stimulation is equated with pleasure, delight, goodness.

These interactions between mother and infant are introjected by the infant to form scattered "good" and "bad" memory islands, which proceed to integrate into progressively differentiated self- and object-images. The mother thus conveys, in innumerable ways, a kind of "mirroring frame of reference", to which the primitive self of the infant automatically adjusts.

A further complicating factor may be that certain environmental relations, which are effective in maintaining stability in and constancy of the environment, may lend themselves easily to projections of internalized sources of anxiety, which are repressed. For example, parameters of perspective indicating distance or depth, occlusion of space, rapidity and direction of movement of objects in space, as in expansion and contraction, but also parameters indicating emptiness or isolation, darkness or the blotting out of orientation cues which otherwise provide a foothold, and so on.

When environmental parameters are conducive to or invite such projections of disturbed self-orientations in certain individuals, their effects might well be more impelling than when these give no occasion to such projections. In the susceptible individual a vicious circle of invidious interactive effects might then be set up, which may yield – among other negative effects such as mounting anxiety, loss of (self-) control – frequent distortions in the perceptual field. It is not difficult, then, to understand why the afflicted person will seek to avoid situations in which these experiences are undergone, or may be anticipated.

On the other hand, if the degree of self-denial or self-rejecting orientations is so mild that the person is able to maintain relatively stable control of environmental structure, no phobia should develop; even though familial conditions may induce chronic states of stress in such a person.

Nor should phobia develop in someone who is characterized by a self-asserting or self-accepting orientation; even though he or she is subject to hallucinatory experiences, and evinces at times a labile control over the environment (as, for instance, in the case of epilepsy, or under the influence of hallucinogens). However, matters may not be so clear-cut when one gets down to a consideration of individual cases. Few personalities are as narrowly definable as this; and, as implied above, one person's denial or rejection of self may differ much from another's. Given such variability, mixed syndromes will necessarily be found in certain individuals.

Still, if support can be found for these ideas, this could mean that more coherence exists in the "structure" of phobia than is supposed; and, despite its protean appearance and multiple origins, that it may be less elusive in character.

An Outline of the Study

In the context of this study on perceptual control, only the aspects concerned with environmental relations and perceptual interactions will be investigated. Not only would an attempt to do more at this point be infeasible, it may not be necessary. Given the ample evidence in the literature, few theorists now doubt that phobia is characterized by disturbances of physiological function, in particular, by hyperventilation and by disturbances in the emotional systems.

There is growing evidence too to support the hypothesis that the phobic personality, in general, can be characterized in terms of self-denying or self-rejecting orientations.

In contrast, the evidence for a greater instability in the control of environmental relations and inconstancy of structure in the phobic, as compared to the normal, experience is still sketchy. Nor is it clear which specific relations in the environment are the crucial ones in phobia, in spite of a quite general acceptance that such relations play some part in the complaint. How these environmental conditions may interact with perceptual systems to bring about perceptual transformations of the world, and which produce greater instability in the phobic experience, is still a matter for debate. This study aims to provide some answers to these questions.

In Chapter II, in elaborating on the concept of control in some theories of perception, specific attention is therefore given to defining the parameters of environmental stimulation which are deemed essential to a successful and stable organization of the world, and which play an important rôle in the regulatory and adaptive responses of the organism to the natural environment. Hypotheses about the perceptual processes involved in these activities are described, and their weaknesses and strengths noted.

In Chapter III, the psychodynamic approach to neurosis, and particularly to phobia, is reviewed from the standpoint of the rôles that perceptual and ego control play in the origin and maintenance of the phobic reaction. Freud's theoretical assumptions form the starting-point for these considerations.

Part One is concluded, in Chapter IV, by an attempt to integrate theory and empirical findings reviewed in the preceding chapters; and, in considering various implications, the stage is set for a proper understanding of the possible relevance of my empirical work with phobic and normal persons which ensues.

In Part Two some empirical relations are explored between environmental structure, organismic process and phenomenal experience as these pertain to the perception of phobic persons and normal controls.

In Chapter V, five studies are described, designed to try and pin-point the characteristics of environmental structure that are effective in phobia.

Chapter VI is concerned with analyses of the *individual responses* from these experimental data, which seem to show that individual differences exist in strategies of perceptual control. In discussing these data, differences in perceptual control between phobic and normal persons, and between phobics in different categories of complaint, are postulated to exist.

In Chapter VII similarities and differences between phobic and normal people in perceptual control, specifically when control fails, are described. Their experiences of perceptual disorientation, derealization and depersonalization are discussed on the evidence of analyses of rating-scale responses.

Chapter VIII is a little intermezzo on the differences between phobic and normal people in the experience of time, with possible far-reaching implications.

In Chapter IX the inner world of the phobic person in relation to the experience of spatial relations is illustrated by vignettes from interviews with individual phobic patients. In this is described the phenomenal experiences of environmental structure, of one's orientation of self (and body) in space, and of perceived (lack of) control over self-in-environment. This information helps to support the main hypothesis of a direct and systematic relation between the effective components of environmental structure (spatial relations), strategies of perceptual control, and phenomenal experiences of phobic patients.

The study is concluded, in Chapter X, by a discussion of the empirical work in the light of the theoretical premises in Part One.

The empirical bases for the theoretical assumptions on the perceptual nature of phobia, as set forth in this study, are summarized in Chapter XI.

II

Concepts of Control in Theories of Perception

Philosophical Antecedents

Earlier the term *perceptual control* was introduced to apply, on the one hand, to the constraints imposed on perceptual systems by the nature of environmental stimulation and, on the other, to the regulatory activities arising in the organism following information thus acquired.

This statement, clear and plausible as it may seem, contains tacit assumptions on the nature of perception as the first source of knowledge about the world. Assumptions which, despite centuries of philosophical and psychological inquiry, have found no definitive resolution. A systematic review of this inquiry would take us well beyond the scope of this book. However, since the unresolved issues still plague theories of perception, some of these will be briefly touched upon in the discussion of concepts of perceptual control.

The problem of control in perceptual theory addresses three issues. First, what is the nature of the information available to perceptual systems in the environment? Secondly, by which process is perception achieved? Thirdly, how is information thus acquired able to control perceptual action?

In attempts to resolve these issues, two distinct schools of thought arose which became known as the Rationalist and the Empirical traditions. (Strictly speaking, those issues concerned the relation between the world and Mind.) In the Rationalist tradition, of which Descartes, Spinoza, Leibniz and Kant were the main proponents, knowledge of the world is said to be obtained through thought, observation and sensory experience. A real world is assumed to exist but is essentially unknowable (the *noumenon*). But its properties and that of human life can be logically deduced from self-evident axioms. *A priori* categories of mind – the categories of Pure Reason (i.e., substance, relation, extension and number, space and time) are postulated. From these, knowledge about external things and events are inferred. Matter is something knowable, if at all, by inference from what is known of mind. Since what appears to the senses is merely a reflection of mind, knowledge by the senses is necessarily more or less confused. In this view, sensible intuition is guided by intellect in conformity with a real world that is itself inadequately experienced (Russell, 1949, 1974).

In the Empirical tradition, of which Locke, Berkeley and Hume were the main proponents, a contrary stance is adopted. All *a priori* knowledge is denied. Instead, the senses become the source of knowledge of the external world, and visual perception the link from light to mind (Gregory, 1981). Locke, who is rightly called the founder of this tradition, held the mind to be a *tabula rasa*, and perception "the first step towards knowledge, and the inlet of all the materials to it". Our ideas are derived from two sources; (a) sensation, and (b) perception of the operation of our own mind, which he called the "internal sense". In this view, mind is regarded as passive, somewhat like a seal accepting impressions. The senses give simple ideas of sensation, and complete ideas by reflection. In perception we experience sequences of "simple ideas" (such as sensations of colour). The characteristics of perception are in the world, not in us, our perceptions merely reflecting the world as mirrors reflect things (Russell, *ibid.*).

Contemporary Theory on Perception

The present state of affairs is such that as many theories of perception exist as there are theorists. During the sixty years or so since psychology entered the field of science, she has witnessed the launching and, in many cases, flourishing of as diverse theories of perception as Gestalt theory (Kohler; Wertheimer), topological field theory (Lewin), cell-assembly and phase-sequence theory (Hebb), sensory-tonic field theory (Werner & Wapner), probabilistic functionalism (Brunswik) and the closely allied transactionalism (Ames, Kilpatrick & Ittelson), adaptation level theory (Helson), directive state theory (Bruner & Postman), theory of information pickup (Gibson), hypothesis theory (Gregory), many other cognitive and learning theories (Neisser; Hull; Tolman), and cybernetic or systems theories (McCulloch & Pitts; Simon; Pribram) with perceptual offshoots.

The focus of this study, however, is not on the merit or charm of these theories. For the sake of coherence (and brevity), the diverse models will not be separately considered here. Excellent reviews of some of these may be found in Allport (1955) and, more briefly, in Pronko, Ebert & Greenberg (1966). What is of interest here is the fact that, despite their apparent divergences, all of these theories, when their specific details are ignored, subsume under two rivalling schools of thought deriving from the Rationalist and Empirical traditions.

In the first school of thought are those theories in which perception is viewed as an inferential activity, the process of perception described in terms of (isomorphic or non-isomorphic) internal representations of an (essentially unknowable) external world, and the perceiver viewed as a passive or active processor of information, a manipulator of symbols, who constructs the perceptual world from the products of this mediation process.

In the second school of thought are those theories in which perception is viewed as essentially a non-inferential activity, the perceptual process described in terms of a direct pickup of information from an objectively existing, in principle knowable, and highly structured world. The perceiver in this view discovers, rather than constructs, the persisting and changing relations therein and what these afford, attuned as are his, her or its perceptual systems by genetic heritage and evolution to do exactly this.

All current information-processing models, whether passive or active, belong to the first school of thought; and, in fact, embody the traditional, and established position (e.g., Hebb, Neisser, Broadbent, Gregory, Piaget, Pribram, to name but a few of the prominent theorists in the field). To the second belong the dissenting, and increasingly articulate minority whose orientation is distinctly ecological (e.g., Gibson, Shaw, Mace, Turvey). Still, though all may make use of the tools of empiricism, not all are (avowed) empiricists. And few, if any, would nowadays defend radical empiricism, that is, the view that the mind of man is at birth a *tabula rasa*, and that all psychological abilities can be traced to the individual's learning experiences. Also, in both viewpoints phenomenalism is rejected, all postulating that knowledge of the world entails more than the phenomena we experience.

In spite of this common ground, though, no unification of perceptual theory is in the offing. Also, because of the radicality of viewpoint on both sides, the logical implication seems to be that if one accepts the viewpoint of the one, the other must be rejected (cf. Michaels & Carello, 1981).

In describing the what and how of perceptual control, viewed from the representational and ecological standpoints, I shall try to clarify the positions by contrasting the theoretical ideas and assumptions of Gregory (1973–1981), as prototypical of the former standpoint, with those of Gibson (1966–1979), the originator of the latter approach.

The representational viewpoint of perception (and knowledge) is generally taken to be the correct one; so it is not easy to bear in mind that in fact its central hypothesis, on which the rest stands or falls, is still unproven. The ecological alternative hypothesis, if it should find support under empirical inquiry, might have far-reaching implications for theories of cognition. Small wonder that the debate has become a spirited, even a heated one.

On how so Little Information Controls so Much Behaviour: *Richard L. Gregory (1973, 1974, 1981)*

Gregory originates in the Cambridge school made famous by Bartlett (1932, 1941) and Kenneth Craik (1943, 1966). In an article of the same title given to this section (1974, p. 590), he notes that Craik was the first to state clearly that the nervous system may symbolize reality. In his *The Nature of Explanation* (1943, p. 61), Craik wrote:

> "If the organism carries a 'small-scale model' of external reality and of its own possible actions within its head, it is able to carry out various alternatives, conclude which is the best of them, react to future situations before they arise, utilize the knowledge of past events in dealing with the present and future, and in every way react in a fuller, safer, and more competent manner to emergencies which face it."

This statement, in fact, also sums up Gregory's theoretical standpoint succinctly. In the following, by quoting only from his own large body of work, in particular the monumental *Concepts and Mechanisms of Perception* (1974), his views on the issues involved in perceptual control are presented.

The Nature of the Information Available to Perceptual Systems

Perceptions, according to Gregory, are constructed by complex brain processes from fleeting fragmentary scraps of data signalled by the senses and drawn from snippets of the past. In this view, normal everyday perceptions are not part of, nor even directly related to, the world of external objects, but are essentially "fictions" or "guesses" based on past experience selected by present sensory data (1974, p. xviii). The sensory inputs are not simply physical patterns of stimulation but rather patterns bearing information (p. 199). The retinas receive flat mosaic patterns of light, the ears ever-changing patterns of frequency and amplitude of vibration; but what we see are solid objects lying in three-dimensional space (p. 50).

Not shape or colour but non-optical properties are of importance; whether the object is useful, a threat, or food (p. 57, p. 599). These non-optical symbols evoke internal models, which have developed by handling objects so that non-optical features have become associated (p. 599).

Eye and brain thus combine to give detailed knowledge of objects beyond the range of probing touch. Just how this is achieved remains in many ways mysterious. Apparently specific features of objects are selected and combined to give an internal account of an object (1973, p. 50).

Perceptual Models and Perceptual Processes

From such snippets of information derived from the external world the brain develops internal models of reality. This must surely require processes of the utmost complexity: calling up its stores of memory data; requiring subtle classifications, comparisons and logical decisions for sensory data to become perceptions (1973, p. 50). These perceptual models are aggregates of data about objects, and about how objects behave and interact in various circumstances (1974, p. 599).

Perceptual models bear a resemblance to hypotheses in science. We may think of sensory data suggesting, testing, and sometimes modifying perceptual models in much the same way that scientific data suggest, test and modify theory and hypothesis in science (*ibid.*).

The notion of perception as predictive hypotheses going beyond available data is apparent even without considering particular experiments. For example, when you trust your weight to the floor, or your mouth to a spoonful of food, you have not monitored the ground's strength or the food's palatability: you have acted on trust, on the basis of the past. You have acted according to probabilities, based on generalizations from past events. But neither generalizations nor probabilities exist, except in brains, for these are not properties of the world of events, though derived from them. Yet on this basis decisions about the world and action are taken (1974, pp. xxiv–v).

If, then, behaviour is not guided by "stimuli" but by guesses about the world, this must require an internal "fiction" of the world, and these internal fictions ("perceptual hypotheses" or "object hypotheses") must be flexible and adjustable to reality (p. xxv).

To perceive, then, in Gregory's view, is to read the present in terms of the past to predict and control the future (p. xix). In fact, the current perception *is* the prevailing set of models (p. 596).

Perceptual Control

Control is not direct (except in the special case of reflexes), but is via these internal models of reality. Generally predictive, and so essentially correct, they may sometimes be inappropriate, thus driving us into error. Mechanism error can be due to malfunction of physiological systems (transducers). Transducers convert signals, represented with one kind of physical energy (e.g., electromagnetic radiation), into equivalent signals of a different physical kind (e.g., electrical changes which serve as signals). The neural system has many kinds of such transducers (in the retina, and in skin, muscle, joints, etc.), and all of these, except for pain, readily adapt to maintained stimuli. This calibration upset, if not corrected, generates error – and illusion (1973, pp. 56–7).

Perceptual models are adjusted by "size scaling" visual features, such as perspective convergence of lines, though not always appropriately. Perception of depth, for instance, is not completely determined by texture or perspective. In impoverished environments the observer's perceptions and his "set" can be important (1974, p. 354).

When scale-setting sensory information are available these modify the models; but when this information is inappropriate to the prevailing reality, then perception is systematically distorted. Examples of this are the familiar perception distortion illusions. Pictures and illusion figures having marked perspective features seem calculated to upset the perceptual systems in just this way. Distortion will occur if these features, when misleading, cannot be ignored or rejected (1973, p. 76; 1981, p. 395).

This idea of setting scale directly, by typical depth features, is an example of scaling "upwards" from data. In the absence of available scale-setting data, perception is determined by average, sizes and distances. Scaling can also be "downwards", from currently held perceptual (or "object") hypotheses, changing with change of hypothesis. Whether "upwards" or "downwards", scaling should generate distortion illusions, when inappropriate.

We may describe "upwards" scaling as given by rule-following (for example, accepting the rule that converging lines should produce expansion to counter the shrinking of retinal images with increasing object distance). Scaling "downwards" from hypotheses is not given by such rule-following, but evidently by "scale constants" stored in certain object hypotheses. When the hypothesis changes, the data shifts (1973, pp. 76–78). As in science, so in perception.

Evidence for this comes from what happens when depth-ambiguous objects change apparent orientations, such as wire cubes whose faces apparently switch in depth. The apparently farther face always looks the larger – although there is no change in sensory input (signals) with shifts of perceptual hypotheses. This change is purely "central", yet it produces completely systematic size changes. This can even take place against stereoscopic information (1974, pp. 348 and 374).

Gregory also speaks of "primary constancy scaling" to refer to scaling set by perspective or other features normally associated with distance (that is, "upwards" scaling); "primary" because it seems to be primitive, and to be mediated by neural systems situated early in the perceptual system. "Secondary scaling" (that is "downwards" from hypotheses) is set simply by apparent distance, and this may be a function of previous knowledge and is not necessarily tied directly to visual information (1974, p. 348). Of these early stages of perception we have, however, no awareness, so that intellectual knowledge of such perceptual situations does not always correct perceptual errors. In other words, perceptual hypothesis-making is not under intellectual control.

Illusions, then, can be produced by inference-procedure and rule-following generating systematic departures from fact. Divergence from accepted fact may not, though, be in error. It could turn out to be largely or wholly true. Certainly it is a requirement for the generation of novelty (1973, p. 94).

Other experimental findings which show that current data (or "stimuli") are simply not adequate to control behaviour directly in familiar situations come from the well-known human tracking experiments, where behaviour remains appropriate though there is no sensory input, and continues to do so through long gaps in sensory data. This seems to imply that these characteristics are inferred from the past (1974, p. xx).

Evidently, then, the visual internal model system is largely autonomous, though it is partly under the control of other systems. Visual size and distance can be set by other senses, especially touch. It is also worth noting that size scaling follows not only currently available sensory information, but also changes in the internal model. Generally, the internal model is reasonably appropriate and complete, but an incorrect model may always be selected, and even if appropriate it may be wrongly scaled. We know from perceptual experiments in situations where only minimal information is available that both selection and scaling can be quite wrong. So it is a small step to say that in the absence of any sensory information entirely wild models might be called up, as could be the case in dreaming, or in drug or fatigue-induced hallucinations. Such states might call up internal but inappropriate models, either by increasing cortical noise or by reducing the threshold criteria for acceptance of the stored models (1974, p. 597). Beside such possibilities, the biological systems employing internal models can always be fooled, for example, when characteristics which they accept for selecting a model occur in *atypical* situations. Also, other errors can result when a model is selected on purely visual data, but once selected it is used for non-visual predictions (p. 593).

In short, the chances for error in selection or scaling, thus yielding perceptual distortion, are much greater than one might imagine, given the generally correct approximations of reality on which we base decision and action.

Advantages and Disadvantages of Internal (Perceptual) Models

To conclude this brief reflection of Gregory's theoretical standpoint, a few advantages and disadvantages of internal models which make use of the redundancy in space and time (whether these are biological or computerized) are noted by him (1974, pp. 592–593). Advantages lie in the fact that:

(a) An internal model can achieve high performance with limited transmission rate. The gain results because perception of objects (which is always redundant) requires identification of only certain key features of each object. Since human transmission rate is estimated to be only about 12 bits/second, this would be an important advantage.
(b) Being essentially predictive, in suitable circumstances reaction time can be reduced to zero.
(c) In the temporary absence of any input, or when the input changes in kind, continuous functioning is possible.

(d) Provided a particular situation is similar for what a "model" was developed, behaviour will be generally appropriate ("positive transfer").
(e) If the internal models are highly redundant, the effective signal-to-noise ratio can enormously improve, since these can be called up with minimal sensory information and signals can be extracted from "noise" in the system.

Such a system does have a few unfortunate disadvantages, however. These lie in the fact that (a) when the current situation is sufficiently similar to past ones which have been selected and combined to give an internal model, but differ in crucial respects, then the system will be systematically *misled* by its model ("negative transfer"); (b) also, being essentially conservative, it will show inertial drag to change, for it must reflect the past rather than the present. This implies that rapid change of environment or social groups will be biologically dangerous, favouring only the younger members of the group.

The Ecological Approach to Visual Perception: *James J. Gibson (1966, 1970, 1975, 1979)*

From his earliest work on visual perception before and during World War II studying visual components of aviation, particularly the activity of landing aeroplanes, Gibson had felt that the first priority of theories of perception "should be to do justice to the everyday perceptual accomplishments that contribute to the survival of the species ... (and) ... the problem of guiding ourselves is primarily a problem of veridical perception" (Gibson, 1958; Mace, 1977). Traditional theories of space perception seemed to offer no help in the practical problem of understanding visually guided locomotion.

Looking back on his prolonged dilemma, Gibson writes (1979, p. xiii):

> "Vision is a strange and wonderful business. I have been puzzling over its perplexities for 50 years. I used to suppose that the way to understand it was to learn what is accepted as true about the physics of light and the retinal image, to master the anatomy and physiology of the eye and the brain, and then to put it together into a theory of perception that could be tested by experiments. But the more I learned about physics, optics, anatomy, and visual physiology, the deeper the puzzles got. The experts in these sciences seemed confident that they could clear up the mysteries of vision eventually but only, I decided, because they had no real grasp of the perplexities."

I have chosen to present Gibson's ideas from 1966 on, because before this time his theorizing and interpretation of his empirical work fit quite well into the traditional paradigm, although there were hints of increasing frustration. With the publication of *The Senses Considered as Perceptual Systems* (1966), it became clear that his ideas on the nature of perception had taken a radical turn. Most of his colleagues in the field, though, chose to re-interpret his meaning so that this could still fit into the traditional one. In 1970 he then re-stated his radical standpoint in an article (*The theory of information pickup*) which left little room for any further misunderstanding. In this article he rejected clearly the need in the perceptual process for retinal images, stored memories, inferences, past and future expectancies, or whatever else the representationists needed to buttress their arguments.

It was at this point, as Gregory notes (1974, p. 296), that he was forced to part company with this renowned theorist who, with his wife Eleanor, had "held his position, and argued so well". This parting of the ways is not surprising seeing that Gregory maintained then, and still maintained in 1981, that Von Helmholtz (1866) is "essentially right" in his argument that a great deal of "unconscious inference" may be involved in perception. And unconscious inference implies stored memories to allow for inferences from the past to the future. Gregory, who considers the study of illusions to be the royal road to an understanding of perception, could hardly have been less chagrined to learn that Gibson considered these to be peripheral to the problem, though intriguing phenomena in themselves, and thus of relatively little use in understanding veridical perception in real life.

Although my own work on perception in a clinical setting has taken place within the traditional conceptions, most of the findings, to my mind, can be better understood in terms of Gibson's theory. For this reason I shall quote at greater length from his work. I shall rely mainly on his last book, *The Ecological Approach to Visual Perception* (1979), in which he motivates and clarifies this radical approach, leaving no room now for misinterpretation or misunderstanding. Since these selections are made inasmuch as they relate to the issues of perceptual control as here defined, justice is hardly done to the richness and originality of thought of this remarkable man, whose work is a tribute to the Cornell school.

The Nature of the Information Available to Perceptual Systems

The environment in which organisms live, move and have their being is not, in Gibson's view, that of space and time, as conceived by the physicists. Space, he notes, can be visualized but cannot be seen; events are perceivable but time is not (1966, 1975, 1979). Environment refers to the surroundings of organisms that perceive and behave. The environment of every animal (human or otherwise) is at a size-level that is neither that of the physical world of atoms and their ultimate particles, nor that of the astronomical world of stars and galaxies, but is the intermediate one that is measured in millimeters and meters (1979, pp. 8–9).

At this level the terrestrial animal's environment can be better described in terms of a *medium* (air), *substances and surfaces* that separate them (substances such as rock, soil, sand, wood, oil, water, minerals, metals, tissues of plants and other animals), and surfaces of substances. All of this has been strikingly constant throughout the whole evolution of life. Organismic life is properly understood when considered as ecological systems and subsystems, animals being more or less perfectly adapted to perceive and interact with their environment, having evolved within this over innumerable centuries. These different components of the environment afford different possibilities for the behaviour of animals. Air, being an insubstantial medium, affords respiration or breathing; it permits locomotion; it can be filled with illumination so as to permit vision; it allows detection of vibrations and detections of diffusing emanations; it is homogeneous; and it has an absolute axis of reference, up and down.

Substances are solids and liquids that vary in composition, and in resistance to change. Generally opaque (that is, reflecting and absorbing, but not transmitting light, except in very special cases), these are more or less impenetrable by solid bodies and more or less permanent in shape. They are compounded and aggregated in extremely complicated ways, and do not tend to homogeneity.

This hierarchy of substances is not categorical but full of transitions and overlap, and tends to be repeated over the whole surface of the earth, not in a metrical, but with a stochastical (that is, probabilistic) regularity.

Surfaces (of substances) have characteristic texture, reflectances and layout. *Layout* refers to the persisting arrangement of surfaces relative to one another and to the ground. The ground itself is structured at various levels of metric size, these units being nested within one another (1979, p. 12). Surfaces are especially important, for that is where most of the action is, for example, from which light is reflected, what touches the animals, where chemical reactions take place providing interesting smells. Surfaces also have characteristic shapes, sizes and colours, are resistant to deformation and disintegration, hide or disclose other surfaces, and so on (*ibid.* pp. 16–32).

All these possibilities and opportunities describe the *affordances* of the environment, a word coined by Gibson from the verb "to afford".

Part of the radiant light from the sun is scattered by being transmitted through the atmosphere that is never perfectly transparent, and re-scattered when it strikes textured ground, reflected back to the sky, each reflection further dispersing the incident rays and thus enabling some light to penetrate into shelters (enclosed spaces) that are not open to the sun or even the sky. (This reverberating flux of light in the medium is called by Gibson the *ambient* light). It is at any point in the medium *structured*, that is, containing information specifying characteristics of the surfaces from which it is reflected (*ibid.*, p. 49).

Only stimulation that comes in a structured array and that changes over time specifies its external source (p. 56). (To be an array means to have an arrangement, specifying structures of surfaces; an array is therefore heterogeneous.)

In ambient light that is unstructured in one part and structured in an adjacent part, such as the blue sky above the horizon and the textured region below it, the former specifies a void and the latter a surface. In the case of unstructured ambient light, an environment is not specified and no information *about* the environment is available. (For if the light is undifferentiated, it cannot be discriminated, p. 52.)

Gibson makes a distinction between the ambient array at an unoccupied point (that is, light surrounding a position in the environment that could be occupied by an observer but is not), and the array at a point that is occupied by an observer, human or other. In the first case the information is there, but is not picked up; in the second case information about the surroundings is available to the observer (and thus pickup-able), but also contains information about the body of the observer. That is, at any occupied point in the environment, two kinds of information are available at one and the same time: information specifying characteristics of the environment and of the self-in-environment. Both go together. This is what the ambient optic array contains (p. 75).

But a stationary point of observation is only a limiting case. In real life the point of observation is never stationary, but a moving one, and the path of locomotion taken through the environment goes with flowing and non-flowing perspective structure in the ambient array, which specify relations between surfaces, substances and the medium, as well as locomotion and rest. The particular instance of flow specifies the particular path of locomotion, the *course* of the flow being specific to the *route* taken through the environment (*ibid.*, p. 75). This flowing perspective is centrifugal in half the array and centripetal in the other half, but these two hemispheres are not invariant (and not to be confused with the permanent hemispheres of earth and sky). They shift around. A focus of centrifugal outflow is always accompanied by another focus of centripetal inflow at the opposite pole of the sphere. This axis is the line of displacement of the observer. Hence, the focus of expansion is the direction in which one is going, and the focus of contraction is the direction from which one is coming.

The invariant structure of the array that specifies the persisting world *underlies* the changing perspective structure. The pattern of outflow and inflow is *superposed*, as it were, on the nonchanging features of the array (the earth-sky contrast at the horizon, and the texture of the earth). There is then not only a static perspective of the array but also a motion perspective, the former specifying the unmoving terrain, whereas the flow pattern specifies the observer's locomotion with reference to the terrain (p. 122).

The earth's surfaces are usually cluttered, the main items of clutter being *objects*, both attached and detached, *enclosures*, *convexities* such as hills, and *concavities* such as holes, and *apertures* such as windows. These features of surface layout give rise to the *separation* of occluding and occluded surfaces. Any face or facet, any surface of the layout that is progressively hidden during a displacement is progressively unhidden during its reversal. Going out of sight is the inverse of coming into sight. Hence, occluding and occluded surfaces interchange. One should also make a distinction between surfaces going out of sight and surfaces that disappear, for the two cases are profoundly different. In the first case the event is reversible, whereas it is not in the case where disappearing means ceasing to exist, as, for instance, by evaporation, destruction, or desiccation (p. 79).

Objects and surfaces of the terrain also move around. Some surfaces often flow or undergo stretching, squeezing, bending and breaking in complicated ways. *Ecological events in the ambient optical array* are specified then by a *disturbance* in the invariant (persisting) structure of the array. Different kinds of disturbances will give rise to different kinds of events, but events in the world are not literally replicated in the ambient light by a copy or simulacrum. The beginning and the end of the disturbance in the light correspond to the beginning and the end of the event in the world, and that is about as far as the correspondence goes (1979, p. 107).

Examples of ecological events in this Gibsonian sense are *transformations*, *permutations* and *fluctuations*. A progressive deletion and accretion of units on one side of a contour, for instance, specifies the displacement of an object against a background. The shearing or slippage of optical structure specifies the rotation of an object, e.g., a disk. Foreshortening and its opposite specifies the turning of the face of an object by perspective transformation. Magnification to the limit of an object and minification specify approach and recession of an object, and so on. These optical transformations, or *invariants under transformation*, are "formless"; they are invariants of structure (p. 178).

Perceptual Systems and the Perceptual Processes

The theory of *information pickup* states that the perceptual systems are able to detect *directly* persistence (invariants) and change (variants) in the environment. The perceiver *separates* the change from the nonchange, *notices* what stays the same and what does not, and *sees* the continuing identity of things along with the events in which they participate. This is done by extracting the invariants of structure from the flux of stimulation while still noticing the flux. For the visual system in particular, the person tunes in on the invariant structure of the ambient optic array that underlies the changing perspective caused by his movements (p. 247). Information in this sense refers not to the specification of the observer's receptor or sense organs but to the specification of the observer's environment.

But how is this done? Gibson asserts that the old idea that sensory inputs are converted into perceptions by operations of the mind, from images projected on the retina, is a false one. Our misconceptions about the perceptual process are partly due to our misconceptions about the nature of perceptual systems. We take it for granted that one sees the environment with one's eyes. But vision is a whole perceptual system and not a channel of sense (1966, 1979, p. 205).

In this view, the visual system is not only the eyes and the brain to which it is connected, but the eyes-in-the-head-on-the-body-resting-on-the-ground. Natural vision depends on all these components of the complete visual system, the brain being only the central organ. When no constraints are put on the visual system, we look around, walk up to something interesting and move around it so as to see it from all sides, and go from one vista to another. All the components are engaged in this activity. The body explores the surrounding environment by locomotion, the head explores the ambient array by turning, and the eyes explore the two samples of the array, the fields of view, by eye movements. These might be called *exploratory adjustments* of the visual system. At the lower levels, eyelid, lens, pupil and retinal cells make what might be called *optimizing adjustments*, the retinas registering invariants in the information (1979, p. 219).

The perceptual capacities of the organism thus lie in systems with nested functions. That is, the five perceptual systems correspond to five modes of overt attention. They have overlapping functions, and they are all more or less subordinated to an overall orienting system. A perceptual system in this sense is an active one that can orient, explore, investigate, adjust, optimize, resonate, extract and come to an equilibrium, whereas a sense cannot (p. 245).

The brain can be treated as the highest of several centers of the nervous system governing the perceptual system (1970, p. 663). The nervous system is part of any perceptual system, and the centers of the nervous system, from lower to higher, participate in its activity. Organ adjustments are probably controlled by lower centers, selective attention by intermediate centers, and conceptual attention by the highest centers (p. 666).

The visual system, in this view, *hunts* for information and comprehension, and does not rest until the invariants are extracted from information in the ambient array. A motionless observer is a special case. He *can* see the world from a single fixed point of observation and thus notice the perspective of things, that is, the natural perspective which refers to a set of surfaces that create visual solid angles in a frozen ambient array. But (except in psychological laboratories), the normal state of affairs is a moving observer. Moving, one sees the world at no point of observation and thus, strictly speaking, *cannot* notice the perspective of things. Seeing the world at a travelling point, over a long period of time for a sufficiently extended set of paths begins to be perceiving the world at all points of observation. Each object is seen from all sides, and each place as connected with its neighbour. The underlying invariant structure emerges from the changing perspective structure (1979, p. 197).

Gibson suggests that this is not only the way in which animals and humans see the environment, but that they may even see it better this way than when motionless. One should bear in mind that all the perceptual systems are *propriosensitive* as well as *exterosensitive*, for they all provide information in their various ways about the observer's activities as well as about the environment. The optical information too specifies the self, including the head, body and arms, information which accompanies specifications of the layout of the environment. Distance, for instance, is specified as a gradient of decreasing optical size and increasing optical density of the features of the ground, and having a limit at the horizon where all visual solid angles shrink to zero. The gradient is also anchored at another limit by the forms projected from the nose, body and limbs. The nose projects at the maximum of nearness just as the horizon projects at the maximum of farness (p. 117).

When the head turns, this is also registered by vision, as well as by the semicircular canals in the vestibule of the inner ear. Head turns are specified by the *sweeping* of the field of view over the ambient array, and the *wheeling* of the field over the array during head tilts. The sweeping and wheeling are not simply "motions" but deletions and accretions of optical structure (p. 118).

Each sample (of the ambient optic array) is a segment that overlaps with earlier and later segments. Moreover, it is a changing segment with elements being progressively included and excluded at the margins. And in a sufficiently long sequence of these segments, the whole structure of the array is specified (p. 118).

Up to this point most perception psychologists would agree that, by the proper specifications of the information available in the environment to the perceptual systems, Gibson has cleared up many puzzles and done us a great service. Some are even willing to acknowledge that, at least in part, the perceptual process may be direct. After all, other ecological subsystems (e.g., lungs, heart) function directly and smoothly in interaction with the environment without recourse to inferential procedures. Though recent knowledge of Yoga techniques shows that these may be brought under the control of Mind and their processes modified at will, this is not the general case. Surely more active and more specialized systems might have this capacity too?

If, in fact, as the representationists would have it, the perceptual systems depend and operate on vastly inadequate "snippets of information" from the external world, which have to be enriched, enhanced and interpreted before adequate perceptual action can be taken, then more than one miracle happens a day. And the greatest wonder of all is that we are not a race of stumblers, misperceiving and mislocomoting at every turn.

What most of Gibson's critics find hard to accept are not these specifications of the information available in the environment, but certain implications following from his assumptions that perceptual systems are geared to higher-order variables, as postulated in his theory of affordances, and pick these up directly.

The affordances of the environment, Gibson goes on, are what it offers the animal, what it provides or furnishes, either for good or ill. The complementarity of animal and environment becomes particularly clear here. If, for example, a terrestrial surface is nearly horizontal (instead of slanted), nearly flat (instead of convex or concave), and sufficiently extended (relative to the size of the animal), then the surface *affords support*. Different layouts afford different behaviours for the different animals, and different mechanical encounters. Terrestrial surfaces are climb-on-able or fall-off-able or get-under-able or bump-into-able relative to the animal. Knee-high for a child, for instance, is not the same as knee-high for an adult, so the affordance is relative to the size of the animal. The other animals afford, above all, a rich and complex set of interactions, sexual, predatory, nurturing, fighting, playing, cooperating, communicating, and so on (1979, p. 128).

All these benefits and injuries, these positive and negative affordances, are properties of things *taken with reference to an observer* but not properties of the *experiences of the observer*. They are not subjective values, they are not feelings of pleasure or pain added to neutral perceptions ... They are invariant properties of the environment, and thus always there to be picked up ... (.) The object offers what it does because it is what it is (pp. 137–139).

In fact, these affordances, being invariant combinations of variables, are probably easier to perceive than it is to perceive all the variables separately. Gibson suggests that "the affordance of an object is what the infant begins by noticing, long before the substances and surfaces, the color and form are seen as such." In this view, "phenomenal objects are *not* built up of qualities, it is the other way around. Those features of a thing are noted which distinguish it from everything that it is not" (1966, p. 286). Perception is economical. It is never necessary to distinguish all the features of an object and, in fact, it would be impossible to do so (1979, p. 135). The infant begins by thinking that these affordances are available only to herself, and the task of socialization is to make her aware that these are available to others as well.

The process of pickup is postulated to be very susceptible to development and learning. The opportunities for educating attention, for exploring and adjusting, for extracting and abstracting are unlimited. Also, according to pickup theory, "information does not have to be stored because it is always available" (p. 250), anywhere and everywhere, a whole life long.

Perceptual Control

The theory of affordances implies that to see things is to see how to get about them and what to do with them. If this is true, visual perception serves behaviour, and behaviour is controlled by perception. Not only does locomotion depend on perception, but perception depends on locomotion inasmuch as a moving point of observation is necessary for any adequate acquaintance with the environment. So we must perceive in order to move, but we must also move in order to perceive (p. 223).

In this theory, if information is picked up, perception results. But the information may be inadequate or of a conflicting nature, in which case misperception will result. An example of the latter is the well-known visual cliff experiments (Gibson & Walk, 1960). The glass-floor apparatus provided information to specify an adequate surface of support; but this was contradicted by the optical information which specified a falling-off brink of a cliff. The babies tested would pat the glass with their hands but would not venture out on the surface. But if a textured surface was placed under the glass they would go forward over the virtual cliff. The other terrestrial animals would invariably choose the shallow edge instead of the deep one.

At the time these results were usually discussed in terms of depth perception and the traditional cues for depth. But to Gibson now, they seem more intelligible in terms of the perception of layout and their affordances, and of the innate capacity to notice falling-off places in terrestrial animals (p. 142).

One of the first studies which suggested to Gibson that information might be directly picked up concerns the perception of motion in depth (Schiff, Caviness & Gibson, 1962). In these studies, a small, dark silhouette was projected at the centre of a large, translucent screen and with the point of observation close to the screen. At intervals of several seconds the silhouette was magnified. After the shadow filled the screen, observers experienced the virtual object as coming out of the screen, as visually colliding with them. The object's form was indefinite, did not seem to get larger but there was a direct perception of approach-of-something. Observers would blink their eyes, duck or dodge involuntarily. The accelerated portion of the sequence was called "looming" by the investigators, and it specified impending collision. The rate of magnification was proportional to the imminence of the collision.

The apparatus was modified by Schiff (1965) and used to test the responses of monkeys, kittens, chicks, frogs and fiddler crabs. All showed avoidance or withdrawal behaviour analogous to the ducking and dodging of the human observer. A control condition (minification of the shadow, the temporal reverse of magnification) either induced no response or one of "curiosity". Darkening or lightening of the screen, or stabilization of the silhouette, produced no response either. But when the magnification was not symmetrical but skewed, the animal (a crab) would dodge appropriately to the left or right, as the path of the virtual object moved to right or left of the animal's position. The fact that a fiddler crab behaved as if it perceived the same event as the vertebrate animals and the human observers was very suggestive to Gibson, because the crab does not have a camera eye or a retinal image but a compound eye constructed of tubes pointing in different directions. Retinal image optics cannot then be applied to it, but ecological optics can (Gibson, 1966, p. 280; 1979, pp. 175–176).

Another study that seems to bear Gibson out in his contention that perception and locomotion are interdependent systems is that of Held & Bauer (1974). These investigators found that monkeys reared from birth in a device that fitted tightly around the monkey's neck (a cloth bib), which kept them from seeing the hands and body but not from feeling them move and touching things, acted at first when freed from the device as if they could not reach for or grasp an object, but had to grope for it. In Gibson's view, the opaque shield had eliminated visual kinesthesis, and had thus prevented the development of visual control of reaching and grasping.

In the theory of information pickup, the pickup may fail when the available information is inadequate, and misperception will result; as it also will when the information is adequate but not picked up. Examples of inadequacy of information are found under conditions of minimal energy (e.g., blackout), blurring of structure (e.g., white-out phenomena), masking of structure, conflicting information; and in almost all laboratory conditions when the array is narrowed down (e.g., to a single point), by interval cutoff (as in tachistoscopic experiments), or by operations on structure.

In real life, when the information is inadequate, the perceptual systems hunt. They try to make sense of what little information they can get. With conflicting or contradicting information, a search for additional clues begins, which will reinforce one or other alternative. When the information is masked or hidden, search over the whole array takes place. And if detection fails, the hunt goes on more and more widely and over a longer period of time. The perceptual systems test for what remains invariant, trying out different perspectives. If the invariants still do not appear, a whole repertory of poorly understood processes variously called assumptions, inferences or guesses comes into play (1966, p. 304).

And so we come full circle. In considering Gregory's and Gibson's ideas and assumptions on the nature of perception and perceptual control, one cannot avoid the impression that their differences are partly due to the fact that the same object of investigation is being viewed under different conditions and from different perspectives, and that they are basing their generalizations on these. In fact, in what Gibson says in the passages just quoted, there is a hint that he is aware of this; unless his remarks are to be taken only as sarcasm. But their differences also seem to be partly determined by deeply entrenched philosophical positions which inspire and guide their theoretical formulations. How far this may be so will become clear when some of the arguments made by other investigators for or against the representational and ecological approaches are reviewed later.

"Where the Perceiver Meets the Perceived": An Alliance of Critical Realism to Rationalism?

In this section, in reviewing the criticisms levied at the state of perceptual theory, and at the theorists from which this derives, in relation to problems of perceptual control, I shall follow the same sequence as before in presenting the theoretical standpoints.

Gibson is given high marks by antagonists and protagonists alike for his elegant research and theory on environmental relations as these affect terrestrial animals, including human beings. Gregory, who disagrees with him on almost every other issue, says of this (1981, p. 376):

> "Gibson has made several notable experimental contributions, by stressing the importance for perception of features of what he called the 'ambient array', which he supposed is selected and picked up to give visual perception according to principles of 'ecological optics'. He hoped to find simple mathematical relations between features of the ambient array of light and corresponding features of perception. In this quest he found evidence of the importance of ... stimulus features, such as gradients of density of texture, and 'optical flow' and dynamic parallax with observer motion. Gibson rightly criticizes the emphasis of much perception work on pictures, viewed by a static observer, with a single eye, while neglecting observer motion through the world of normal objects lying in three-dimensional space ... Gibson's emphasis on ... patterns of stimulation ... has proved useful and has inspired much valuable research."

Fodor & Pylyshyn (1981), in their rebuttal of Gibson's rejection of the need for indirect perception and inferences, give Gibson some left-handed compliments:

> "There is a way of reading Gibson which permits the assimilation of many of his findings

into the general framework of Establishment psychological theorizing. Moreover, given this conciliatory reading, much that Gibson says is seen to be both true and important; and it does indeed differ in significant respects from both what has been generally assumed by psychologists who accept the information processing framework ... (.) But Gibson does not want to be read in a conciliatory way. And for good reason: if the program as he presents it were to succeed, it would constitute a conceptual revolution on the grand scale. Many of the deepest problems in cognitive psychology and the philosophy of mind would be bypassed, and the future of research in both disciplines would be dramatically altered" (p. 141).

Epstein (1977), who is quite appreciative of the worth of Gibson's contribution, though differing with him on some points of interpretation of experimental findings, cites even his earlier theoretical standpoint (Gibson, 1950) as a notable exception, in questioning the doctrine of equivocality regarding distal-proximal relationship of stimuli. The claim that proximal stimulation cannot specify the properties of the distal situation is an assumption held by almost all twentieth century theoreticians, regardless of their differences (p. 3). And Epstein goes on:

"In general, acceptance of the doctrine of equivocality has encouraged theories that emphasize the contributions of extra-stimulation factors such as selective principles of organization or cognitive-like algorithms that structure the perceptual world. In other words, the equivocality of the distal-proximal relationship has seemed to call for the identification of mechanisms that disambiguate, supplement or organize the proximal input ..(.). Gibson has been a notable exception in pointing out that earlier writers have been misled by faulty specification of both the distal and the proximal stimulation, and it is this claim concerning the specificity of the distal-proximal relation that constitutes Gibson's special contribution" (p. 4).

Unfortunately, Epstein's tardy appreciation of Gibson's contribution comes a little too late to do Gibson any good, since Gibson's subsequent emphasis on perceptual systems actively obtaining stimulation forced him to abandon the sensori-motor dichotomy and, therefore, the proximal-distal distinction (see Gibson, 1966, p. 4; Reed & Jones, 1982, p. 365).

Hamlyn (1983), a philosopher who has keenly followed psychological advances on perceptual and learning issues, is lavish in his praise of Gibson for the specifications of the information available to the perceiver. Although he agrees with him on the essentials of his theory, he doubts whether it is as complete as Gibson thinks it is:

"Gibson has done immense service to the subject in pointing out how complex an amount of information is available to the perceiver in the optical array itself, and particularly in what is invariant in the transformations that this undergoes ... (p. 58). My main criticism of Gibson's theory is that it is not complete in the way that Gibson seems to think it is. That, however, is not to say that it is wrong in its essentials, and I would like to end ... with a tribute to one of the best pieces of psychological theorizing for many years."

Fodor & Pylyshyn (1981), well aware of the threat that Gibson's theory holds for the establishment, are critical of all aspects of it. Though they find his specifications of "stimulus features" in the environment a vast improvement on the established version, in their view the properties of Gibson's ecological optics are not suitably constrained. Without proper restrictions on the notions of "invariant" and "pickup", Gibson's case becomes a very weak one indeed. And this would leave the establishment's theory as the sole winner in the field since, as they note: "Gibson and the Establishment agree that pickup and inference exhaust the psychological processes that could produce perceptual knowledge" (p. 141). In what they call "the trivialization problem", Fodor and Pylyshyn's gambit is to show that only the representational model can appropriately constrain the notions of "invariant" and "pickup". This prejudice is stated clearly at the outset: "To put the same point the other way around, our argument will be that the notion of 'invariant' and 'pickup' can be appropriately constrained only on the assumption that perception is inferentially mediated" (p. 141). Unfortunately, their bias tricks them into making assertions about Gibson's statements which do not tally with what he has been at such pains to elucidate; and, in trying to undermine the part of the theory which they admit is superior to establishment theory, they resort to gambits which do more than "trivialize" Gibson's formulations. Let us follow them in three of these attempts:

> *First gambit.* Only the ecological properties of the environment are directly perceived. .... If the notion of an ecological property is to serve to constrain the notion of direct perception, then it cannot be stipulated to embrace all properties that are "perceptible by animals like ourselves". For if all properties that can be perceived are *ipso facto* ecological, then the claim that perception is the pickup of ecological properties is vacuously true; and what is needed is some criterion for being ecological other than perceptibility. This Gibson fails to provide (p. 141).
>
> *Second gambit.* Only the projectible properties of ecological optics are directly perceived. .... The projectible ecological properties would be the ones which are connected, in a lawful way, with properties of the ambient light. It would thus be in the spirit of much of Gibson's text to suggest that it is the projectible properties, and only those, that are the possible objects of direct visual perception ... but ... Not all the properties that Gibson wants to be directly perceptible are plausibly considered to be projectible; in particular, affordances usually are not projectible. There are, for example, presumably no laws about the ways that light is structured by the class of things that can be eaten, or by the class of writing implements, though being edible or being a writing implement are just the sorts of properties that Gibson talks of objects as affording.
>
> The best one can do in this area is to say that things which share their affordances often (though, surely, not always) have a characteristic shape (colour, texture, size, etc.) and that there are laws which connect the shape (etc.) with properties of the light that the object reflects. But, of course, this consideration does Gibson no good ... (pp. 147–8).
>
> *Third gambit.* Only phenomenological properties are directly perceived.
> (We will omit their considerations on this, since Gibson leaves no room at all for misunderstanding on this point.)
>
> *Fourth gambit.* What is directly perceived is whatever "perceptual systems" respond to. .... Gibson is right to claim that reparsing the system of perceptual organs provides for, or at least permits, a new census of directly detected properties. It follows that *if* Gibson had a motivated criterion for deciding what is to count as a perceptual system, he would *ipso facto* have a principled way of constraining the notion of direct pickup. But Gibson provides *no* criterion for identifying perceptual systems or even for circumscribing which organs can in general be regarded as parts of the same perceptual system. For example, it is notable that Gibson's enumeration of the parts of the visual system does not include *the brain* (1981, p. 152).

Although Fodor & Pylyshyn are right to require appropriate constraints on the notions of "invariant" and "pickup", if Gibson's theory is to be a valid alternative, it is clear that their gambits contain misreading and misrepresentation of Gibson's formulations, which only serve to weaken their arguments. These pertain to his position on the rôle of the brain in governing perceptual systems (cf. Gibson, 1970, 1979); as also to what affordances are, and why they may be considered, as combinations of higher-order invariants, to be projectible properties of ecological optics (cf. 1970, 1979); and finally with regard to his distinction between environmental properties that are ecologically significant and those that are not (cf. 1979). Small wonder that Gibson was constrained to carry in his (1966) book a reproach in a quotation from J.L. Austen (1962), which read: "There is nothing so plain boring as the constant repetition of assertions that are not true".

After having written this, it was brought to my attention (Van Heerden, personal communication) that Turvey, Shaw, Reed & Mace (1981) have published an extensive reply to these and many other points of criticism made by Fodor & Pylyshyn. The interested reader is referred to this publication.

Mace (1977) commends Gibson for his recognition of the necessity for appropriate constraints on the stimulus for perception, and for his serious work to remedy the state of perceptual theory by proper specification of this:

> "The new insight Gibson provided .(.). was that the stimulus for perception is just as much a problem for research and theory as are the mechanisms of perception. In fact, once the appropriate description of stimulation becomes a scientific problem, one might well presume that it is logically and strategically prior to any detailed proposals about processing (Mace, 1975) ... By specifying the accomplishments of the system first, one can gradually limit the classes of plausible mechanisms for perception to those that satisfy the job description" (1977, p. 44).

Mace goes on to point out that it was Gibson who argued that just as units of structure can be sought at many levels of analysis in the light, so perceptual mechanisms functioning as units might be analysed at corresponding levels of analysis. "His suggestion that the functional organization of perceptual systems must be analysed with respect to corresponding levels of stimulus patterning is a serious constraint that more detailed theories must consider (Gibson, 1966). Surely imposing constraints to be satisfied by possible mechanisms is a key part of any effort to understand what mechanisms are actually at work" (Mace, 1977, p. 44).

What are these brain mechanisms? In the following we will consider the main ones that are postulated in different perceptual theories: constancy mechanisms, including the mechanisms of tuning or resonance.

Detecting the permanence of objects, and of the objective environment behind barriers or outside the momentary field of view or behind one's back is, according to Piaget & Inhelder (1956), entailed in the fact of intelligent behaviour. It is a central thesis of Piaget's later work, *The Mechanisms of Perception*, that perception is not the clue to the nature of the world that it is sometimes thought to be. "Perception is likely to be responsible for deformation in our view of the world. Objectivity comes through intelligence, which is active. Objectivity (1969, p. 364) is constructed on the basis of, and in proportion to, the activities of the subject" (Hamlyn, 1983). He summarizes Piaget's view as follows: "Through the study of 'primary perceptual illusions', Piaget arrived at the thesis that the overestimation of some feature of an object like its length is due primarily to centration or fixation of the object, and that the reverse effect which takes place when an illusion decreases with age or practice is due to co-ordination of centrations. This is explained on a model which presupposes 'encounters' between elements of the perceived figures and elements of the sensory receptors together with 'couplings' or correspondences between such encounters" (p. 118).

The details of this theory will not concern us here. What is important is Piaget's postulate that the child *constructs* reality instead of detecting information. He has shown that this ability to attend to features of objects and events develops in graded stages. Epstein (1977) maintains that although he differs in important respects from proponents of a strict empiricist approach, Piaget also subscribes to the doctrine that touch educates vision (cf. Gregory, 1974):

> "Hence (size) constancy makes its appearance ... after the coordination of vision and prehension ... the size of an object is variable to the sight but constant to the touch ... It is no accident, then, that constancy of size makes its appearance after and not before the coordination of vision and prehension; although of a perceptual nature, constancy thus depends upon the overall sensori-motor schemes" (Piaget & Inhelder, 1968).

Piaget & Inhelder, he goes on, "assert that 'constancy' of size makes its appearance at about six months. Once the child has been trained to choose the larger of two boxes, he continues to choose correctly if you move the larger box farther away so that its retinal image is smaller (Piaget & Inhelder, 1968, p. 31). This assertion was apparently based on the work of Cruikshank (1938, 1941), which led Piaget to believe that perceived constancy of size develops before object permanence but after the beginnings of coordination of vision and prehension" (Epstein, 1977, p. 298). But Cruikshank's experiments and others (e.g., Misumi, 1951), which tried to remedy the defects of Cruikshank's procedure, suffer, in Epstein's view, because of the inadequacy of the reaching response. "Differential reaching for objects of different sizes at a near distance may not be exhibited at a greater distance, not because the apparent size has changed but because the greater distance may inhibit reaching" (p. 299).

In similar vein is the criticism of Gregory (1981) on Piaget's decentration experiments:

> "In Piaget's best known experiments on what he calls 'decentration' (1956) he set up three model mountains, which are distinguished by colour on one, snow on another and a house on the third. The experimenter produces a doll, which he places at one side of the mountains, so the doll would have a different view from the child, who is asked what the doll would see. Because a verbal description would be difficult, even for an adult, the child may be given pictures of the model taken from various positions, and asked which of these is the doll's view of the mountains. There are other variants of the experiment, but all children under about nine years of age do markedly less well than adults. Children of six or seven choose the picture corresponding to their own viewpoints. This has been held by Piaget to show that children up to this age cannot visualize or conceive the world apart from their own viewpoint. It is, however, argued by Margaret Donaldson (1978), following extensive experiments, that the children do not understand the instructions; and when the situation is arranged so that they can understand what is required of them, they perform much better than Piaget claimed" (Gregory, 1981, p. 36).

Piaget, as Vuyk (1981) notes, is often faulted, and more often than not unjustly so, for his far-reaching assumptions about the child's competencies which are based on simplistic experiments, experiments on concrete operational structure which show failure of the children that is not due to a lack of understanding but to unfavourable variables of the tasks (p. 413), and for underestimating the social activity of the young infant (p. 409), etc. But in the three-mountain experiment, for example, "Piaget and Inhelder were primarily interested in the child's conception of space. Whether the child can understand a situation seen from different perspectives, and not whether he can see them from the perspectives of different persons, is the fundamental issue" (Vuyk, 1981, p. 112).

The constancy hypothesis, as Gregory and other representationists assume, postulates that, at least over the range of phenomena where it applies, perception is based on sensations. Thus where the hypothesis cannot get application, the deviations that are apparent cannot be due to anything sensory, and must therefore be explained by reference to processes that are not sensory. Von Helmholtz stated this as an explicit principle, and it forms the basis for Gregory's postulation of "perceptual hypotheses" or "object hypotheses", to explain systematic deviations from fact, as we saw earlier in this chapter.

In Piaget's theory, object permanence is a function of the stage of cognitive development of the child, and is specified by the structure of intellectual activities, and thus conserved in thought. Since, in his view, perceptions are not accurate reflections of the world, perception is subject to distortions which must be compensated by intellectual activity.

Gibson (1966) argues that the constancies in perception depend on the infant's (or the individual's) ability to detect invariants in the environment. This ability "depends on development insofar as the invariants of input have to be differentiated from one another in the nervous system. But the registering of invariants is something that all nervous systems are geared to do, even those of the simplest animals. The visual perception of 'depth', for example, is surely not dependent on a gradual process by which the brain learns to interpret local sensations of color. Constancy is learnable to a degree but not by a process of associating, organizing, or remembering" (Gibson, 1966, pp. 284–285).

Piaget, however, takes a radically different stand. In his view, Gibson's assumptions could never be correct since "we do not know the world as it is. Even in the case of physical knowledge arrived at by empirical abstraction, objects are no more than 'observables' which only get a meaning or signification for the subject by being assimilated into his schemes" (taken from Vuyk, 1981, p. 50). In fact, as Vuyk points out, Piaget goes so far as to agree with what the physicist Foerster said in a lecture at Geneva: "the environment contains no information. It is what it is, period" (Piaget, 1977, p. 59). For Piaget reality does exist but cannot be known as such by the subject, but only through the assimilation to action schemes.

Gibson rejects this assumption entirely and, as we have seen earlier, makes a plausible case for assuming the contrary. On the matter of the origin of the child's perception of permanence of objects, he says:

> "Does it have to depend on some kind of intellectual understanding of the causes of the child's impermanent sensations? Piaget (1954) and many others have assumed so. David Hume asserted (1739) that senses 'are incapable of giving rise to the notion of the *continued* existence of objects after they no longer appear to the senses. For that would be a contradiction in terms' (Part IV, Sec. 2). Hume was quite right; the awareness of the continued existence of a thing after it has been hidden by the edge of something else cannot

be derived from the visual sensation after it has been wiped out. But it *can* be explained by the detecting of stimulus information for occlusion, that is, the property of transformation that we call 'wiping out', which is quite distinct from the transformation that we call 'fading out' (Reynolds, 1966). The child must distinguish, or learn to perceive when a thing merely goes out of sight and when it vanishes but he does not have to 'construct' reality out of impermanent sensations (Piaget, 1954). Nor does he have to associate tactual sensations with visual ones in order 'to understand that the objects in his environment have a continuous and consistent identity entirely detached from himself'" (Vernon, 1952, p. 10).

Furthermore:

"The occlusion of a surface can be nullified, whereas the destruction of a surface cannot. Occlusion can be canceled by a movement of the body, head, or limbs in the opposite direction. Destruction, although it can sometimes be remedied, cannot simply be canceled by an opposite movement. It seems to me that young children must notice the optical transitions that can be nullified and those that cannot. How could they fail to pay attention to them? They play peek-a-boo, turn their heads, and watch their hands, all cases of reversible occlusion, and they also spill milk, break the glass, and knock down the tower of blocks, things that cannot be reversed. But this hypothesis has not been tested with babies, because the only experiments carried out are in the spirit of rationalism promoted by J. Piaget, which asserts that children must form a concept of persistence or permanence and emphasizes what children believe instead of what they see (for example, Bower, 1974, Chapter 7)" (Gibson, 1979, pp. 194–195).

Bower's (1979) experiments show that very young infants are far more competent than can be explained by Piaget's constructivism. New-born infants do not appear to live in a state of adualism, as Piaget assumed, but are already quite competent in their interaction with the environment. They "are aware of intermodal properties of objects; seen objects can be touched, heard objects can be seen and touched, etc. ... (.). There is evidence that infants perceive three-dimensionality, defend themselves against oncoming objects, distinguish figure-ground, etc. They are also capable of imitation in which perception and motor behaviour are integrated, imitating the mother when protruding her tongue, and so on" (Vuyk, 1981, p. 403). Infants as young as six weeks produced a greater change in heart-rate by the non-appearance of a stationary object from behind a moving screen than from its reappearance. This observation suggests that the infant is aware of the continuing existence of the object. However, the conclusion that some permanence is involved is not supported by studies using manual search responses until a much later age (Bower, 1971).

Though Bower's findings with infants would seem dramatically to support Gibson's contentions and undermine Piaget's assumptions, some caution is advised before reaching such a conclusion. First, because his findings have been much criticized, either because the results could not be replicated (see Dodwell, Muir & Di Franco, 1976), or because of methodological flaws (see McGurk, 1974, cited in Vuyk, 1981, p. 403). Second, because these early competencies seem to disappear after some time, and to reappear in a much more complex form late in the "sensori-motor stage".

Bower found that infants under five months of age make all sorts of mistakes, but that around five months of age there is an important change. All of this would seem to suggest the development of operational structures. If Bower's findings can be replicated, then the very early (i.e., immediately after birth) appearance of such competencies in the infant would suggest that Gibson may be right too in his assumption that perceptual systems are geared to detecting higher order variables in the (social) environment; though it is puzzling why these integrations of perceptual and motor functions should then disappear after a while. Though Bower himself was originally inclined to reject Piaget's constructivism on the basis of his findings, recently he has developed his own theory which is interactional-constructivist, though differing on essential points from Piaget. As I will return to some of the problems concerning object permanence (constancies) in Chapter IV, when considering how pathological relations become established in the mother-child interaction, I will conclude these considerations with a brief opinion based on other experimental data.

Epstein (1977, pp. 321–375) reviews the experimental data on the phenomena of constancy and comes down heavily on the side of the hypothesis that unconscious inference plays a part in the perception of constancies, but also in other perceptual phenomena (e.g., of subjective contour, Kanizsa, 1955/1974; Gregory, 1972, 1973; stroboscopic movement, Sigman & Rock, 1974; and other phenomena). He concludes:

> "Concerning all of these facts, it was suggested that the taking-into-account hypothesis is essentially correct for all constancies and moreover is based on a process of unconscious inference. In spatial constancies perception results from a process analogous to syllogistic reasoning. The major premise consists of certain 'known' rules concerning transformation of the proximal stimulus (e.g., the law of the visual angle). It is not necessary to assume that these rules are acquired by experience. The minor premise consists of the present input, one component of which leads to a percept in the proximal mode (e.g., perceived extensity), and the other of which leads to other correlated perceptions (e.g., perceived distance). In achromatic color constancy perception is based on 'knowledge' of the rule that nearby regions in a plane receive equal illumination. Evidence was presented from other areas of perception supporting a cognitive theory" (1977, p. 369).

If we allow Gibson the last word, he says: "Efforts to answer the question of why the world looks upright, stable, and unbounded despite all the vicissitudes of the retinal input are still going on. Up-to-date knowledge of this research can be obtained by reading *Stability and Constancy in Visual Perception* (Epstein, 1977). This is an admirable book if you accept its premises" (Gibson, 1979, p. 116).

Finally, some remarks on Gibson's concept of *tuning* or *resonance* at higher centres of the nervous system which lands us right in the middle of the problem of perceptual control, as defined by Gibson, and for that matter, Piaget too, in terms of the interdependency of perceiving and acting. When Gibson first formulated this concept, he was somewhat vague about it, due to lack of any solid evidence from research in this particular field.

> "The 'resonating' or 'tuning' of a system suggests the analogy of a radio receiver. This model is inadequate because there would have to be a little man to twiddle the knobs. A perceiver is a *self-tuning* system. What makes it resonate to ... (information)? The answer might be that the pickup of information is *reinforcing*. This is essentially the answer Woodworth suggested twenty years ago, in a paper on the 'reinforcement of perception' (1947). Clarity in itself, he asserts, is good, is valued. A system 'hunts' until it achieves clarity. The process can occur at more than one level. First, the pickup of information reinforces the exploratory adjustments of the organs that make it possible. And second, the registering of information reinforces whatever neural activity in the brain brings it about. We know something about the adjustments – e.g., the accommodation of the eye

where the clarity of detail is somehow 'satisfying' to the ocular system. We do not know much yet about the neural action of resonance at higher centers, but it too may prove to be the reaching of some optimal state of equilibrium" (Gibson, 1966, p. 271).

Pribram (1977), who agrees with Gibson on his major premises, regarding perceptual systems being geared to pick up invariants in the environmental structure and to do so directly, and regarding his concept of "tuning" in neural centres, disagrees with him, however, in his intransigence in rejecting that perception can be both direct and constructional, his negative views on "images", and his ultimate philosophical position (p. 89). On the mechanism of tuning in cortical centres, he mentions some of the experimental evidence for this:

"The fact that the cortex becomes tuned to environmental invariances rather than just to the retinal image is borne out dramatically by a hitherto unexplained discrepancy in the results of two experiments. In both experiments a successful attempt was made to modify the orientation selectivity of the cortical neurons of cats by raising them from birth in environments restricted to either horizontal or vertical stripes.

In one experiment (Blakemore, 1974) the kittens were raised in a large cylinder appropriately striped. A collar prevented the animals from seeing parts of their bodies – so they were exposed to only the stripes. However, and this turns out to be critical, the kittens could observe the stripes from a variety of head and eye positions. In contrast, in the other experiment (Hirsch & Spinelli, 1970), head and eye turning was prevented from influencing the experiment by tightly fitting goggles onto which the stripes were painted. In both experiments cortical neurons were found to be predominantly tuned to the horizontal or vertical depending on the kittens' environment, although the tuning in Blakemore's experiments appeared to be somewhat more effective.

The discrepancy arose when behavioral testing was instituted. Blakemore's kittens were consistently and completely deficient in their ability to follow a bar moving perpendicular to the orientation of the horizontally or vertically striped environment in which they had been raised. In our experiment, Hirsch, despite years of effort using a great number of quantitative tests, could never demonstrate any change in visual behaviour! The tuning of the cortical cells to the environmental situation which remained invariant across transformations of head and eye turning was behaviorally effective; and the tuning of the cortical cells to consistent retinal stimulation had no behavioral consequences.

These results are consonant with others obtained in other sensory modes and also help to provide some understanding of how brain processing achieves our perception of an objective world separated from the receptor surfaces which interface the organism with his environment ... (See also Von Békésy's work (1967) on auditory and somatosensory perceptions) ...

Gibson and his followers are correct, perception is direct. They are wrong if and when they think that this means that a constructional brain process is ruled out or that the percept invariably and directly gives evidence of the physical organization that gives rise to perception" (Pribram, 1977, p. 94).

A viewpoint which parallels this argument closely is that of Marr (1982). He accepts the value of ecological optics but asserts the need for algorithmic explanations of how properties of the optic array are detected:

"Gibson's important contribution was to take the debate away from the philosophical consideration of sense-data and the affective qualities of sensation and to note instead that the important thing about the senses is that they are channels for perception of the real world outside, or, in the case of vision, of the visible surfaces. He therefore asked the critically important question. How does one obtain constant perceptions in everyday life on the basis of continually changing sensations? This is exactly the right question, showing that Gibson correctly regarded the problem of perception as that of recovering from sensory information 'valid properties of the external world' (p. 29).

Although one can criticize certain shortcomings in the quality of Gibson's analysis, its major, and, in my view, fatal short-coming lies at a deeper level and results from a failure to realize two things. First, the detection of physical invariants, like image surfaces, is exactly and precisely an information processing problem, in modern terminology. And second, he vastly underrated the sheer difficulty of such detection" (Marr, 1982. p. 30).

Marr's approach to these problems is in a framework of a "computational" theory from which algorithms for perceiving are derived (Marr, 1976–1982). His alternative approach, while paying great attention to Gibson's insights about the importance of surfaces and optical flow patterns in perception, attacks from a representational standpoint the difficult and extremely complex issues involved. His is still far from a definitive resolution, and it would take us too far from our main thesis to discuss his theory and experimental work at any length. The interested reader is referred to his own publications, and also to a recent, introductory work (Bruce & Green, 1985) in which an overview is given of both Gibson's and Marr's theories and empirical work. These are compared and contrasted from the point of view of their relevance for perception and action in human beings and animals, and of their merits or shortcomings in understanding physiological aspects of vision.

Returning briefly to the question of tuning, it is only fair to the ecological standpoint to point out that some work of a more sophisticated nature has been in progress since 1977. Turvey (1977 onwards) describes how tuning in higher and lower order brain centres could be brought about. If, as he argues, "the constancy function in perception is achieved in ways fundamentally different from the constancy function in action, then the construction of theories of how we identify events (cf. Neisser, 1967) – theories of the perception concept – can proceed virtually independent of the construction of theories of the action concept. On the other hand, if the constancy function is treated in the same way in both perception and action, that is, if there is only one class of appropriate structures or only one class of appropriate procedures for achieving constancy, then the theory of identification and the theory of production ought not to be considered separately" (p. 214). In other words, a perceptual account of constancy must be potentially translatable into an action account of constancy.

Assuming this to be the more plausible case, he suggests that "co-ordinative structures which devolve on separate neuroanatomical systems (i.e., reflexes and functional combinations of reflexes) ... may be the mechanism through which the interjection of environmental details ('topological properties') is brought about, and to which the initial representation of the action plan is related" (p. 257). These "topological properties" Turvey identifies with "invariants of a higher order, for example, those which specify the identities of objects and their possibilities of transformation" (cf. Gibson, 1979). "We hypothesize that the properties of the optic array interlace with the representation of an action plan in a systematic fashion: different properties map different representations. We have ... already implied that this might be the case in arguing that the specification of action plans and the tuning of structure correspond to different properties of stimulation ... Of the properties of optical stimulation relevant to the control of action, those of a higher order are realized as tunings in higher domains and those of a lower order are realized as tunings in lower domains of the action hierarchy" (Turvey, 1977, p. 257).

This work shows that ecologists are not, by definition, averse to considering brain processes; but I introduce it here mainly as an example of a follow-through of Gibson's suggestions, which seems to clarify his concept of tuning and give more precision to his ideas about this mechanism.

In his major new work *Brain and Perception. Holonomy and Structure in Figural Processing* (1991), Pribram gives a sophisticated analysis of the concept of tuning and tuned frequencies in perceptual processing. I quote very briefly from this important work:

> "When a harmonic analysis is taken as the approach, the elongated receptive field organization of cortical neurons suggests that neurons act as 'strings' tuned to a limited bandwidth of frequencies. The ensemble of strings compose resonators or active filters as in musical instruments. A century ago, Helmholtz proposed that sensory receptors are akin to a piano keyboard; that a spatially isomorphic relation is maintained between receptor and cortex as in the relation between keys and strings of a piano, but that each cortical 'unit' responds (resonates) to a limited bandwidth of frequencies as do strings to the pianos sounding board ...(.). The details of the neurophysiological data ... show that features such as oriented lines, movement and color are best conceived as identifiable emergent characteristics of form because they are already conjoined in the receptive field. Furthermore such features become activated *either by sensory input or by central process to configure a percept*. This evidence makes the 'resonating string metaphor' more reasonable than the feature detector approach.
>
> There are four critical reasons for preferring tuned frequencies to detected features: (a) Neurons in the visual cortex respond to several features of sensory input and there is no evidence that the different features are represented by separate neurons, as would be required if it acted as a detector; (b) the receptive field properties of such neurons can be accounted for by considering them as spatial and temporal differentiations of tuned frequency; (c) tuned frequencies provide a potentially richer panoply of configurations (e.g., texture, parallax); and (d) perceptual research has clearly shown that lines (and therefore line detectors) composing contours are inadequate elements with which to account for the configural properties of vision.
>
> Rock (1983) summarized the evidence and argument as follows: The emphasis on contour detection is entirely misplaced because, as far as form is concerned, a contour simply marks or delineates a location. What matters for form perception is the set of all such locations; and if these can be delineated without contours, contours are not necessary. That is why, in addition to depth, we perceive regions of particular *shapes* in two random dot patterns viewed binocularly despite the absence of any physical contours (Julesz, 1971). Illusory contours ... also support this conclusion. (p. 43)
>
> Rock provided the results of innumerable experiments to document his insight that the configural properties of vision are due to a 'process of directional integration' (p. 47). The most critical is the demonstration that 'the perceived direction of a point with respect to ourselves...is a joint function of retinal locus and eye position' (p. 46) ....(.)
>
> In summary, cortical receptive fields are considered analogous to resonating strings in a piano. The functional relationship among strings (among the receptive fields of the sensory cortex) and with the keyboard (with the sensory receptors) is spatially organized and provide a macrolevel of perceptual processing. The functional relationship among resonant frequencies, characteristic of overlapping functions of the receptive field of the cortical neurons, provides a microlevel of perceptual processing. It is this cooperative

microprocess that allows one to assume that indeed a specific brain process is coordinate with the richness of experience that is perception" (1991, pp. 15–16).

To do justice to all, one should also note that in 1976 Neisser had already abandoned his earlier (1967) ideas on how events are identified, and moved much closer to Gibson's standpoint. As he wrote:

> "A generation ago, the primary dispute between 'stimulus-response' and 'cognitive' theories of animal learning was about whether behavior was controlled by reinforcement or expectancy. I now believe that both sides were right in that dispute, just as I believe that both J.J. Gibson and the hypothesis-testing theorists are right about perception. Indeed, there is a striking parallel between these theoretical confrontations. Gibson, like the radical behaviorists, hopes to explain activity purely in terms of the structure of the environment; all hypothetical explanatory constructs (including 'schema'!) seem dangerously mentalistic. Extreme versions of information processing or constructive theories, on the other hand, pay little heed to the kind of information the environment actually offers. They leave the perceiver lost in his own processing system, just as the older cognitive theories were said to 'leave the rat lost in the maze.' Perhaps if the present attempt to reconcile these views in terms of the perceptual cycle has any merit, it may suggest how to reconcile the older questions about behavior as well" (p. 51).

Some older work on perception, in which feedback theory (servo-system theory, cybernetics) is applied to psychological concepts (Powers, 1973), points the way to a clear understanding of some of the issues involved in perceptual control, which might be especially relevant to some of the empirical work with phobics. For this reason I mention it here.

In his book *Behavior: The Control of Perception*, Powers builds up a deceptively simple and testable model on behaviour based on negative feedback relationships between organism and environment. His thesis is that our perceptions are the only reality we can know, and that the purpose of all our actions is to control the state of the perceived world. In his own words:

> "All behavior is oriented all of the time around the control of certain quantities with respect to specific reference conditions. The only reason for which any higher organism acts is to counteract the effects of disturbances (constant or varying) on controlled quantities it senses. When the nature of these controlled quantities is known together with the corresponding reference conditions, variability all but disappears from behavior" (p. 47).

In his view, perceptual signals are continuous functions of something outside the nervous system; and perceptions do not arise mainly from brief stimuli or changes in stimulation. Some receptors emphasize rates of change; and all habituate to some extent so that the zero of the perceptual scale may wander. Perceptual signals (neural signals) are compared with reference signals from reference conditions within the individual, through comparator functions which yield zero error when perceptual and reference signals match, but larger and larger error according to how much discrepancy there is between input and reference signal. The error of this matching or comparing process is what drives the output systems (e.g., muscle tensions). Powers postulates an hierarchical organization in orders of perception, each a function of lower-order perceptions. Intensity, magnitude of stimulation of the sensory receptor, or energy flow reflects the state of the immediate environment impinging on the sensory receptors on a continuing basis, and constitutes the first order of control. Sensation control, that is, quality of intensity, constitutes the second order; configuration control (of object, pattern, arrangement, or invariant of the present moment) the third; transition control (e.g., space-time changes) the fourth; control of sequence or event (i.e., a fixed succession of lower-order elements; ordering) the fifth; control of relationship (i.e., a regularity in the simultaneous space-time behaviour of two or more independent lower-order elements) the sixth; and control of programs, principles, and system concepts the seventh, eighth and ninth orders of perceptual control, respectively. As far as the mechanics of his model go, these seem to accord well with other models of control in contemporary control theory of behaviour, so I will omit consideration of this here.

What is of more interest, and possibly relevant to phobia, are his ideas on the nature of conflict and control in higher organisms, from a perceptual standpoint:

> "A person is said to be 'in conflict' when he wants two incompatible goals to be realized at once ... Conflict *itself*, not any particular kind of conflict, represents the most serious kind of malfunction of the brain short of physical damage, and the most common even among 'normal' people. The basic mechanism behind conflict is *response to disturbance* .... Conflict is an encounter between two systems ... which attempt to control the same quantity, but with respect to two different reference levels. For one system to correct the error, the other system must experience the error. There is no way for both systems to experience zero error at the same time. Therefore the outputs of the systems must act on the shared controlled quantity in opposite directions. If both systems are reasonably sensitive to error, and the two reference levels are far apart, there will be a range of values of the controlled quantity (between the reference levels) throughout which each system will contain an error signal so large that the output of each system will be solidly at maximum. These two outputs, if about equal, will cancel, leaving essentially no net output to affect the controlled quantity; certainly the net output cannot change as the 'controlled' quantity changes in the region of the reference levels, since both outputs remain at maximum. This means that there is a range of values over which the controlled quantity cannot be protected against disturbance any more. Any moderate disturbance will change the controlled quantity, and this will change the perceptual signals in the two control systems.
>
> As long as neither reference level is closely approached, there will be no reaction to these changes on the part of the conflicted systems. When a disturbance forces the controlled quantity close enough to either reference level, however, there *will* be a reaction. The control system experiencing lessened error will relax, unbalancing the net output in the direction of the *other* reference level. As a result, the conflicted pair of systems will act like a single system having a 'virtual reference level,' between the two actual ones. A large dead zone will exist around the virtual reference level, within which there is little or no control" (Powers, 1973, pp. 254–255).

He gives an example of this, in terms of real behaviour:

> "Consider a person who has two goals: one to be a nice guy, and the other to be a strong, self-sufficient person. If he perceives these two conditions in the 'right' way (for conflict) he may find himself wanting to be deferential and pleasant, and at the same time wanting to speak up firmly for his rights. As a result, he does neither. He drifts in a state between, his attitude fluctuating with every change in external circumstances, undirected. When cajoled and coaxed enough he may find himself beginning to warm up, smile, and think of a pleasant remark, but immediately he realizes that he is being manipulated and resentfully breaks off communication or utters a cutting remark ... (.) He can react only

when pushed to one extreme or the other, and his reaction takes him back to the unconscious middle ground.

In theory and in reality, conflicted reference levels seem to have two major consequences: they define a fixed and restricted range within which behavior will keep the controlled quantity, and they destroy control *within* that range. The behaviors that do occur are always negative in their effects; they cause a strong avoidance of either reference level. Thus conflict frustrates the purpose for which either system was set up.

Conflicted pairs of control systems may exist anywhere in the hierarchy. However, conflict is highly unlikely to occur except between systems *of the same order*. Systems of different order control different classes of perceptions and are unlikely to share a single controlled quantity ... Conflict is only possible when perceptions define mutually exclusive states of lower-order sets of perceptions. Systems of order lower than the conflicted systems therefore behave normally ... If nothing disturbs the controlled quantity of a conflicted pair, an equilibrium will be reached somewhere between the reference levels. The result will be a fixed virtual reference level for a given lower-order system. ....

Higher-order systems are affected by conflicts at lower orders in two main ways. Sending reference signals to the conflicted systems will *not* result in appearance of the corresponding present-time perceptions; something unintended will be perceived. Fixity of lower-order reference signals will create the other main effect: unwanted lower-order avoidance of certain perceptual states, or almost equivalent lower-order behaviors that interfere with achievement of the higher-order goal. ...

One of the important features of higher-order compensations must be avoidance of situations in which a perception drifting in the dead zone between conflicted reference levels is forced to approach either reference level. Such an event will make the presence of conflict strongly felt, as explained above. As long as the controlled quantity remains safely in the dead zone the conflicted systems seem quiescent (in reality they are both producing maximum output, but the outputs cancel). A disturbance that brings the controlled quantity very close to one of the conflicted reference levels unbalances the conflict and meets strong resistance, a pseudo-avoidance reaction that is caused by relaxation of the output that was aiding the disturbance.

If that 'disturbance' is nothing more than a result of one's normal behavior, that behavior will be disrupted by an automatic resistance to some aspect of it. This resistance is felt as a reluctance to carry out the behavior leading to some goal, even a total inability to perform the required actions. ....

Severe conflict involves abnormally large error signals, and I think there is reason to consider that condition, occurring anywhere in the hierarchy, as an intrinsic error condition. The state of chronic large error is felt as anxiety, a state which seems universally unwanted. Thus a likely result of chronic conflict is *reorganization*. If that reorganization alters perceptions or choice of goals, all is well, but unfortunately nature does not guarantee that a reorganization will have good long-term effects. In many situations the chronic error can be largely corrected by means that leave the conflict in full effect: avoiding situations requiring the use of the conflicted systems, substituting imagined information for the uncontrollable perceptual signals from the conflicted systems, or even altering one's rules of logic in ways that are temporarily useful but in the long run will create even worse intrinsic errors. All these temporary but eventually dangerous methods are well known to the therapists; they are called *defenses*. What the system defends itself against is not anything external, but the threat of experiencing error due to conflict" (Powers, 1973, pp. 256–258).

This contribution takes us right to the subject matter of the next chapter. But before going forward, let us take a moment to reflect on a fundamental problem of all perception theories of a representational nature, as this one is too.

The problem of perception and perceptual control revolves and has revolved around the question of whether or not the perceptual process is direct. This question brings us back to the philosophical antecedents of perception (and psychology). For, as we have seen, perceptual theories are drawn across battle lines separated by this issue. Up to the last decade or so, theorists postulating a representational theory hardly seemed aware of the fact that such a model may be conceptually misleading insofar as it presupposes a basic dualism between intracerebral perceptual events and extracerebral stimulus objects (see, e.g., Tibbetts, 1969, 1972, who argued strongly against the use of representational theories of perception in experimental psychology, because of the epistemological dualism entailed).

Recently, however (e.g., Fodor, 1980, and others), there is much wider recognition of the serious problems involved for representational theory. As Tibbetts said, this "invariably commits its defenders to an epistemological dualism between a perceiving subject and external stimulus objects ... thereby 'locking us up' within the brain, with perceptual processes standing on one side of the nervous system and the external world on the other. Some sort of medium is then required to allow for communication between the two. Historically, this medium has successively been termed impressions, sensations, sense-data, neural impulses, and sensory information" (p. 408). Nor did Kant's "Copernican Revolution", although a serious attempt to reconcile the incompatibility of the axioms of rationalism and empiricism, as Needleman (1975, p. 11) carefully points out, transcend this dualism. Mind, in his view, "is not utterly separate from nature, true; nor is our contact with nature limited exclusively to a passive subjection to its influences." Knowledge being "the union of the active, organizing (constitutive) function of the mind with its more receptive and passive function ('sensibility')", leaves this dualism of mind and nature intact; for we can know phenomena but are forever barred from having knowledge of the noumena (things in themselves).

To my mind, Gibson's specifications of the information available to perceptual systems are unparalleled in psychology. But his great contribution lies in making us freshly aware of this dichotomy in our conceptions of reality, which had crept into our psychologizing from its philosophical past. For in showing us that we are not at all separate from the world but, willy-nilly, immersed in it, we come to realize that only when we recognize this fully, not just pay lip-service to it, will our understanding of the perceptual process increase, and our theoretical conceptions of the world, and of ourselves in it, mature.

Perhaps we should not ask, then, whether or not perception is direct, but approach the problem a little differently, as Mace (1977) suggests by the amusing title to his article promoting Gibson's strategy; a title which is undoubtedly inspired by parody of the title of McCulloch's article (1965), *Why the Mind is in the Head.* "Ask not what's inside your head but what your head's inside of." To this problem, but in another version, I now turn.

III

Psychodynamic Conceptions of Neurosis and the Origins of Phobia

In this chapter I shall explore some of the relations that may exist between psychical or psychological structures of the person and aspects of environmental stimulation from the point of view of disturbances in these relations which lead to formation of symptoms and to pathological behaviour.

First, I shall describe Freud's original ideas on the relation of the mind to environment, and on neurosis and phobia. Then I shall elaborate on his ideas by introducing Matte-Blanco's (1975) clarification of Freud's theoretical formulations on the characteristics of the unconscious. In this context the question arises of whether anything is added to our understanding of behaviour in pathological states by his postulate of an unconscious as a topographic system underlying consciousness. Or whether the unconscious is better understood in terms of "something which can only become known through the translating function of consciousness, or as something conscious after it has undergone transformation" (Freud, 1915, p. 166; Matte-Blanco, 1975; and also Van Heerden, 1982, p. 147, who seems to hold a similar view).

Matte-Blanco argues that Freud's conceptions of cognitive and emotional (dys) functioning can be clarified, and made more precise (and thus open to falsification), in terms of logico-mathematical principles taken from symbolic logic, in particular, by describing the unconscious-consciousness functions in terms of symmetrical-asymmetrical relations. In showing how this might be so, his conceptualizations lead him to the postulate of the unconscious as constituted by infinite sets.

The chapter is concluded by a brief consideration of some of the ideas of one other psychodynamically-oriented clinician, whose extensive work on theory-forming and clinical intervention on the phenomenon of phobia was renowned in the Netherlands. With his untimely death, Johan Barendregt's *Phobia project* (1966–1982) suffered some reverses. This study draws sustenance from his ideas. In this chapter Barendregt's last comments (1982) on the nature of phobia in terms of a "desperate attempt to re-organize the experienced chaos in consciousness (repersonalization)" are seen in the light of Matte-Blanco's clarifications.

In the following chapter the issues of interest in this and in the preceding chapter are taken up again in reconsidering the functions of "ecologically relevant optical structures and visual events" in normal and pathological behaviour. The work of Mahler et al. (1968, 1975) and of Winnicott (1960, 1982) serve to illustrate some of these relations, in showing how the young child makes use of the "potential space" between the mother (or caretaker) and him- or herself, and the uses of "transitional objects". In a reconsideration of some of the experimental results with children (e.g., Bower, 1971, 1976) the problem of perceptual control comes once more to the fore, and we return to the issues earlier explored. The stage is then set for considering the possible significance of the findings from my laboratory work with normal and phobic persons that ensue.

Freud and the Discovery of the Characteristics of the Unconscious: Freud, the Natural Scientist

As Ellenberger (1970) reminds us, the discovery of the existence of the unconscious is not due to Freud, for prior to his work, "Charcot pointed to the existence of unconscious 'fixed ideas' as nuclei of certain neuroses, a concept which was later developed by Janet and Freud" (p. 102). In fact, many of the concepts attributed to Freud do not derive from him. "Freud took from Fechner the concept of mental energy, the 'topographical' concept of the mind, the principle of pleasure-unpleasure, the principle of constancy, and the principle of repetition" (p. 218). Even the concept of defense (*Abwehr*) was taken from Meynert, although Ellenberger does concede that "there was definitely something new in the way Freud used it (1894) to mean the 'forgetting' of painful memories or ideas" (p. 486).

Sulloway (1980, p. 270) notes that Freud scholars have long known that Freud was greatly indebted too to Hughlings Jackson (1835–1911), the English neurologist, not only for the general concept of regression but for several aspects of his theory of mind, such as Jackson's conception of the human mind in terms of a hierarchical series of functional levels, with "higher", voluntary functions over-laying and "keeping down" the more involuntary, "lower" ones (1884: p. 58). He was also indebted for his understanding of a general reversal of the evolutionary process in senescence and in various neurological diseases. Jackson called these phenomena, after Herbert Spencer, "dissolutions" in mental functioning. "He also taught that the lower functional levels of mind – dynamically and subconsciously present in all healthy individuals – are temporarily unleashed during states of sleeping and dreaming (1894: 412, 415 n). 'Find out all about dreams,' Freud later quoted Hughlings Jackson as saying, 'and you will have found out all about insanity'" (p. 270).

Those, like Roazen (1969, p. 88), who claim that "the theme of plagiarism (that) can be found almost everywhere one turns in Freud's career", do him an injustice though. If Freud was sometimes remiss in acknowledging the value of the contribution of others or the debt he owed to them (e.g., in the case of Albert Moll's (1862–1939) contribution to sexual theory), most of his critics acknowledge his supremacy in the boldness of his conceptual syntheses of the assumptions of his scientific generation. Sulloway (p. 497) formulates this as follows:

> "Few thinkers took the step from a physiological to an evolutionary theory of mind more ardently than did Sigmund Freud, with his conceptual syntheses of the biogenetic law; the unconscious as the phylogenetically archaic in man; the primacy of early experience and the power of fixation, regression, and the inherited past; the theory of psychosexual stages; the dichotomy between primary (impulsive) and secondary (inhibitory) psychical systems, and, above all, evolutionary solutions to his three psychoanalytic problems (pathological repression, the choice of neurosis and Why sex?)".

But even if his contribution to science revealed "a supreme boldness in conceptual syntheses", this can hardly be seen as his main service to science. Binswanger (1975) conceives this in the way Freud himself evaluated it:

"Just as the notion of the psychic apparatus is a theoretical epitomization of the actuality of experience, so 'experience' is a theoretical verification of that epitomization ...(.).. The theoretical manner in which experience is approached is such that between theory and experience there exists an open, mutual correspondence. Freud correctly estimated that this theory was his main service to science. He did not attribute major significance to the 'practical task' of interpreting symbols but rather to the 'theoretical task' of explaining the supposed 'operations' of the particular modes of functioning of the psychic apparatus ...(.) What singles out Freud's doctrine is his attempt to demonstrate *what follows as a mechanical necessity from the given conditions of man's natural organization and the impact between these conditions and environmental factors*" (pp. 164–65).

The essence of man for Freud is "... *homo natura*, man as nature ... and that unknown that binds Freud's homo natura to the primal source of all life and that, more than any other biological conception of man, distinguishes and stamps Freud, namely, the instincts" (p. 151). As Freud says:

"Psychoanalytic investigations show ... that the deepest essence of man is instinctual impulse, whose elemental nature is the same in all men and which directs him to the satisfaction of certain primal needs" (GS X, 322 f).

Reasoning from this premise, Freud in genuine natural-scientific spirit and using a reductive dialectic, constructs his theory of man, "the pure specimen of homo natura: bodily instinct, the gaining of pleasure (sacrificing a lesser for a greater gain), inhibition because of compulsion or pressures from society (the prototype being the family), a developmental history in the sense of ontogenetic and phylogenetic transformations of outer and inner compulsions, and the inheritance of these transformations" (Binswanger, 1975, p. 153). Thus the sexual instincts (and, to a lesser degree, the aggressive instincts), which are of primary importance in the survival of the species, become those elemental impulses that motivate behaviour. The postulate of an (unrepressed) unconscious or *id*, as the deepest, most primitive psychic reality, as their source becomes necessary in order to fulfil their rôle of reducing the phenomena.

Explaining the Operations of the Modes of Functioning of the Psychic Apparatus: Freud's Theory of Mind

According to Ernest Jones (1956), as a student Freud went through a phase of radical empiricism and held throughout his life a deterministic view of man. Like most scientists of the time, he adopted the prevailing general scientific attitude of empiricism, and subscribed to the view that "the mind is the only source of information about the outer world, including the body itself, but that its perceptual data concerning the outer world need have no close correspondence with the essential nature of the latter".

Freud believed that all thought, will and action accord with laws as definite as those which govern the physical world. In this context, he held the opinion that "there was no evidence of psychical processes occurring apart from physiological ones; that physical processes precede psychical ones: information reaching the mind, whether from the outer world through the sense organs or from the body through the chemical stimuli it provides, must begin as a physical excitation" (Jones, 1956, p. 403).

Although he realized that the essential nature of mind and matter was probably intrinsically different in kind, and that it would therefore be a logical error to translate the description of the processes of the one into terms of the other, nevertheless he was greatly intrigued by the correlation between mental and physiological processes. In fact, following in the footsteps of his teacher Exner's (1894) attempt to explain psychical processes in physiological terms, he tried (1895) his hand at the same game. Though he abandoned his attempt at a relatively early stage in his career (circa 1900), calling it an "aberration", he did so more because he could find no satisfactory solution to the problems that arose, than because he ceased to believe in the relevance of such an attempt.

Much has been written about the different aspects of his metapsychological theory of mind but relatively little about this neurophysiological model, in part because his attempts have not survived in a complete form. His metapsychological theory is too well-known to bear repeating here, but the physiological theory is of interest because, first, in it are prefigured all the principles which would later be translated into psychological ones, and which give a clearer insight into what lay behind these ideas (that are expressed in language relatively unfamiliar to psychologists). Secondly, because it is his clearest statement about how he conceptualizes the interaction of sensory and perceptual systems with psychical-mnemic ones.

In the *Project for a Scientific Psychology* (1895, 1954), Freud outlined a theory of mind in which psychical processes are specified as quantitatively determinate states of material elements. The material elements are represented by neurones, each of which is separated from its neighbours by "contact-barriers" ("synapses"). These neurones can be "filled" or "empty" according to the flow of energy ("quantity') in them, a conception he later (1900) replaced by the more psychological one of "cathected ideas". The flow of energy through these neurones ("nervous excitation") might either be resisted or facilitated according to the state of the "contact-barriers" between the different neurones. The function of the nervous system is subject to two general and closely related principles: "Inertia", which stated that neurones tend to get rid of any quantity they contained. (In later years this was replaced by the "pleasure-unpleasure principle".) And the principle of "constancy", which was defined by Breuer & Freud (1892) as: "The nervous system endeavours to keep constant something in its functional condition that may be described as the 'sum of excitations'". Reflex movement, where a sensory excitation is followed by a motor discharge, is seen as the primary function of the neuronic system; nothing matters but the discharge in any direction. A secondary function comes into play when paths of discharge are chosen that put an end to the stimulation – "flight from excitation".

The external world is linked to the internal world through the stimulation of sensory neurones, which allow a current of excitation to pass through without affecting any change (the nuclei of afferent nerves). These are connected to psychical-mnemic neurones by intermediate, perceptual ones. The psychical-mnemic neurones (which form the nerve cells of the brain proper) are concerned with stimuli arising from within the body, and retain permanent traces of any stimulation affecting them. The function of the perceptual neurones is to transform energy ("quantity') into qualitative ideas.

Consciousness is neither a mere appendage of the physiological-psychical processes nor the subjective aspect of all psychical processes, but rather the subjective aspect of a *part* of them, the perceptual process. The psychical-mnemic neurones do not involve consciousness until they become associated with speech associations.

The arrangement of the peripheral nerves acts as a screen against the stream of stimuli from the external and internal world, but their "contact-barriers" are helpless against painful stimuli. Flight from pain is then postulated as a primordial tendency of the nervous system, and the memory itself of the object that had evoked the pain causes unpleasure. This conception of the breaking of barriers Freud later linked both with the importance of the part played in psychopathology by trauma as with the theory of fright and the warning signals of anxiety.

The stimulation of the nuclear neurones of the sets of psychical-mnemic ones by instinctual processes manifests itself as the Will, and supplies the motive power for the whole machinery. This necessitates some action in the outer world. Of this path of discharge Freud added that it "thus acquires the highly important function of establishing human contact, and it is the early helplessness of human beings that provides the original source of all moral motives" (1950, p. 402). It anticipates his later account of the part played by human relationships in the transition from the pleasure to the reality principle. The ego is described as an organization of neurones charged with a constant reserve of "quantity", with fairly free communication between themselves. An essential function of it is its capacity to inhibit incoming excitations; this is accomplished through part being diverted to "side-cathexes", that is, charged neurones connected through simultaneity with the first neurones stimulated; they are always available.

Freud made a distinction between what he called "primary processes" and "secondary processes", a conception he later extended. In this theory the difference lies in the flow of discharge in the two processes. In the primary process the flow is an uninhibited one; in the secondary process, which distinguishes between an external and an internal stimulus, the flow is an inhibiting one, and the level of energy lower. The distinction is thus between "free, mobile" energy and "tonic, bound" energy.

The working of the apparatus can suffer in two ways. With a wish clamouring for satisfaction the excitation may, after stimulating the memory image of the satisfying object, revert to perceptual neurones, thereby evoking an hallucination that is biologically futile; an indication is needed to distinguish between this and the perception of the real object. A criterion of reality is similarly needed in the second case, that of a "hostile" memory associated with unpleasure; when it is present a defensive flight can occur, whereas otherwise the excitation would evoke the full amount of unpleasure. (Freud, 1900, p. 757, termed a "wish" a current of accumulation of excitation in the apparatus, starting from unpleasure and aiming at pleasure.) The criterion of reality is afforded by the inhibiting powers of the ego.

Freud also distinguished between a "primary defence" against pain and "repression", the latter being an exclusion from the processes of thought of an idea which would cause unpleasure in the ego, an idea that takes its origin in a sexual impulse. In this model the concept of Attention played a prominent rôle (although Strachey, 1976, notes that it played a very small part in later writings). Freud described how the ego neurones respond to an external stimulus not simply passively, but by actively directing a charge of energy to the perceptual neurones. This happens particularly when consciousness is present (Jones, 1956, p. 429).

In his metapsychological theory of mind Freud points out that an hallucinatory wish-fulfilment is an occurrence familiar in the psychoses and also highly characteristic of the processes of dream formation. Sooner or later this in its turn fails to relieve the situation and the unpleasure persists. Herein lie the beginnings of thought.

> "Among those wishful impulses derived from infancy, which can neither be destroyed nor inhibited, there are some whose fulfilment would be a contradiction of the purposive ideas of secondary thinking. The fulfilment of these wishes would no longer generate an effect of pleasure but of unpleasure; and it is precisely this transformation of affect which constitutes the essence of what we term 'repression'" (Freud, 1900, p. 764).

The preconscious is nearly equivalent to what Freud later calls the ego, though the ego extends into both the unconscious proper and consciousness. The important inhibiting function of the preconscious on the original free flow of energy is the distinguishing mark of the secondary system. There is a sieve-like barrier between the unconscious and the preconscious, and also between the preconscious and consciousness. Ideas can traverse these barriers only when certain conditions are fulfilled, the pleasure-unpleasure principle being the regulating one. Freud saw these barriers as functioning as "censors".

The preconscious has no qualitative, only quantitative attributes. In this it differs from consciousness, which derives qualities from three sources: the release of either pleasure or unpleasure; from association with speech memories, which have a quality of their own; and, more directly, from perception. Freud therefore defines consciousness as "a sense organ for the perception of psychical qualities" (1900, p. 776).

Consciousness can be brought into being through a perceptual stimulus emanating from the outer world or through the evocation of pleasure or unpleasure from the preconscious. In both the physiological and metapsychological theories then three different aspects appear: the economic aspect (in the equating of any accumulation of tension with unpleasure and any diminution with pleasure). This aspect implies also the principle of constancy (the keeping constant of the "sum of excitations" in its functional relations). Both principles together imply the dynamic aspect of the theory, which conceives mental phenomena in terms of psychical forces which may conflict, inhibit one another, or combine, and so on. Finally, inherent in the hypothesis of an unconscious part of the mind underlying the preconscious and conscious parts, the topographical (or structural) aspect is outlined.

In the years between 1917–20 some revisions of this theory appeared. The essence of these revisions lay in (a) the stressing of the importance of a biological tendency in the organism to restore earlier states of being – this was explained in terms of the formulation of "life" and "death" instincts, which are as fundamental as the sexual and aggressive ones – and, (b) the formulation of the threefold differentiation of mental processes in terms of the agencies, regions or realms *id, ego* and *superego*. Also, in dealing with the fixation and lack of plasticity characteristic of neuroses, Freud postulated still another fundamental principle, the principle of repetition, which could explain the tendency towards repetition observed in his neurotic patients, and sometimes too in ordinary, normal functioning.

Anxiety and Symptom Formation in Neurosis and Phobia: "Struggle and Conflict as Mental Paradigm"
(The Phrase is from Sulloway, 1980)

In earlier work, Freud held to the assumption that anxiety and symptom formation could be explained in terms of a primal trauma of a sexual nature. The excitatory processes arising in the id as a consequence of this but which could find no discharge in the external world brought about a transformation of affect. This transformation constituted the essence of repression (1900, p. 764). In his later formulations (1926–36), he reveals a much more sophisticated approach to the whole problem. Though he never entirely relinquished his postulate of symptom formation as due to sexual trauma, he broadened the basis for his assumptions. In these formulations the problem of "transformation of affect" too, which had not been satisfactorily resolved, is more plausibly explained. In *Inhibitions, Symptoms and Anxiety*, Freud now identifies anxiety (and symptom-formation) as due to "a reaction to a traumatic situation in the past, the essence of which is an expectation of *helplessness* on the part of the ego in the face of an accumulation of excitation, whether of external or internal origin, which cannot be dealt with" (1926, p. 80). This formulation allows for trauma to be understood not exclusively in sexual terms. The fear of being abandoned by the mother is for the infant just as traumatic. In fact, even the act of birth, as the individual's first experience of anxiety, can have become incorporated in the mind as *the* primaeval traumatic experience, thereby giving a certain characteristic form of expression to subsequent affective states. Which is not to say that, in an outbreak of anxiety, something like a re-enactment of the situation of birth goes on in the mind.

The ego is now seen to be the actual seat of anxiety. Normally, by keeping any undesirable impulse from the id from becoming conscious by inhibiting or deflecting it, it exerts a powerful influence over id processes. By its connections with the perceptual system, which is bound up with the phenomenon of consciousness, it receives excitations from outside and within. When the ego is opposed to an instinctual process in the id, it gives a "signal of unpleasure" to the id, and represses it using its own energy to do so. But, "since it is intimately bound up with the id, it can only fend off an instinctual danger by restricting its own organization, and by acquiescing in the formation of symptoms in exchange for having impaired the instinct. If the rejected instinct renews its attack, the ego is overtaken by all those difficulties which are known as neurotic ailments" (p. 70).

The ego then is engaged in a constant struggle with the id, and under the influence of external reality to find a *modus vivendi* acceptable to both agencies. It is therefore obliged to guard against those instinctual impulses which it knows from contact with reality can find no adequate expression, and to treat them as dangers. An undesirable instinctual impulse can be aroused by some external perception, but also internally without any such provocation (e.g., sexual excitation directed towards a forbidden object, or aggressive impulses).

When repression fails, in greater or lesser extent, the instinctual impulse finds an outlet for satisfaction in a substitute; but because of the interference of the ego in its struggle against this satisfaction, it has to make do with a substitute which is very much reduced, displaced and inhibited, and which is no longer recognizable as a satisfaction. When the substitutive impulse is carried out, there is no sensation of pleasure. On the contrary; its carrying out has the quality of a compulsion. Since the ego does all it can to prevent it having an external outlet, this substitute often takes first form as alterations in the subject's own body (for example, physiological symptoms such as heart palpitations, and fainting, and other psychosomatic symptoms, even conversion hysteria).

As a rule, the instinctual impulse to be repressed remains isolated, for the mental process which has been turned into a symptom is kept outside the organization of the ego. But the initial act of repression is often followed by a tedious and interminable sequel in which the struggle against the instinctual impulse is turned into a struggle against the symptom (p. 11). The ego copes with this defensive struggle by trying to bind or incorporate the symptoms into its own organization, and on the other hand by "adapting" to the symptoms and exploiting them so as to appease the demands of the superego or refuse some claim from the external world. Thus the symptoms become representative of important, secondary interests.

Freud distinguishes between three forms of neurotic anxiety:

(1) freely floating anxiety which readily attaches itself to any available or suitable object, and is characterized by an "anxious expectation" or general apprehensiveness;
(2) anxiety which is bound psychically to and attached to particular objects and situations. The majority of phobias belong to this group;
(3) anxiety in cases where the connection to threatening danger is completely lost to sight, as in obsessional states.

A phobia can arise after a first anxiety attack, for example, in a street, public vehicle, or in solitude. The anxiety is held under ban by projection onto the situation in which it was first felt, and by thereafter avoiding this, and similar situations. In this way the phobia serves as a means of defending oneself against the instinctual impulse which is the driving force behind the anxiety; and as long as the protective condition (avoidance) is maintained, it may remain in abeyance. Phobia, in this view, is then defined as "a projection in that it replaces an internal, instinctual danger by an external, perceptual one ... and in the last resort is merely that one danger is replaced by another" (1926, p. 40).

One can now see how important a rôle the external situation plays in helping the person to avoid the instinctual danger, the re-occurrence of the debilitating experience of helplessness. Also, how anxiety functions as a signal to warn of and ward off such an attack. It becomes clearer how an internal and external danger situation come to be linked, for by localizing the source of one's unease in the external situation, a situation which is in general much more easily controlled than the terrifying instinctual danger situation, one may hope to avoid the latter. Besides, an external situation often has the advantage of alleviating one's dependency needs through the help proffered by sympathetic others, so that facing up to the real source of danger can be postponed.

Since, in Freud's view then "human beings fall ill of a conflict between the claims of instinctual life and the resistance which arises within them against it" (1933, p. 88), it might be worth our while to take a second look at the mechanisms and characteristics of the id, "a province as foreign to the ego as the external reality is".

The Mechanisms and Characteristics of the System Unconscious (Ucs) Reconsidered: Freud; Matte-Blanco

Through his self-analysis, the interpretation of his dreams and those of his patients, Freud discovered that dreams have a compromise-structure, which is similar to the compromise-structure found in neurotic and psychotic symptoms. In his analysis of the process of dream-work he distinguished five mechanisms, four of which are peculiar to the id: condensation, displacement, representation and symbolization. Condensation is the process through which different elements that have any point of contact are condensed into new units, like images superimposed on one another to form a new constellation. Displacement is the process by which a shifting of accent takes place, as when cathexes or affects of two separate ideas are displaced onto something else, a common intermediate. Representation is the process through which unconscious thoughts become modified so that they can be expressed in a predominantly visual, and to a lesser extent, a verbal or conceptual form. Symbolization is the process through which the symbols that already exist in the unconscious are made to stand for or depict some unconscious wish, which in less disguised form might meet with disapproval or resistance from the ego. (The fifth is the replacement of external by psychical reality.)

All these mechanisms may contribute to the typical dream-distortion with which we are familiar. The importance of this finding was increased by the discovery that the same mechanisms are operative in the construction of neurotic symptoms.

From this Freud concluded that the dream is a "pathological" product, though a harmless one in that, in the state of sleep, the turning-away from the real, external world is willed and temporary, and the dream-psychosis disappears when relations with the external world are resumed. This recognition that an extensive part of mental life is normally inaccessible to the ego, the processes involved being in a truly dynamic sense unconscious, led him to postulate a "system" of the unconscious (Ucs) distinct from a "system" of the preconscious (Pcs), and from consciousness (Cs). At different times he would speak of mental provinces, regions and realms, particularly in describing the id, ego and superego functions. These delineations were conceptualizations of the ego and superego as having areas which are unconscious, although the repressed parts of the ego are potentially retrievable to consciousness. To get around this dilemma, he compared these partially overlapping systems and structures of mental life by the analogy between these and countries and their peoples. The countries stay put but the people (the inhabitants) are wont to move around from country to country, and intermingle at will.

The use of metaphor and analogy to describe dynamic functions of the mind has obvious advantages but many limitations too; not least of these is the danger that by frequent usage, the metaphorical or analogical aspect tends to become lost to sight, as one begins to think of these systems or functions as having real, substantive being. Though Freud was well aware of this danger, like most explorers he tended to underestimate his own susceptibility to it; to say nothing of those who came after him.

On a suggestion of Groddeck (1923), from then on he used the term *id* to describe "the impersonal part of the province of the mind that is alien to the ego" (Freud, 1923).

He described its characteristics as follows:

> "... a chaos, a cauldron full of seething excitations ... it has no organization, produces no collective will but only a striving to bring about the satisfaction of the instinctual needs. ... The logical laws of thought do not apply to the id, and this is true above all of the law of contradiction. Contrary impulses exist side by side, without cancelling each other out or diminishing one another; ...
> ... There is nothing in the id that could be compared with negation; ... There is nothing in the id that corresponds to the idea of time; there is no recognition of the passage of time, and no ... alteration in its mental processes is produced by the passage of time ... Wishful impulses which have never passed beyond the id, and impressions too which have sunk into the id by repression, are virtually immortal; after the passage of decades they behave as though they had just occurred ...
> The id ... knows no judgment of value; no good and evil, no morality ... Its energy ... is far more mobile and capable of discharge, otherwise the displacement and condensation would not occur ... We are in a position to attribute to the id characteristics other than that of its being unconscious, and ... recognize the possibility of portions of the ego and superego being unconscious without possessing the same primitive and irrational characteristics ..."

The characteristics of the actual ego, on the other hand, are quite different:

> "... The ego is that portion of the id which was modified by the proximity and influence of the external world ... The relation to the external world has become the decisive factor ... It must lay down an accurate picture of it in the memory-traces of its perceptions ... The ego controls the approaches to motility under the id's orders; but between a need and an action it has interposed a postponement in the form of the activity of thought.
> ... The relation to time ... is also introduced into the ego by the perceptual system; ... But what distinguishes the ego from the id quite especially is a tendency to synthesis in its contents, to a combination and unification in its mental processes ... It alone produces the high degree of organization ...
> The ego develops from perceiving the instincts to controlling these ... The ego stands for reason and good sense while the id stands for the untamed passions" (Freud, 1933, pp. 106–109).

In his book *The Unconscious as Infinite Sets*, Matte-Blanco (1975) evaluates these characteristics or laws of the unconscious and preconscious systems as Freud's unique, essential and most creative contribution to our understanding of mental life. The results of a lifetime of clinical work as a psychoanalyst (and theoretician), dealing mainly with schizophrenic patients, have convinced him that Freud's formulations of the special characteristics of the system Ucs "reveal to us the operation of a logic peculiar to this system, whose fundamental distinguishing mark is that it treats as symmetrical relations which in scientific logic are not so considered". Freud himself realized, when he wrote "the logical laws of thought do not apply to the id", that he was onto something most peculiar in the functioning of this part of mental life, and he even spoke of it as the Realm of the Illogical (1940, p. 168). His perplexity is clearly evident in the fact that, although these characteristics are systematically described, he states also that it is "a chaos ... with no organization". Matte-Blanco points this discrepancy out, and goes on, "if the system Ucs. were a chaos, then nothing would be predictable, and Freud could not have found the characteristics he described" (p. 37). Therefore, argues Matte-Blanco, "if the laws of the system Ucs. exist, if the system has discernible characteristics that can be systematically described, it must also have an organization that is not chaotic but different from the system of consciousness, which conforms to principles of scientific (or Aristotelian) logic".

In studying the thinking of schizophrenics, he reached the conclusion that a type of their thinking is no different from normal thinking (that is, conforms with scientific logic), but another type conforms to the thinking Freud described as characteristic of the Ucs, that is, the replacement of external by psychical reality. "In psychiatric terms, this is sometimes referred to as 'the literal interpretation of metaphor'". In one and the same mental product of these patients, both types of thinking could be discerned. To Matte-Blanco it seemed as if in unconscious thinking two principles of (symbolic) logic were operative, namely, the principle of generalization and the principle of symmetry. He goes on to show that, taken together, these principles predicate the characteristics discovered by Freud in the system Ucs: (1) absence of mutual contradiction, (2) absence of negation, (3) absence of time (and space), (4) condensation (5) displacement, and (6) replacement of external by psychical reality (or the literal interpretation of metaphor). In his view, "the principle of generalisation is representative of conscious normality ... and is also representative of the system Ucs. For the system Ucs. treats an individual thing (person, object, concept) as if it were a member or element of a set or class that contains other members. It treats this class as a subclass of a more general class, and this more general class as a subclass or subset of a still more general class, and so on ... Also, we find this principle is frequently applied according to another principle which predicates it, which may be formulated as follows: In the choice of classes and of higher and higher classes the system Ucs. shows a preference for those propositional functions which in one aspect constitute increasing generality and in others keep particular characteristics of the individual thing from which they start" (p. 38). So far, so good.

But the system Ucs also treats the converse of any relation as identical with the relation. In other words, it treats asymmetrical relations as if they were symmetrical. For those of us who are not students of logic, a simple illustration will show what is meant: "If John is the brother of Peter, the converse is: Peter is the brother of John. The relation which exists between them is symmetrical, because the converse is identical with the direct relation. But if John is the father of Peter, the converse is: Peter is the son of John. In this case the relation and its converse are not identical. This type of relation which is always different from its converse is called asymmetrical ... What the second principle (the principle of symmetry) affirms, ... (as applied to the system Ucs.) is, that the system Ucs. tends to treat *any* relation as if it were symmetrical. In the example given: If John is the father of Peter, then Peter is the father of John ... In scientific logic this is absurd; in the logic of the system Ucs. it is *normal*" (p. 38).

Matte-Blanco asserts that this formidable departure from the logic on which all our scientific and philosophical thinking is based is found constantly in operation in schizophrenic and unconscious thinking. The main thesis of his book is to show that not only are these two principles of symbolic logic sufficient to generate all the laws of the Ucs. that Freud discovered, but that in this approach the need for the delineation of mind in topographic systems, realms, regions or agencies disappears. It also has some surprising implications for our understanding of infantile logic, the logic operative in neuroses and psychoses, in our emotions, as well as in science and art. In this context I will explore only those implications which may be relevant to my own thesis.

From the principle of symmetry follows certain fundamental consequences which are important in this context. According to Matte-Blanco, these are:

"1. When the principle of symmetry is applied there cannot be succession. Succession of moments is actually a serial ordination, and if asymmetrical relations are barred, then, according to symbolic logic, there cannot be such ordinations; and therefore there cannot be time in the physico-mathematical sense.
2. When the principle of symmetry is applied the (proper) part is necessarily identical to the whole. For example, an arm can be said to be a proper part of a given body. If the principle of symmetry is applied then the relation 'the arm is part of the body' is identical to its converse 'the body is part of the arm'. In the same way that time disappears, there is no place for any difference between the proper part and the whole. In other words, the proper part is treated as though it were an improper part. By virtue of it, the total (and therefore the potentialities of the total) is included in any part, which results in any part being identical to the total, and in consequence identical also to any other part. This applies to the parts or constituents of any set or class, aggregate, whole, concept, person, object or situation."

Three particular types of examples of this application are mentioned by him (pp. 39–40):

"(a) When the principle of symmetry is applied, all members of a set or of a class are treated as identical to one another and to the whole set or class and are therefore interchangeable with respect both to the propositional function which determines or defines the class and also with respect to all the propositional functions which differentiate them, and owing to which functions, according to Aristotelian logic, the members of the class are not identical with one another.
(b) When the principle of symmetry is applied, certain classes whose propositional functions are of the type *p* and not-*p* and which, therefore, are empty by definition, may be treated as not empty. For example, if we call *p* 'being alive', then not-*p* is 'not being alive'. One variety of not being alive is being dead. In symbolic logic a class whose propositional function is 'being alive and being dead' (intersection) is by its very definition an empty class, because according to the principle of non-contradiction there cannot be *p* and not-*p*. But being alive and being dead are subclasses of a higher class whose propositional function may include all possibilities regarding life. It follows then from the application of the principle, stated under 2, that being alive is identical to being dead. From this a new class may be formed, that of those who are alive and dead. (In fact, schizophrenics and the system Ucs. or id actually treat this empty class as though it were not empty. Note that such procedure does not conform to the principle of non-contradiction.)
(c) When the principle of symmetry is applied there can be no relations of contiguity between the parts of a whole. (Matte-Blanco notes that this is especially important if applied to material objects) ... For example, take the pages (parts) of a book. If the whole book is contained in each page, there can be no relation of contiguity between the pages. The same can be said of any material object, because our conception of material objects contains contiguity as an essential element. So, it follows by virtue of the principle of symmetry, that both space and time vanish."

Returning now to the characteristics of the id, as described by Freud, and in the light of Matte-Blanco's assumptions, these may now be understood as follows:

"The lack of mutual contradiction, for instance between two impulses, which appear incompatible to scientific logic and their union in one expression, which is accomplished in condensation, suggests that both are treated either as going in the same direction, or as being parts of a more general whole, parts that would not be mutually exclusive. This suggests (a) the formulation of more inclusive classes; (b) treating the subclasses of each of these classes as identical to one another; and (c) perhaps even treating as identical various different concepts which in scientific logic are mutually exclusive. In other words, the operation of the principle of generalization and the principle of symmetry. In condensation we see that a given object may suggest more than one meaning or represent more than one person. If we keep in mind that according to the principle of symmetry each part contains the potentialities of the whole and of any other part, then it becomes perfectly understandable that an element may have more than one meaning or represent more than one person; and it becomes comprehensible that two impulses symbolised by two material (i.e., spatially extensive) objects 'do not diminish each other or cancel each other' (Freud, 1933).

The absence of negation, about which characteristic Freud was not consistent and explicit in his different works, might be an indirect implication of the absence of the logical principle of non-contradiction, to which Freud seems explicitly to refer when he says, 'the logical laws of thought do not apply to the id, and this is true above all of the law of contradiction'.

— The absence of time, and the lack of alteration in its mental processes is a consequence of the fact that the processes of the system Ucs. are not ordered in time, and this in turn is a consequence of the principle of symmetry operating in the Ucs.

— Displacement is a fundamental characteristic of the functioning of the Ucs. It is at the base of projection, sublimation, transference, the return of the repressed and the division of objects. All these mechanisms are in some way examples of displacement ... In displacement we see the simultaneous action of two different processes. (An example will clarify this) ... When an individual displaces, he treats the primitive object and the object towards which he displaces as elements of a class which has a certain specific characteristic, which is perhaps not striking to conscious thinking, but is to his unconscious. For example, if he feels his chief to be a dangerous father it is because he considers that both have the same characteristic, dangerousness. If this is expressed in terms of symbolic logic we may say that in his unconscious he treats both as elements of a class; it may also happen that he treats one as an element of another class, but in this case both classes are always subclasses of a more general class. For example, a mother who feeds belongs, let us say, to the class of women who feed materially; a professor who teaches belongs to the class of men who feed mentally. When on account of a process of displacement an individual feels the professor as a mother who feeds he is, first of all, treating both classes as subclasses of a more general class, that of those who feed, either materially or mentally. This is the first process visible in displacement, clearly the operation of the principle of generalization. But this principle alone would not suffice for the understanding of displacement. There is yet another aspect. When displacing (for instance, from mother to professor) the unconscious does not treat both only as possessors of something in common, but treats them as identical. And this shows the operation of a consequence of the principle of symmetry. Displacement is then the result of the joint operation of that aspect of scientific logic described as the principle of generalization, and a logical consequence of the principle of symmetry. If displacement is viewed in this light, then one can see that its name, which seems appropriate if referring to cathexes or charges of energy (a certain amount of energy goes over, or is displaced, from one process to another) is no longer justified. For, from a logical point of view, nothing is displaced. The original and the displaced aspect are simply both treated as being identical. Put in another way, we can only speak of displacement if we view the workings of 'symmetrical logic' from an 'asymmetrical' vantage point (1975, p. 43).

> — Replacement of external by psychical reality is now seen to be a particular example of displacement ... Consider as examples the identity established by the unconscious between mental cannibalism and real cannibalism, between the aggressive desire and an aggressive accomplishment, between the emotion described as bursting with rage and a real bursting, etc. It is obvious that in every one of these examples the essential process at work can be described as follows: First, the unconscious treats both as elements of the same class or as elements of different classes which themselves are subclasses of a more general class; then it treats the two as if they were identical. These are precisely the two processes at play in displacement."

That the unconscious does not deal with individuals but only classes or propositional functions which define the class, is one of the main themes of Matte-Blanco's work: "Of course, this is only from the point of view of outside observers. The unconscious does not follow or worry, to use an anthropomorphic expression, about the logic anymore than our digestive tract worries about the chemistry of the enzyme ... This is only a logical way of describing the indescribable, the experience of being which cannot be grasped in her totality. But one might say, from this point of view, that symmetrical being is the normal state of man, and the colossal base from which consciousness or asymmetrical being emerges" (p. 101).

That the symmetrical mode of being (or the id) cannot be apprehended as such but only through the distortion it creates in the asymmetrical mode of being ("consciousness"), was already realized by Freud (1915, p. 166), who wrote: "How are we to arrive at a knowledge of the unconscious? It is of course only as something conscious that we know it, after it has undergone transformation or translation into something conscious. Psychoanalytic work shows us every day that translation of this kind is possible". See also Van Heerden's work (1982), *De zorgelijke staat van het onbewuste* (*The precarious state of the unconscious*), who explores the concept "Unconscious" from philosophical and psychological viewpoints. Matte-Blanco underwrites this proposition: "The Ucs. proper without its unfolding function can never be apprehended as such, but only through the distortion it creates in the asymmetrical mode of being. Whereas in the case of 'repressed' ideas, ... which, having been conscious, are ordered in a spatio-temporal way (so that bringing them back into consciousness is comparable to shining a light on something already 'there') ... in the unconscious mode of being there are no asymmetrical relations *within* it. Consciousness therefore picks 'bits' here and there and gives them order in time (and, in fact, also in space). In other words, it behaves as though it were transforming symmetrical being into something which symmetrical being is not ... by describing, for instance, as a disorder something which in itself is neither order nor a disorder. It is a task similar or identical to that of describing something immaterial by means of material images ... This is the function of translating, which cannot by the nature of things, ever be successful (p. 110). Words, or rather their meanings, are the asymmetrical tools of the translating, unfolding function".

The two modes of being in man can only be conceived as given together. When mental manifestations begin to make their appearance in the infant, the so-called primary and secondary processes appear together. In logical terms, "the primary process can be seen as the unavailability of asymmetrical relations". But mental activity would not be possible with symmetrical being alone. Mental activity implies the establishment of relations, and ordering these in space and time (which is the way

Freud defines the secondary process). "The mind is structured in such a way that in every one of its direct manifestations we can, if we look for it, detect the activity of its various levels, from the asymmetry seen in conscious thinking to the great proportion of symmetry of the deepest levels (p. 161)". A few simple examples to illustrate this. If we put ourselves in the mind of the new-born baby (which, in this view, is largely that of symmetrical being) we can imagine that the breast, or rather, its functions of feeding, warming, caressing, and so on, are the only thing the baby feels or knows. The total person (the mother) is for the baby what we might call an immense "breastness". And, immersed as it is in symmetrical being, its world that of the Eternal Now.

By the same logic, we might say that the toddler who tells his mother that "I don't want to be you anymore, I want to be me" is, in giving vent to feelings or longings for separatehood, showing some recognition of increasing emergence from symmetrical being into an asymmetrical mode of being.

If our mental life is described by these two modes of being, then in all our manifestations of life (thought, emotion, action) these must be intermingled, the proportion of symmetrical to asymmetrical being determining the depth and density of feeling, thought, and so on. The more symmetrical is our thinking, the less discriminable will be the elements contained in it, but the greater the feelings of "ineffability" perhaps. By contrast, the more asymmetrical is our thinking, the greater may be the clarity contained in it, but from the point of view of symmetrical being, the more superficial must be its content.

The notion of intrapsychic conflict can be seen in a new light from this vantage-point of the bipolarity of symmetry-asymmetry. According to Matte-Blanco, the effect of psycho-analytic therapy has been attributed to the fact of "making the unconscious conscious". The assumption underlying such an assertion is that the sole fact of something being unconscious is already a source of pathology. But it has never been clear how and why this should be so. "If symmetrical being is 'the true psychic reality' (the source of all that is), then inasmuch as we are symmetrical beings we are not independent from others because we are a unity with others. For asymmetrical being, in contrast, this absence of individual limits is inconceivable. Consequently, whenever such an absence becomes omnipresent, and therefore imperative, this is felt by our asymmetrical aspect as a loss of our identity as individuals, and a danger of annihilation. Such a contrast between both modes of being would constitute the deepest source of conflict (p. 319).

If we consider actual cases of neuroses and psychoses, such a view seems justified ... For instance, in the case of phobia, in which the dangerousness of a parent is 'repressed' and 'displaced' onto an external object. In conformity with the principle of symmetry, the individual is identified with all other individuals in the class, and with the class. Seen from this angle, the fear of the external object, which becomes invested with characteristics which, asymmetrically speaking, it does not have. The danger is felt, deep down, as infinite, in conformity with the nature of emotion which tends to consider its object as an infinite set. And the actual danger becomes multiplied in a completely fantastic way ... At the root of neurosis, and psychosis then lies the strange interaction between the all-expanding tendency of the principle of symmetry and the limiting tendency of asymmetry, whereby very concrete entities become invested with the power of infinite sets" (p. 320).

It will come as no surprise, then, to hear that Matte-Blanco, though a great admirer of the early Freud, sees from this point of view neither need for "the extremely vague concept of mental energy" to explain psychical relations, whether "bound" or "freely flowing"; nor for the use of the terms "primary" and "secondary" processes to describe them. "This can be quite misleading if defined, as Freud sometimes did, in terms of the 'so-called charges of energy or cathexes', or alternatively, as 'the totality of laws which the *processes in the unconscious or id* obey' (1940). For the concept of process with regard to the unconscious implies something that evolves in time. Nor, viewed logically, can exemption from mutual contradiction, or the replacement of external by psychical reality be considered in terms of process ... Also, the adjective 'primary' refers to a chronologically earlier process, and this makes no sense if symmetrical and asymmetrical relations go together". Symmetrical being without its unfolding (asymmetrical) functions cannot be known, in the same way that asymmetrical being divorced from its content ("its bags of symmetry of which it forms the wrappings"), cannot comprise any reality, psychical or otherwise.

In this view too the threefold conception of mind (id, ego and superego) can hardly be understood except in terms of a self or person who exercises such *functions*. "Seen as provinces, which separate three entities, is to see these as split-off parts of the self or person, an extreme state of affairs when things have become intolerable" (p. 123).

Finally, Matte-Blanco notes that "instincts, as intentional, purposive strivings (desires, wishes) are already highly asymmetrical concepts, so that the zone of contact between instincts and the self is not at the most symmetrical, deeper zone of self but at a more superficial one ... Hence, these can hardly be considered to be "the deepest essence of man ... whose elemental nature ... directs him to the satisfaction of certain primal needs" (1975, p. 123).

Matte-Blanco's perspective on the workings of the unconscious-consciousness systems certainly seems to clarify much that remained abstruse in Freud's formulations. But the value of his approach depends to a large extent on the validity of his application of logic to the system Ucs., and its characteristics. Without wishing to detract from the exciting prospects which seem to open up in this approach, Van Heerden (1986), in a personal communication, advises some caution on the basis of what is reflected of his work in the foregoing. As he notes, and I quote:

> "Matte-Blanco presents the reader with a puzzling problem. It is not clear whether the Ucs. is treated as an independent logical system or as a reservoir of impulses that seduces the person into making typical logical errors. The text permits both interpretations. On one hand is stated with regularity that the Ucs. is a logical system in which the asymmetrical relation is also symmetrical. On the other hand in the text are found formulations such as 'tends to treat', 'perhaps even treating', 'may have', etc., which imply no logical necessity (as a system). In the first case, the *system* contains a contradiction and therefore further elaboration of certain typical consequences is useless, because in a contradictory system all possible consequences are directly given and derivable. In such case it is unclear how one can *logically* limit oneself to certain typical statements which interest.
>
> If one tolerates shades of meaning (nuances), such as 'tends to treat', in doing so one robs the system, as logical system, of its imperative character. This is allowed only if the Ucs. is *not* conceived as an independent logical system but as a set of statements which the 'patient' makes, and which peculiar errors (e.g., infringements of the law of non-contradiction, or of treating asymmetrical relations *sometimes* as symmetrical ones,

etcetera) the patient makes under pressure of certain (unconscious) impulses; but in that case the Ucs. is no longer a logical system.

The ontological status of 'the system Ucs.' is also unclear. When, as is said 'In fact (...) the system Ucs ... actually treats ...', is this to be understood as a personification? (see page 55 in this book, under b.). The second paragraph (on page 57) seems to support this: the Ucs. as independently thinking body. But that is quite another thing than a logical system, which does not think, deal or 'worry'.

In sum: what is the Ucs.? A part of the person? A logical system, that therefore does not deal, think, condense, etc.? A personified system where the personification is merely a heuristic tool? A manner of thinking that is characterized by certain infringements of formal logic which can *sometimes* take place? I would opt for the last."

Whether one should take Matte-Blanco literally, and what the metapsychological consequences are, is thus unclear. Nevertheless, the perspective of being able to describe the operation of the unconscious (Ucs.) in logical terms is certainly clarifying; and shows that, at least in the effects, there is lawfulness.

Since this was written, Matte-Blanco has extended his concepts in a new book *Thinking, Feeling and Being* (1988), in which he further elaborates on some of his ideas regarding the bi-logical stratified structure of our internal world. He views all processes of thinking (and for that mattter, emotions too) as having a certain structure, as sets endowed with various relations between their components ... In the introduction to the book his editors summarize some of his ideas:

"The logical structure of thinking may be compared by considering how they differ in the way bivalent and symmetrical logics intertwine with one another...Matte-Blanco suggests that our everyday ideas, thoughts, and feelings about people, things, and their relationships mean different things to us at what may be considered deeper and deeper zones or *strata* in our minds, conceptually differentiated according to the degree of symmetrization routinely present at that level. He suggests that at the deepest levels (in our unconscious) we all experience a unity, between ourselves and everybody and everything else. There is no asymmetrical thinking, and there are no distinctions. However, this is not incompatible with recognizing differences at less deep, more conscious, or more superficial levels. In these terms human experience can be conceived as structured by the existence of up to an infinite series of strata in which our capacity to recognize differences declines as the amount of symmetrization increases. At the limit, the deepest levels, is what Matte-Blanco calls the indivisible mode" (p. 27).

In this book Matte-Blanco clarifies his ideas about the different strata, giving substance to these ideas by concrete examples from clinical practice. The interested reader is referred to this book, which is considerably more accessible than his former work.

The Nature of Phobia Reconsidered: Barendregt's Model of Phobia as "Repersonalization", Seen in the Light of Matte-Bianco's Clarifications

In his last weeks of life, Barendregt (1982) clarified and extended his earlier statements on the nature of phobia (see his essential definition, 1974). According to him, "phobia derives from the *depersonalization* phenomenon, and is in fact *one* form that a desperate effort to re-organize the chaos that is experienced in consciousness may take, when the person is threatened by or overwhelmed by the strange or ominous feelings characteristic of this syndrome. The patient who often can find no suitable words to describe these feelings of impending disintegration, doom, strangeness, uncertainty about what is happening to him or her, interprets this as anxiety, and the situation in which it occurs as dangerous, to be avoided. In a given situation, the person experiences feelings of falling-short, of the inadequacy of his repertoires (whether perceptual, cognitive, or emotional) to deal with the situation, to process it or respond to it in an orderly way. Chaos in consciousness then arises, and depersonalization is the result. But the elusiveness of the experience of depersonalization, often denoted by the patient as 'it', is so unreal, so absurd that the need is felt to clamp onto something tangible. This support is found by re-organizing these experiences in terms of feelings of fear. For fear is preferable to the nothingness of 'it'. However, since fear itself is a very negative experience, so-called 'coping'-mechanisms come into play to canalize and rationalize this fear"(p. 171).

In schematic terms these relationships can be described as follows:

$$\text{situation} \rightarrow \text{chaos} \xrightarrow[d]{} \text{“it”} \xrightarrow[r]{} \text{fear} \rightarrow \text{coping}$$

where d: depersonalization
r: repersonalization

In his elaboration of this model he makes a number of observations which, in the light of Matte-Blanco's ideas, are particularly enlightening. "Though the depersonalization experience is part and parcel of many psychiatric syndromes, it is also common to many normal experiences. The only difference lies in its being coded differently, giving it a literary or philosophical name, for example, existential anxiety, or feelings of alienation, feelings of 'Nothingness' (Sartre), falling into a black hole (the abyss of the Soul in mystical writings), or the Big One (Rilke) ... One patient with a philosophical bent even described this 'it' experience as 'the loss of the belief in the illusion of the I' (p. 167) ...(.). The content of the experience of 'it' is vaguely and indirectly described because 'it' consists of the lack of definition ...(.) 'It' is the experience of the lack of available repertoires, or schemata with which to order the awareness of and responses in a meaningful way; ...(.) to see relations between things or persons and to act functionally; ...(.) it is the experience of disorganization, or rather more extremely stated, of lack of reason (irrationality). In each of these formulations lies contradiction (p. 168) ... it is not irrationality that is described, but the experience of ... the awareness or consciousness of that is described, and that is no longer the irrational".

Paraphrasing one of his favourite writers, Musil, he says: "In the state of depersonalization the person does not lose his qualities, rather it is the qualities that have lost the person" (p. 169).

"The chaos in the perceptions of the person should not be understood as the chaos of an untidy room. Rather it is as if in the perception of the room, besides the objects in the room (tables, chairs), the molecules and atoms of which these are made are also perceptible. Or better still, ... as if the sets of coloured planes which go to make up the perception of a chair are perceived, but the idea 'chair' is temporarily lost to view ... In the repersonalization of 'it' into fear, one does not see the perceptual levels and perceptual structures as such as intermingled but one interprets it faultily. (...) The reality level of these re-interpretations can differ. One can say that it is 'as if' ...(.) or that it *is* so. Between the 'as if' experience and the delusion, there is a continuum of possibilities ...(.) One tries to structure the disorded perception through language. That is another reason why there are so many and varied descriptions and experiences of 'it' ...(.) Since one can repersonalize in different ways, the number of possibilities becomes larger (p. 172).

In phobia, in contrast to psychosis, the chaos is not complete ... nor is attention dispersed over separate sensations. On the contrary; it is fixed on the lack of relationship (p. 168) ...(.) The experience of 'it' is often of very short duration, varying from a few seconds to seldom longer than an hour (p. 168).

Once repersonalization of 'it' has become fear, then one has to learn to live with it. This is done by means of the so-called 'coping-'mechanisms. In the ban of fear one seeks support in: (1) remedies (e.g., alcohol, tranquillizers); (2) other persons (spouses, doctors); (3) compulsive acts or thoughts (avoidance of the phobogenic situation; feelings of doom). It is mainly these coping-mechanisms which make the phobics so difficult to live with, for themselves and for others. Coping can take on an independent rôle, pushing the original fear into the background ...(.) Anxiety and fear are hardly felt anymore but the situation has become unliveable" (p. 173).

Although Barendregt avoids using the concept "unconscious" in elaborating on his model, these selections from his last publication show, without any doubt, that the described experiences of "it" coincide with what Matte-Blanco calls "irruptions of the symmetrical mode of being" onto concrete situations, and with Freud's conceptions of the id, as "the true psychic reality". Compare Barendregt's formulations: "It" is the experience of the lack of available repertoires, or schemata with which to order the awareness in a meaningful way ... (the inability) to see relations between things or persons and to act functionally; and "it" consists of the lack of definition, with Matte-Blanco's formulations: In logical terms, the "primary process" can be seen as the unavailability of asymmetrical relations ...(.) Mental activity implies the establishment of relations, and ordering these in time and space. Again Barendregt: The chaos in the perceptions of the person ... is as if in the perception of the room, besides the objects (therein), the molecules and atoms of which these are made are also perceptible ... or better still ... the sets of coloured planes which go to make up the perception ..., compared to Matte-Blanco: Consciousness ... picks "bits" here and there (of symmetrical being) and gives them order in time and space ... (.) it behaves as though it were transforming symmetrical being into something which it is not ... by describing, for instance, as a disorder something which is neither order nor a disorder. It is a task similar or identical to that of describing something immaterial by means of material images ...(.) This is the function of translating ... Words, or rather their meanings, are the asymmetrical tools. Barendregt: One tries to structure the disordered perception through language. That is another reason why there are so ... varied descriptions and experiences of "it".

How much the conceptions of both scientists (who may not have read each other's work) coincide can be seen in the alternative forms of repersonalization/relations between symmetrical and asymmetrical modes of being, which they use to bolster their points of view. Both see psychosis and neurosis as different forms (rather, different degrees) of efforts to assimilate the irruptions of the "it" into consciousness. And both consider the experience of falling in love and its rationalizations, and the experiences described by various philosophers and poets as Non-being, as prototypical of the same condition in normal, everyday experience, "translated" or "coded" differently (e.g., Sartre's "Nothingness" as opposed to "Being"; Kierkegaard's "Sickness unto death" or existential doubt; Rilke's "Courage de luxe" in the face of the Big One -- Barendregt, 1982, pp. 177–78; Matte-Blanco, 1975, pp. 184–85 and pp. 460–61, for example).

In pointing out limitations of other models of phobia to give a completely satisfactory explanation of its origins and maintenance, Barendregt is careful to show the lacuna in his own model. According to him, the conditioning-model fails to account for the fact that in most phobias that which is so greatly feared has never actually been experienced (e.g., few persons with a phobic fear of dogs have ever been bitten by a dog). The genetically "preparedness"-model (Seligman), which states that (the acquisition of) fears which are now irrational were once evolutionary useful, is not borne out by the experimental evidence, using Seligman's procedures. The psychiatric model in terms of depersonalization as (primary and secondary) defense against anxiety does not convincingly explain why phobic responses should be so persistent (pp. 173–75).

A weak point in his own model, Barendregt admits, is the lack of an analysis of which situations (are able to) evoke "it". "Though some situations appear to be more often the focus of phobic anxiety than others, there is so much difference in individual preferences for situations, that this individuality is comparable to preferences in love and art (p. 178). The problem remains unsolved. If only we knew this (he sighed), then we would know how phobia originates, what falling in love is, what art is. Psychology would have progressed" (p. 179).

That is a tall order. Knowing Barendregt as a scientist who was more given to understatement than to exaggeration, I imagine that by this formulation he merely wished to describe the enormity of the problem. So, if in the following chapter (and in Part Two) I assay an answer to the first riddle, by drawing together the skeins of knowledge and integrating them; and if I should arrive at a plausible description of which (structures of) situations trigger the phobic response, and how and why this occurs, I do not by this make any pretense to a better understanding of what falling in love entails, or what art is. But, by following Gibson's suggestion that one perceives better by circumgyrating an object, I shall take heart and approach it in this way, to gain a better perspective.

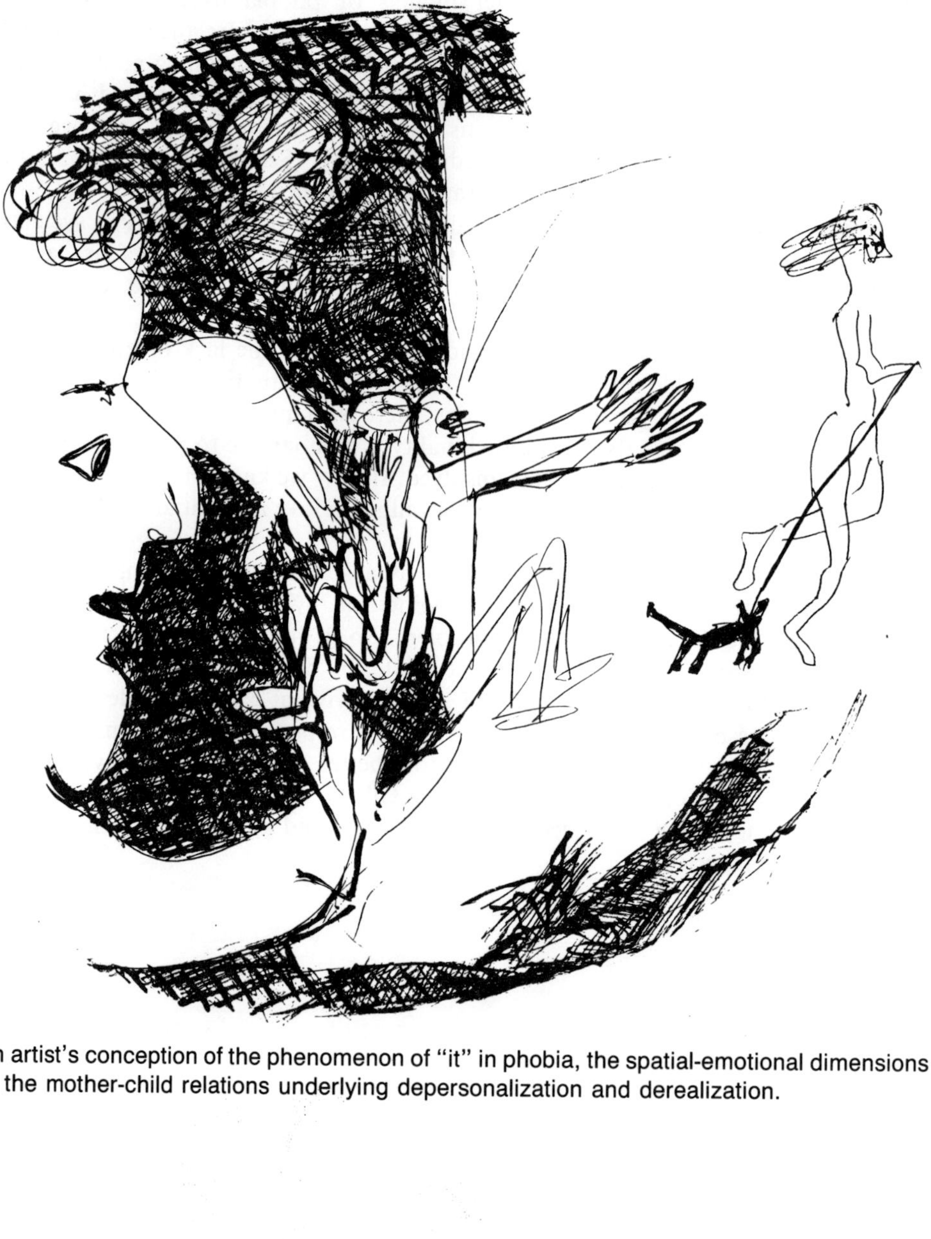

An artist's conception of the phenomenon of "it" in phobia, the spatial-emotional dimensions of the mother-child relations underlying depersonalization and derealization.

IV

The World is All That is the Case: Drawing the Skeins Together

["*Die Welt is alles, was der Fall ist*" – Wittgenstein, 1969]

Once More Around the Field of View: Persistence and Change in Ecologically Relevant Optical Structures and Visual Events

For a long time scientists thought that the world appeared to the new-born as "a buzzing, blooming confusion". But recent investigations of new-borns and infants in the first weeks of life show that this view is erroneous. Already at birth the infant appears to perceive depth (three-dimensionality), defends herself against oncoming objects, and reaches out to touch objects that are seen and heard. If properly supported, the new-born will march along a flat surface, which is an indication of co-ordination of perceptual and motor skills. This implies that the infant sees the surface as a supportable one stretching out in front, and "knows" how to traverse it. An extraordinary capacity to imitate the adult also appears, for instance, in the ability to stick out her tongue in response to the same act by the mother (Bower, 1976).

These behaviours suggest that Gibson may be right in his postulate that the perceptual systems are geared to higher-order invariants and pick these up directly, although the precision with which this is done is dependent on developmental stage and learning.

Other experiments show that the infant can also recognize that an object can go inside another object and still exist. The tracking behaviour (eye-movements), following the moving object into the improvised "tunnel" in which it disappears and beyond to the end of the tunnel, demonstrates this. The greater change of heart-rate when the object fails to reappear seems to suggest some awareness too of "something wrong" (Bower, Broughton & Moore, 1971). Yet at this age the infant has no words, no concepts at her disposal to make known what has obviously been registered by perceptual systems, and which awareness affects the child.

In Gibson's ecological optics the field of view is described by the combined fields of view of the two eyes when one is sitting still in an armchair or, like the baby, lying on one's back in a cot or turned over on the stomach in a playpen. This field of view describes a large visual solid angle with an oval boundary which is vague and indefinite, but still a boundary. It is a frozen sample of the environment which one would have if one moved one's head or walked about. Over time, all these overlapping samples would provide one with a panoramic view of the environment (Gibson, 1966).

This stationary field of view, this frozen sample, with head fixed and eyes mobile, contains only what is in front and to the side. It is bounded on one or more sides by the nose, perhaps overhanging locks of hair on the forehead, and by what can be seen of one's hands, legs, and feet. For this reason Ernst Mach (1886–97) described the field of view as "The Visual Ego".

Its boundaries are in some ways like occluding edges behind which the rest of the environment lies hidden. When the field moves, either because one moves one's head or because objects are moved away by someone, there is an increment (accretion) of optical structure at the leading edge and a decrement (deletion) of structure at the trailing edge. But movement of one's head (or body) and movement in the environment are not equivalent events. For in turning one's head, the surfaces that go out of sight with one movement come back into sight with the opposite movement, and the reversible occlusion is not part of the world but of one's own movement. When an object in the field of view disappears from sight, however, it may only have gone out of sight temporarily (like the mother moving about in the room of the child), or it may have disappeared permanently (either because it has moved permanently out of one's ken, or permanently out of the world by destruction). In both cases, this movement is independent of one's movement but the visual events are different. The mother moving in and out of the field of view is seen as an object displacing itself against a stable background, a faster element that brings about an accretion and deletion of structure that is reversible, whereas the person or object which moves permanently out of the field of view is seen as a vanishing or vanished structure. Which changes in the optic array are reversible, and which are not, is learned in the first few weeks of life, for these optical transformations, and the visual events to which they give rise, are repeated endlessly. Long before the child has learned even a basic vocabulary, it has learned to differentiate them.

That this is so is clear from the different emotions accompanying these observations. For instance, the infant playing peek-a-boo with her own fingers or with her mother's face gurgles and coos with pleasurable tension, and reacts with little or no distress to her mother coming into sight and going out of sight, if these reversible events are characterized by very brief intervals. But if the mother goes out of sight and takes a long time coming back, or comes and goes at irregular intervals, emotional distress and interruptive behaviour (agitated flexion of limbs and crying) are observed. Bearing in mind the very short time span of the infant at this stage, such disappearances are no doubt perceived as mother "gone forever", vanished.

Other changes in the optic array that are laden with meaning are the visual events "coming up close", and its inverse "vanishing into the distance". In the first case, the expansion of the object is accompanied by a progressive occlusion of other structures in view, and in the latter, the shrinking of the object by a successive disocclusion of the surrounding structures. If these changes take place in a leisurely, gradual way, experiments show that infants and animals reach out to, and are attracted by, the event or object. If, however, these events take place in a rapid, haphazard or irregular way, emotional distress is shown. Where the object "looms" into sight (that is, approaches rapidly), evasive or withdrawal action is taken (Schneirla, 1965; Gibson et al., 1962; Schiff, 1965). These responses seem to be "innate" in different species of animals.

The optical transformations too that the elastic surface of the human face undergoes when a person smiles, laughs, cries, becomes angry, is tired and so on, are easily picked up by the infant and soon differentiated. Their different meanings (affordances), for instance, the smooth, soft surfaces of the tenderly smiling caretaker and the crinkledup, furrowed surfaces of the angry or tired face, are either immediately perceived or quickly differentiated, since different behaviours ("good" or "bad" for the infant) generally go together with these different elasticities. At the same time, the infant receives additional information, some of which is redundant, through other perceptual systems, as she smells and is smelled, touches and is touched, hears and is heard, tastes the milk of her mother and experiences her care.

The sweeping of the field of view and its wheeling with head turns and head tilts are also registered by the perceptual systems, as well as the spinning and swirling of the world when the infant is tossed by the parent into the air in a playful spirit and caught before she falls. That these optical transformations are picked up and have a peculiar fascination for the infant and young child can be seen in the conflicting emotions of terror and excitement with which these are greeted, and the clamouring for more of the same.

All these different transformations that permanent structures in the field of view undergo – the progressive covering and uncovering of surfaces, the foreshortening and lengthening of form as an object turns, the shearing and stretching of elastic surfaces, the coming into sight and going out of sight and, in some cases, the coming into and going out of existence, the magnification to the limit with approach and minification with recession, the sweeping and wheeling, the spinning and swirling of the optic array with head turns, head tilts, body tosses – all these optical transformations are noticed and differentiated, even before the infant can sit up unaided and walk around. What stays the same and what changes is apparent to the infant even at this early age.

Most likely the infant notices too that the changing and unchanging world "out there" is bounded by herself "here". But what developmental psychologists remark is the fact that in the first days and weeks of life, snuggled down in the mother's arms with her nipple in mouth, suckling, the mother's breast covering one's cheeks, the world there and the infant here merge into one, undivided Being. This is the state or the mode of symmetrical being, in which the world has become "an immense Breastness" (Matte-Blanco), with asymmetrical Being temporarily in abeyance. This is the oceanic feeling of having merged into all that is (the infinite), from which the omnipotence arises that the infant has when the mother satisfies her needs, and about which poets will sing in nostalgic longing for the lost paradise in later years.

In every satisfying cuddle, holding close, feeding, this experience is repeated and reinforced, strengthening the infant's ego. The different optical transforms, specifying different faces of the world and different meanings, are incorporated and experienced as being part of the One, each aspect identical with each other and with oneself, conform the nature of symmetrical being. But with eyes and ears open and hungry again, looking around and perceiving the variety of transforms of the unchanging world, asymmetrical being (or the ego) emerges, as the infant attempts again and again to master these. Winnicott (1960, pp. 145–6) describes the same relations in the following words:

> "The good-enough mother meets the omnipotence of the infant and to some extent makes sense of it. She does this repeatedly. A True Self begins to have life, through the strength given to the infant's weak ego by the mother's implementation of the infant's omnipotent expression ..(.) and in consequence the infant begins to believe in external reality which appears and behaves as by magic ..(.) and which acts in a way that does not clash with the infant's omnipotence ..(.) The True Self ..(.) has joined up with the world's events."

Still largely confined to the field of view, the infant is taken out in her perambulator and exposed to the greater world outside. If not asleep all the time, she will experience not only kinaesthetic sensations of being moved along passively, but will see the world now rolling, wheeling and sweeping by, people and animals looming into sight and vanishing as quickly, houses and trees passing more slowly, but cars and autobuses more speedily. Sounds, sights, smells and colours of such variety are encountered that, had the infant not already gained some perceptual mastery (differentiation, stabilization and constancy of objects despite their optical transformation), she would be worn to a frazzle within minutes of these encounters. In fact, most infants take such adventures in their stride, either sleeping through them with a grand insouciance, or smiling imperturbably at these strange goings-on. Evidence perhaps that perceptual systems are what Gibson supposes them to be: highly adaptable, active, organizing, functional units geared to such transformations.

Put out on the grass under a shining sun, the infant may perceive a shimmering, a sparkle of all the objects around her, and experience new delight. Or if the rays of the sun are too intense, the infant may experience pain and glare, and perceive the blurring and masking of all environmental structure, which must in itself be a frightening experience.

But if conditions are more congenial, she may notice that the earth affords support, and that the sky is a blue canopy overhead. The earth, cluttered with people and animals and things, the sky relatively uncluttered, except for a few birds flying and clouds floating by. These events too will make her acquainted with wind and showers of rain, substances and surfaces not encountered in the small confines of the nursery.

With sudden nightfall, the world is blotted out in an instant. This disappearance of the world by darkness is so alarming that although it is a regular occurrence and wholly predictable, young children find it difficult to become accustomed to. Thoughtful parents often ease then the transition from day to night by providing a small night-light, or a small toy (teddy-bear, doll, a piece of blanket) to hold fast and close. For not only is the world blotted out but the mother also leaves for a long period of time, to sleep herself. Thus does the "transitional object" come into being. The ideal "hold-fast" should smell of mother as well as of self, if it is to be effective as solace, one of the reasons why the washing of such objects is strenuously resisted by the child.

If no such hold-fast is provided against the terrors of the night, or the disappearance of the world, the infant will often provide herself with one, her fingers or fist, objects which partly seem to belong to one's own body, partly to the world "out there". Sucking on these extremities, the infant falls asleep. Developmental psychologists (e.g., Winnicott, 1971, 1982) see these transitional objects as substitutes for the mother's breast, bridging the illusion that self and world are united in one extensive Being.

This might be the point at which symbolization begins, in the sense that Freud too understood this, in stressing the body as referent of symbol formation, the symbolic process bridging the inner and outer world (the "I" and the "non-I").

Whatever the case, it is probably in these very early weeks of life that the ground for impaired functioning at later ages is laid. For the same optical transformations which specify the visual events described above can undermine the developing sense of "I", as a being separate from mother and able to cope with new experiences, new situations. If the mother or caretaker is unavailable when needed, negligent, or provides the infant with conflicting information about the world in which she is immersed, this will hinder her capacity to deal effectively with the world around her. For example, rapid, abrupt approach to the infant is described by the sudden occlusion of all space, the swallowing-up of all other structures, implies impending collision and hence, annihilation of self. The experience(s) of one's own puniness and inability to control such threat, such alarming disturbances in the world cannot be other than anxiety-provoking. So too is the unexpected vanishing of the mother or caretaker, her shrinking to zero as she disappears in the distance, despite the child's expressed need for her presence. And equally debilitating is incongruency of facial expression with action – the handling of the infant roughly and harsh vocalization with a smiling face, for example – conflicting information that will confuse the perceptual systems with respect to the affordances these actions entail. Freezing behaviour, disorientation, inability to choose between whether to approach or avoid this frightening parent, will be the result. And all these, and other discordances will sink into (be repressed in) symmetrical being, where they will exist, side-by-side, with more congruent experiences and events, without contradiction. In Mahler's (1968) words, they are "introjected by the infant to form 'good' and 'bad' representations of the world" which will be integrated into (un)differentiated self- and object-images. Matte-Blanco may be right: symmetrical and asymmetrical modes of being go together from the very first, although the life of the very young child is probably lived more in the first mode of being than in the second.

Perceptual Control and increasing Asymmetricalization (or Ego-control)

While confined by necessity to the field of view, the infant is more or less wholly dependent on the caring other for support and effective control of (objects in) the world. In pressing her hands against the mother's breast and arching back and away to look at her face, she sees herself "mirrored" in her mother's face, and takes for granted that her mother's competencies are her own. The sense of omnipotence through congruence between mother and child increases. That is, if all goes well. But if the mother's facial expressions and handling of the child are not congruent with the child's, or if the child repeatedly finds a face turned from her own and a mother busy elsewhere, this sense of omnipotence is gradually undermined. Perception of separateness, and feebleness to deal with the world is prematurely instilled, and another pathological germ takes root (see also Winnicott, 1982).

As the child grows, becomes able to climb down from the parental lap and crawl around on the floor, the sense of self and mastery of self-in-world increases. With this increase in mastery, the sense of separateness also increases, and the world divides up into a "self" and "other", as finer and finer discriminations (establishment of asymmetrical relations) are made. (I am assuming here that it is possible for the child to gain perceptual awareness and make discriminations of an asymmetrical kind before she has acquired conceptual knowledge of these relations.)

In this view the assumption is that the infant in her mother's arms is much more aware of optical structures and the perceptual events to which these give rise than was supposed by Freud and others, who place a greater stress on internal (instinctual) sensations as the basis for the perceptions which give rise to consciousness. But this point of view does not rule out that, at about four to five months of age, the infant's attention noticeably expands into increased directed perceptual activity. Mahler, Pine Bergman (1975, p. 54) characterize this subphase as the "hatching process" when, with increasing periods of wakefulness, the infant shows a greater alertness, persistence and goal-directedness. They describe with great poignancy how this sense of separate self comes into being, or fails to do so. Increasing proficiency in ego-control is gradually accomplished by a process of "two steps forward and one step back".

The child who has weathered, more or less successfully, the vicissitudes of the first six to nine months is not, however, necessarily less prone to "regression". Sudden anxieties and terrors may come to the fore, so that the "checking-back" pattern to mother as the toddler explores the environment may deteriorate into a panicky flight back to her safe arms. This flight may last for brief moments, several hours, days, weeks or months.

Among the possible sources of such panics, one that has been generally overlooked by developmental psychologists is explicitly taken into account by Gibson. This is the inflow and outflow pattern associated with locomotion through the environment. As we recall, this inflow-outflow is centrifugal in half the array and centripetal in the other half, and shifts around an axis which is the line of displacement of the moving person. The focus of expansion is the direction in which one is going, the focus of contraction the direction from which one is coming. These inflow and outflow patterns are hardly noticed any more by the adult observer, except when these obtrude on his awareness while fleeing from some danger or, more usually, while being transported in a fast vehicle (e.g., as the car accelerates or decelerates, or at take-off and landing in an aeroplane).

For the young child though, who has only recently graduated from the toddling stage, these flow patterns which seem to follow her progression through space may be quite alarming. One should bear in mind that, at this stage of development, the perceptual mechanisms which control stability and constancy of objects may not yet be operationally stable, so that fluctuations in expansion and contraction of other objects and persons moving in the environment, together with these inflow and outflow patterns generated by the child's own movement, may induce chaotic perceptions which might be quite terrifying. Developmental psychologists have often noticed that young children for no apparent reason will suddenly stop running, freeze all action, and cry or scream for mother while in the midst of exciting play (Mahler, 1975). And not only the children who are dispositionally weak or nervous. Even the boldly exploring, daring little boy or girl who only a few moments before had resisted the protective impulses of the mother, may in the next moment halt, panic-stricken, while running from place to place. Not all of this fear may be due to a sudden awareness of the distance between the mother and child, as is often supposed, although distance and the perspective layout of surfaces are more easily observed standing still. Some of it may well be due to the perception of distortions of the world around and the alarming flow-patterns engulfing the child.

The young child encounters other "affordances" of the environment around this age too: the falling-off places, the bump-into-able objects, the climb-under-able objects, and so on. In this newborn love affair with the world, all that is encountered may not be filled with sweetness and light. If the ongoing acquaintance with the world and self-in-world is to proceed harmoniously and successfully, the child needs a safe place where he can play, fantasize about, rehearse possible responses to the "inner" impulses as well as the "outer" demands of reality. A place where the symmetrical mode of being can be explored and integrated with the asymmetrical mode. This "intermediate zone", which Winnicott calls the "potential space" between mother and child, is vital for healthy development:

> ... "Sitting on the floor, in creative play with toys under the aegis of the mother ..(.) a hypothetical area (that) exists (but can not exist) between the baby and the object (mother or part of mother) during the phase of the repudiation of the object as not-me, that is, at the end of being merged in with the object" (Winnicott, 1982, p. 126).

This is what is meant by the "potential space". And he clarifies this further in the following passages:

> "From a state of being merged in with the mother, the baby is at a stage of separating out the mother from the self, and the mother is lowering the degree of her adaptation to the baby's needs (both because of her own recovery from a high degree of identification with the baby and because of her perception of the baby's new need, the need for her to be a separate phenomenon).
>
> ... In the experience of the more fortunate baby (and small child and adolescent and adult) the question of separation in separating does not arise, because in the potential space between the baby and the mother there appears the creative playing that arises naturally out of the relaxed state; it is here that there develops the use of symbols that stand at one and the same time for external world phenomena and for phenomena of the individual person who is being looked at" (p. 128).

Just as earlier (and still) the transitional objects used by the child to bridge the gap between herself and mother (or greater world) should go unquestioned and uninterfered-with, so this potential space must be unquestioned by the caring adult and uninterfered with; although at the behest of the child the adult can (and should) participate in this play. For a child who grows up without such a potential space that is respected and protected by the adult is not only more prone to disturbed forms of adjustment to reality in adolescent and adult years; but, more importantly, has missed out on the chance at creative playing, with all that eventually adds up to a cultural life. This seems to be the implication of what Winnicott says in the above-mentioned passages. And failure in confidence, and lack of *savoir faire*, arise out of this relative lack and limitation. As Barendregt (1982) describes it, in referring to the phobic person confronted with feelings of disintegration, doom, strangeness and uncertainty, or "it": "It is the experience of feelings of falling-short, of the inadequacy of his repertoires (whether perceptual, cognitive, or emotional) to deal with the situation ... to respond to it in an orderly way". See also Barendregt & Frijda (1982), in which these ideas are elaborated.

To avoid any misapprehension, it might be wise to remind the reader at this point that the ideas about the importance of optical structures and visual events in the early weeks and months of the child's development are my own, formed from Gibson's ideas and by integrating these with psychoanalytic and developmental ideas on these relations. Neither in Mahler's work nor in Winnicott's will one find explicit references to these optical structures or visual events. Yet, as I have tried to show, their formulations seem to imply such relations (or do not at least disqualify them). In a personal communication, Kolk (1986) draws my attention to this: "Object relations theorists ... pay more attention to the investigations of infants on their preferences for human faces and for the known, than for other kinds of perceptual investigations. Your interpretation of the behaviour of the mother, in perceptual terms, is *new*". Indeed; for with the exception of Gibson's work, I found little in contemporary perceptual research which was able to throw much light on the complex interactions between person and world, and pathological interactions in particular. From a clinical point of view, much perceptual research is irrelevant, though of vital importance to our understanding of fundamental issues on information-processing in general.

A perceptual system of probably equal importance to the visual one in our understanding of these relations, and one given extensive consideration by Gibson, is the haptic system and its components. Its importance has been briefly indicated by Gibson (see Chapter II) in showing the close and complementary relations between perceptual systems geared to picking up information from the environment and systems which yield information about the person's activities and impressions (or sensations) during this information pickup. As he says (1966, p. 99) about these two poles of experience – the objective and the subjective – "The fact seems to be that in touching a solid object one can attend either to the external resistant thing or to the impression on the skin ..(.) It is as if the same stimulating event had two possible poles of experience, one objective and the other subjective. There are many possible meanings of the term *sensation*, but this is one: the detection of the impression made on a perceiver while he is primarily engaged in detecting the world". Throughout this chapter, I have implied that both sides of these interactions are important and must be considered.

Perceptual Mechanisms and Processes

Up to this point an attempt at integration of the positions taken by different theorists presents little difficulty since their ideas are congruent, even when expressed in a different terminology. If consensus is a proper criterion for objective knowledge, then the account so far may be considered to be a good approximation of this. Perceptionists on the whole, and no doubt informed clinicians too, agree on the superiority of Gibson's specifications of the information available to our perceptual systems in the environment. Some are also willing to support his contention that perceptual systems (in contrast to conceptual ones) are geared to higher-order invariants and pick these up directly. Pribram (1977), for instance, makes a good case for this standpoint in his evaluation of some recent experiments (p. 94; see also Chapter II, p. 37). Another highly interesting, intriguing, though perhaps not a clinching finding, is the later substantiation by Siegel (1977) and others of the work of Klüver (1926) on hallucinations.

Klüver found that, in the absence of an actual external stimulus, the central nervous system tends to generate form constants of four specific types: (a) gratings, lattices, filigree, honeycomb and chess-board forms; (b) cobweb-like forms; (c) tunnel, funnel, alley, cone-like forms and unusual perspectives; and (d) spirals; as well as combinations of these. These form constants are further characterized by varied and saturated colours, intense brightness and symmetrical configurations. The work of Siegel et al. (1977) shows that these form constants are not peculiar to hallucinatory states in clinical syndromes only (e.g., in psychotic episodes, epilepsy, drug intoxication, advanced stages of syphilis, insulin hypoglycemia), but are also found in almost all states in which consciousness is temporarily abased. For instance, in hypnopompic and hypnagogic states, photostimulation, migraine headaches, dizziness, sensory deprivation, and the delirium of fever. The generation of these form constants is also much alike from one person to another, and across cultures. Like Freud, Siegel supposes that these hallucinatory experiences are due to extreme excitations of the central nervous system. But this finding suggests to me that the central nervous system (or its perceptual systems) may either have an intrinsic prediliction to organize stimulation in certain invariant patterns, or may reproduce under reduced states of consciousness invariant patterns which have been abstracted from the environment earlier, and sank into memory. This tendency to generate form constants, regardless of (external) stimulation, undoubtedly plays a rôle in our dreams too.

An issue on which there is partial agreement is the interdependency of perception and action, although as we have seen, theorists differ on the question of which processes are involved in achieving coordination of perceiving and acting.

No agreement at all is found on the relations of sensation to perception, the mechanisms of these relations, and hence the directness or indirectness of process.

As to the question of the veridicality of perception, the different theoretical assumptions span the whole scale of possibilities: from total rejection of veridicality in perception because of its egocentric nature (Piaget), hence the need for decentration of intellectual operations to achieve objectivity; to the intermediate position (Gregory), which supposes that, in general, perception approximates objective reality but accepting that, given the chances for misperception in selection, scale-setting, classification, interpretation of stimulation, nonveridicality is quite frequently the case; to the standpoint that perception is veridical (Gibson), except under extreme (and inadequate) conditions of information pickup, whether these are due to environmental conditions or conditions in the perceiver.

Gibson also contends that the process of perception is much more straightforward than is assumed; and, despite the fact that psychology has spent much more time studying sensation rather than perception, it is our understanding of sensation that is confused. Sensations, being of a much more subjective nature, and their identification requiring sophisticated processes of learning, are often misperceived. The variables of sensory discrimination are also radically different from the variables of perceptual discrimination:

> "The variables of sensory discrimination are said to be dimensions like quality, intensity, extensity and duration, dimensions of hue, brightness, and saturation, of pitch, loudness, and timbre, of pressure, warm, cold, and pain. The variables of perceptual discrimination are dimensions of the environment, the variables of events and those of surfaces, places, objects, of other animals, and even of symbols ... Perceiving unquestionably depends on sensitivity or the use of the sense organs. To observe, one must sense. But sensation is not perceiving ... and the fact that there is invariance of perception with varying sensations (demonstrates this)" (Gibson, 1963, p. 351).

One might say that sensations are perceptions with subjective reference, or propriospecific stimuli that carry information about the self. They go together with the objective information about the environment, but are not the same. "Sense impressions, far from being original experiences, are very sophisticated ones and depend on having a great deal of past experience" (*ibid.*). Where the process of perception is direct, the perceptual systems being geared to the pickup of higher-order invariants, perception of sensations would be indirect (since these depend on "having a great deal of past experience"). In this view, sensations and conceptual thought would necessarily involve indirect processing, whereas perceptual processes (the pickup of invariants) could be direct, or at least, more direct. The point of view is rendered quite plausible through Marcel's (1983) more recent discussion of the relation between perceptual awareness and sensory cues. From these more inclusive, fresher or more recent viewpoints there might be room for reconciliation between psychological approaches, that is, the representational and ecological; for Gibson does not say perceptual process cannot be influenced by sensations or conceptual thought; only that this influence is not a prerequisite for perceiving. But, even if this were so, the traditional and accepted viewpoint would be in need of revision, a matter which few contemporary representationists seem willing to accept. We will leave these skeins dangling, then, until such a time as fresh evidence from future investigations decides in favour of one or other standpoint.

Of specific concern in this study is the question of constancy or object permanence. Whether or not nonconstancy derives from misapplication in tuning of lower, intermediate or higher perceptual or conceptual schemes with action schemes (see Gibson, 1966, 1979; Turvey, 1977; and even more to the point, Pribram, 1991), or from lack of decentration of intellectual operations (Piaget, 1969), or from a misapplication of constancy scaling mechanisms ("upwards from data" and "downwards from hypotheses", Gregory, 1974, 1981), some kind of constancy regulating device in brain mechanisms must be operative in perception. Otherwise the overwhelming empirical evidence for systematic deviations (over- and under-estimations of stimuli) in perceptual and judgmental tasks becomes incomprehensible (see Helson, 1964, for an excellent overview). Even if constancies depend only on differentiation (Gibson), insofar as the invariants of input have to be differentiated from one another in the nervous system, and therefore to some extent on development and learning, there must be some mechanism or mechanisms which regulate these differentiations. In the earlier work of Bower (1971, p. 62), he concluded from the results of a series of ingenious experiments with infants less than sixteen weeks old that younger infants are not affected by feature differences. For them movement is predominant:

> "They respond to a change in motion but not to a change in size, shape or color. They ignore features to such an extent that I would suggest they respond not to moving objects but to movements. Similarly, I would suggest that they respond not to stationary objects but to places. In contrast, older infants have learned to define an object as something that can go from place to place along pathways of movement. They identify an object by its features rather than by its place or movement. For them different features imply different objects that can move independently, so that the stopping of one does not imply the stopping of the other ...(.) ... According to these studies it seems that infants less than sixteen weeks old live in a world articulated in terms of solids that are stably arranged in space according to their location, with a constancy of existence when they occlude one another ...(.) An object becomes a differentiated object as soon as it moves to a new location".

Clearly, before such complicated issues can be resolved definitively, much more work, and of a sophisticated nature, must be done in investigating the world of the infant and the young child.

The Environment, an (in)Appropriate Substitute for Unresolved Psychic Conflict? Why Optical Structures and Visual Events can Evoke "It"

The reader who has followed the argumentation through the windings of knowledge on perceptual control and psychodynamic issues will hardly be surprised by the conclusion that, far from being an inappropriate substitute for unresolved psychic conflict, the environment should be seen for what it is: a major, and most appropriate representative. In this view, Freud's definition of phobia as "a projection in that it replaces an internal, instinctual danger by an external, perceptual one", may need emendation. For, as Matte-Blanco (1975, p. 43) argues, from a logical point of view, nothing is displaced, nothing projected. And from a perceptual informational point of view there is no projection either.

As I have tried to show, the so-called internal, instinctual danger has its origins in the first perceptual experiences in the first weeks of life when the infant perceives disturbances of optical structure which give rise to visual (and haptic) events that are directly anxiety-evoking. But Freud's commitment to a mechanical view of man and his postulate of the instincts as the primal essence may have biased his early theoretical ideas. In fact, his later formulations, in terms of "a traumatic situation ... the essence of which is an expectation of helplessness on the part of the ego in the face of an accumulation of excitation, whether of external or internal origin, which cannot be dealt with" (1926), seem to agree with this view; or are at least not discordant with it. But he spoke of a traumatic situation *in the past*. Of course, given the over-determination of most clinical syndromes, phobia included, it is quite possible that the first anxiety-evoking, visual experiences of the infant in fact determine the perception of later anxiety-evoking visual events. But there need be no projection, since the present situation that evokes the pathological response is, from the point of view of optical structural disturbance, identical to the old, i.e., when one was a baby-in-arms or a child. It may be that such disturbances in optical structure are only noticed under conditions of abased or reduced consciousness. Also, these may immediately give rise to memories of that long-lost childhood in which one first experienced their frightening and incapacitating effects. But these memories need not be "repressed", nor does one need to postulate an independent repressive mechanism to understand how their effects become so pernicious and long-lasting.

If Matte-Blanco (1975) and Barendregt (1982) are right in their conceptions of neurosis and phobia, as "irruptions of the symmetrical mode of being onto concrete situations ... and the unavailability of asymmetrical relations", or "the lack of available repertoires to deal with the chaos in consciousness, the experience of depersonalization"; and if these persons are those who have missed out on the chance to create a potential (and available) space in which to rehearse and coordinate possible responses to the demands of both modes of being (Winnicott, 1982), then they will be especially prone to disorganization and panicky feelings in situations of a particular kind. These particular situations are those in which disturbances of optical structures give rise to visual events that evoke the characteristics of symmetrical being.

In the view put forward here, this means that *the reversible optical structures, and their concomitant visual events*, will be effective in evoking "it". For these and their converses (or inverses) are experienced as identical with each other and with the whole. These reversible optical structures and visual events are: occlusion phenomena, the accretion and deletion of optical structure as a person or object comes into sight and goes out of sight (lateral occlusion); expansion or magnification of optical structure and occlusion of surrounding structure, as well as contraction or minification of optical structure with concomitant disocclusion of surrounding structure, as persons or objects "loom" or vanish into the distance (vertical occlusion); inflow and outflow patterns which accompany locomotion through the environment, whether one moves actively or is transported passively in a fast vehicle; sweeping, wheeling and whirling of the field of view and the inverse motions; foreshortening and lengthening of structure with turning of objects; stretching and contracting of animal bodies, shearing and smoothing in the elastic surfaces (faces and bodies), especially those which go with "good" and "bad" expectancies simultaneously; extreme darkness and light, which blot out or blur, or eliminate optical structure; and events which portend coming into existence or destruction of existence.

What of the fear of animals? Some animal phobias, for instance fear of snakes, fit in well in this conception. The expansion and contraction of their bodies as they move, and the peculiar stretching and smoothing of the skin of these animals as they glide about might be enough to elicit "it", apart from their strangeness factor, or their dangerousness. But cats and dogs, and birds too are also feared. Though they live in close proximity with us, they all have an element of strangeness which, in periods of lowered consciousness, might be just as effective in eliciting anxiety (Frijda, 1981). Fear of these animals is sometimes attributed too to their unpredictability. But having lived for a number of years with five cats, and the birds outside, it seems implausible, for they are the most predictable of animals. But they seem to share some other attributes which fit in well with characteristics of what is here called "symmetrical being", which are incorporated in the first few weeks of life. Their soft, furry bodies and dependent, gentle and beguiling ways, their tendency to sleep in blissful contentment after feeding, goes together with a fierce scratching, snarling, or pecking destructiveness, when thwarted. In a twinkling of an eye, their friendly, endearing behaviours can change into the opposite. In this sense, perhaps, one might call them unpredictable.

We should not lose sight, though, of the fact that it is not symmetrical being, or the id, that is the cause of the phobia or the neurosis, but the distortion of symmetrical being by the *translating* function of asymmetrical being, or the ego. These psychodynamic clinicians are agreed on this point, whether it is formulated in terms of conflict between the two modes of being or not. It is not the system unconscious itself, but its dominating influence on the conscious and preconscious systems that brings about "the insatiability, the automaticity, and the endless repetitiveness that are the stamp of the neurotic process".

The approach taken here does not imply that phobia can be understood merely from a perceptual point of view. As I have tried to show (chapter I), the tendency of psychologists to lose sight of other important factors while concentrating on those they advocate has slowed up our understanding of these extremely complicated issues. In drawing together the skeins of knowledge, this is also implied. Nor should the bringing together of different aspects of reality be understood as the confusion of one with the other.

"Physical space" is not seen as equivalent to "emotional space", nor are optical structures and visual events equivalent to their emotional attributions. What is assumed is that these aspects of reality are intrinsically bound up together, like two sides of a coin. Psychologists have tended to stare at the "emotional" and "behavioural" sides of things, with relative neglect of the "environmental" side. This study seeks to redress that balance. I have argued that Gibson's great contribution to psychology lies, to my mind, in his refusal to separate person from world, to split up the world into an "inner" and an "outer" component, or into a "physical" versus a "social" and "emotional" life. In the consistency with which he has done so in his theorizing, he has clarified our understanding of their intrinsic relations immensely. That, as I have understood it, is the main message contained in his theory of affordances.

A question that may arise in the reader who can only scan what has gone before is: "If these reversible optical structures and visual events are observed by all infants and young children, why do not all grow up to be phobic to the environment?". At the risk of being repetitive but for the sake of clarity, this question is answered as follows:

Phobia will arise only when certain conditions come together, namely, reversible optical structures which give rise to visual events that are anxiety-evoking (these are described in chapter II, and in this chapter), which events take place when the mother or care-taker is careless, indifferent, absent or unpredictable in her behaviour; when she neglects to provide the child with a potential space in which to fantasize undisturbed about the impulses from within and the events without; overlooks or consistently misinterprets the beginnings of trauma from such events which are signalled by emotional upset or collapse. In other words, when the child has been unable to learn to cope with these conflicting events, which then sink down into the id (symmetrical being) and erupt suddenly in consciousness. In this view, rather than being downgraded, developmental and emotional issues become more important than ever.

A matter that I shall take up, after reviewing the evidence from the empirical inquiry, is the possibility that these disturbances in optical structure may give rise to maladaptation of constancy mechanisms, which maladaptation may be linked to different forms that phobia takes. But this is jumping ahead.

Assuming that the viewpoint put forward here has something to recommend it, and I have understood the profound implications of the theories described, then the puzzle of phobia becomes transparent, its universal occurrence across the ages comprehensible, and its protean appearances indeed mere illusion. But psychologists, to be convinced, need more than a plausible argumentation. Only hard facts will suffice, which can be demonstrated and replicated again and again. In the context of this study, however, only preliminary explorations are offered. Though their results seem to back up this viewpoint in the main, these are only tentative. But intriguing nonetheless.

And though I have no greater understanding of what falling in love is, or what art is, as Barendregt hoped would be the case on solving the riddle of events that evoke "it", I do know that poets and other artists have long had an intimation of these relations, as the English poets John Keats, and Walter de la Mare proclaim:

> "Am I to leave this haven of my rest,
> This cradle of my glory, this soft clime,
> This calm luxuriance of blissful light,
> These crystalline pavilions, and pure fanes
> Of all my lucent empire? It is left
> Deserted, void, nor any haunt of mine.
> The blaze, the splendour, and the symmetry,
> I cannot see – but darkness, death and darkness."
> – John Keats, 1818, *Hyperion. A fragment. Book I, 235–241*

> "Our restless senses leap and say,
> 'How marvellous this! – How ugly that!'
> And, at a breath, will slip away
> The very thing they marvel at.
> Time is the tyrant of their fate;
> And frail the instant which must be
> Our all of actuality.
> (......)
> Ay, once I dreamed of an age-wide sea
> Whereo'er three moons stood leper-bright;
> And once – from agony set free –
> I scanned within the womb of night,
> A hollow inwoven orb of light,
> Thrilling with beauty no tongue could tell,
> And knew it for Life's citadel.
>
> And – parable as strange – once, I
> Was lured to a city whose every stone,
> And harpy human hastening by
> Were spawn and sport of fear alone –
> By soulless horror enthralled, driven on;
> Even the waters that, ebon-clear,
> Course through its dark, raved only of Fear!
> .(.....)
> Two worlds have we: without; within;
> But all that sense can mete and span,
> Until it confirmation win
> From heart and soul, is death to man."
> ....
> – Walter de la Mare, 1942, From *Dreams.*, 43–45

PART TWO

AN EMPIRICAL INQUIRY

General Introduction

In Part Two some empirical relations of a perceptual nature are explored. In considering clinical formulations about phobia, its nature and course (Chapter I), I drew the conclusion that certain perceptual relations which had received scant attention in these formulations might be of more importance in the phobic complaint than was assumed by the different theorists. The implication was that the phenomenon of phobia, at least in part, derives from some not well understood perceptual interactions of phobic persons with relatively permanent structures common to all environments in all ages, forms that these perceptual transformations of structures take, and inadequate control of the situations involved.

In Chapter V, I return to the first part of this assumption. The empirical work with 82 phobic patients and 110 normal controls described in this chapter forms an attempt to pin-point some of the actual structural components of situations and of objects operating in phobia, which seem to trigger anxiety and avoidance responses to these situations and objects.

In Chapter VI, on the basis of an analysis of the individual data from these experiments, specifically from 78 phobics and 88 normals, systematic deviations in the responses of phobics and normals to the varying ratios of stimulation suggest that phobic responses differ in degree and/or pattern from normal ones. If this finding is valid, it may be an indication of the rôle of ratios of stimulation in steering or guiding brain mechanisms that are tuned to or adjusted to varying ratios early in the perceptual life of the person. The different patterns of overestimation and underestimation of low and high magnitudes or ratios of stimulation (dubbed here "strategies" of perceptual control), suggest either systematic malfunction of mechanisms involved in phobic information-processing, or the existence of functional differences in the way that information is processed, which differences may be linked to learning processes in familial contexts, and in the course of early development.

These data suggest, furthermore, that important questions about information-processing, specifically the ins-and-outs of constancy, matters which have occupied Gregory and other representationists, may need to be taken more seriously by the ecologists following in Gibson's footsteps (Chapter II).

A forceful conclusion drawn from the contributions to psychodynamic conceptions of phobia (Chapter III), particularly by Barendregt and by Matte-Blanco, is that the clinical phenomena of depersonalization, derealization and perceptual disorientation are not limited to neurotic and psychotic syndromes, but also occur (or ought to occur) in normal adaptations to the world. This must necessarily be so, given the intrinsic intertwining (or confluence) of conscious and unconscious cognitive systems. Such conclusion, obvious enough to these clinicians, has been overlooked by others, perhaps because of different forms that coding of such experiences take in neurotic (or psychotic) and normal adjustments of individuals. For instance, whereas phobic patients tend to code these experiences negatively and adjust to them with coping mechanisms that alienate them still further from their environment and from themselves, similar experiences in normal persons tend to be coded more positively, explained in terms of philosophical (for example, existential) givens, and adjusted to creatively as sources of inspiration for works of art and science. In the dependency relationships of daily life, these phenomena are often coded too as indications of "being in love".

If this is so, then no systematic differences should be found between neurotic and normal persons in the *occurrence* of these experiences, although neurotic persons might well differ from normal persons in the *frequency* and/or *intensity* of these experiences. In Chapter VII, from rating-scale responses on the *spontaneous* occurrence of perceptual disorientation, derealization and depersonalization experiences in daily life, collected from 188 normal persons and 63 phobic patients, evidence is found that there may be a valid basis for this theoretical premise.

In Chapter VIII, a little intermezzo on the experience of time, some evidence is presented to show that normals tend to differ from phobics in some time attitudes, being significantly more flexible about time perspectives but also more anxious about the passage and control of time. In itself, not a surprising difference. But, taken together with some interesting differences between phobics and normals on spatial experience (Chapters V, VII, IX) suggest a profounder difference in their spatio-temporal orientations. In Chapter IV the assumption was made that certain optical structures, visual and haptic events have great impact on early perceptual adjustments in the infant and young child. This is so because of their "affordances". Their pernicious effects are exacerbated when conditions of parental care that could counteract or alleviate these are inadequate, intrusive or lacking. If these effects go unchallenged or uncorrected, a vicious circle might be set up in the interactions of the young child (and the adult) with his or her world, since these structures appear again and again (and throughout life) in the optical flow. How and why this should be the case was argued by drawing together the skeins of knowledge on perceptual and psychodynamic theory (Chapters II and III).

In Chapter IX, the information obtained from phobic patients during personal interviews, on the nature of their perceptual activity and experiences, certainly implies that the supposed links between these optical structures, visual and haptic events to which they give rise, and anhedonic responses to these, are not hypothetical but securely forged; and the predicted pernicious effects their bitter facts of life. Since neither patient nor interviewer had knowledge of the hypothesis entertained by me on these relations, this information may be quite valid.

In the general discussion, Chapter X, the balance is drawn up. The skeins of the phobic tapestry are taken up again and tentatively interwoven. With some prudence in doing so, because one important link in the chain is still speculative (constancy-scaling or conflict-control), and the exploratory nature of the others, inherent defects in methodology, or in the conclusions drawn from the results, advise such caution. Possible ways in which the built-in defects might be remedied are suggested for future exploration, which might provide sounder bases for the plausibility statements on which this thesis rests.

To avoid a certain dissatisfaction arising in the reader when the promise of the foregoing theoretical analysis of perceptual aspects of phobia remains unfulfilled by the tentativeness, incompleteness or fragility of the evidence to be presented, a warning and a reminder is called for at this point.

As I mentioned briefly in the Preface, in this thesis the empirical investigations do not follow from theoretical analysis, prior to their conception, except for the expectation that perceptions of phobics may well offer clues to their understanding; rather, it is the other way around. When the results from the first, preliminary explorations came in, the puzzles these presented made me aware of the lacunae in my understanding of perceptual process in pathological states, and of the insufficiencies of established perceptual theory to clarify these satisfactorily.

I first sought footholds in contemporary perceptual research with normal subjects, by modelling further search for environmental variables of possible importance in phobia on this work, only to end up with more puzzles. So I returned to basics: What do we actually know for certain about the nature of perception and perceptual control? What about the nature of phobia and psychodynamic conflict in the phobic process? How can one combine knowledge from both fields to gain a coherent picture of perception in phobia? This is what the reader is offered in Part One, Chapters I to IV. Therefore, to follow or appreciate the arguments, and the implications drawn from the results of the empirical work in Part Two, Chapters V to X, he or she should read these in the light of Part One. Otherwise, my conclusions may sometimes seem quite far-fetched, or fail to satisfy.

The reader should also bear in mind that I am well aware of the inherent defects of these explorations, which in hindsight were taken by a blind (wo)man; but despite this, they contain much that is enlightening on perceptual experience and control in phobic and in normal people. Because of these defects, however, no pretension is made to a full-bodied understanding of phobic perceptual process, nor are the conclusions reached definitive. At most I would venture that we now know more about *some of the environmental relations* that help to maintain the phobic reaction to different situations, and have a better understanding of how and why these may be so effective. The rest is tantalizing hint or allusion. Which is not to say that what is suggested by the rationale of Part One and the findings of Part Two, are any more illusory than other contemporary approaches currently masquerading as established fact.

An important clinical issue which receives very little attention in this study is the question of definition of phobia, and of the diagnostic criteria and procedures used in selection of patients for therapy (and research). Beyond the brief comments on definition problems in Chapter I, I have chosen to skirt the issue, for different reasons. When the studies to be described were initiated, little was known about perceptual function in phobic states; so my first concerns were to obtain more knowledge of this, and to worry about definition problems later. As Barendregt assured me (Barendregt, 1975), an implicit definition is as good as any to begin research: [*Onderzoek wordt dan mogelijk, waarvan niet aan het begin maar aan het eind een goede definitie wordt verlangd.*] "Research then becomes possible, whereby a good definition is not required at the beginning but at the end".

Over the years spirited discussions on problems of definition and diagnostic criteria were carried on in the department (see e.g., Chabot, 1975; and Barendregt's reply to Chabot, 1975; Knoppers, 1976; Van Krogten & Schaper, 1976). Yet these seemed to have few consequences for departmental policy, as far as selection of patients for therapy was concerned. Chabot and Ramsay, respectively the psychiatrist and clinical psychologist then in charge of intake procedure, agreed on the criteria (listed below), for soliciting patients from G.P.'s and physicians, and for accepting patients for therapy. Because of this agreement not to use a too narrow definition of phobia, the intake remained remarkably stable over the years in which our explorations were carried out.

Chabot describes the criteria on which both intakers agreed as follows: the patient is offered treatment only when (i) there is evidence of anxiety or an *emotional reaction* presented by the patient as a complaint; (ii) which arises in (relatively) specific situations; (iii) and leads to *avoidance*; (iv) some of which situations may be rôle-relevant (cf. Barendregt's definition, 1974). Furthermore, when (a) physical examination reveals no somatic anomaly and/or anomalies which might require medical therapy prior to psychological therapy (that is, in the judgment of the examining physician), and which might interfere unduly with the offered therapy. Also, that (b) no evidence of (pre-) psychotic characteristics; (c) no evidence of serious suicidal intention; (d) no evidence of a post-concentration camp syndrome; and (e) no addiction to alcohol and/or other drugs is found.

In the same publication he defines the criteria that a person has to satisfy before being given the label "agoraphobic" in this intake-procedure: The patient

(1) either (a) considers the term "anxious" and/or "afraid" and/or "fearful" and/or "panicky" to be applicable to him or her;
or (b) considers the term "tense" and/or "nervous" and/or
"I don't know what to do/where to turn" to be applicable to him or her;
or (c) shows signs of at least two symptoms of hyperventilation as defined (see Chabot, 1975);
or (d) a combination of (a) and/or (b) and/or (c).
(2) The term(s) under (1) are considered by the person to be as a rule applicable to him- or herself in at least one of the following situations:
– (alone) in a square or street or shop or department store; (independent of number of persons present);
– (alone) in a tram or train or bus or boat or aeroplane or car;
– (alone) in a cinema or theatre or in a church or large building or closed shower-bath/toilet;
– (alone) on a bridge or in a tunnel or in a lift;
– (alone) at home or leaving the house alone.
(The term "alone" signifies "without an anxiety-reducer".)

These, then, are the criteria on which the patients in the following studies were accepted for treatment. When I speak, as I shall, of the "agoraphobic", "claustrophobic" or "social phobic" experience in the studies to follow, I mean no more than "as diagnosed by the clinician in question"; and no less than "one of the basic variants of (negative) experiences possible when one adapts to stimulation or spatial relations in certain ways to be described".

V

The Enemy Without: The Information Picked Up by Phobic and Normal Persons under Stationary Conditions

The Effective Structural Components of Environments in Anxiety and Avoidance Behaviour

When the experiments to be discussed in this chapter were conceived and implemented, relatively little was known about the nature of the relations existing between specific classes of stimuli or situations, and approach and avoidance responses, which these seemed to elicit. In an article celebrating the emerging discipline of environmental psychology, Wohlwill (1970) noted that, with a few exceptions, the influence of the rôle of the physical environment on behaviour has been a neglected area, in spite of the fact that psychologists agree on its importance as background and context of all behaviour.

The notable exceptions at that time were the works of Gibson et al. (1950, 1963, 1965, 1966), Berlyne (1957–1968), and of Schneirla (1959, 1965). In his work on the investigation of the aesthetics of experience and affective responses to the environment by normal persons, Berlyne found that stimuli of high uncertainty, complexity and of novelty are especially effective in eliciting feelings of displeasure and anxiety. Schneirla found in his work with neonates and young animals (vertebrates) that stimulation of high magnitude, high intensity and frequency, of irregular arrangement or succession, and of angular or abrupt contour have highest effectivity in evoking distress and withdrawal responses in animals. These authors stressed the functional value of these stimulative effects in the survival of the species.

Before Gibson's pioneering work, however, (especially 1966 and 1979), the importance of surfaces and optical flow in the perception of the real world was hardly recognized. In clinical work, and in accordance with what was known from fundamental research on perception, the focus was on problems of distinguishing form and size, and focal stimuli from the background, of selectivity of stimuli and of anticipatory responses to fear-evoking stimuli. The designs of our experiments were therefore based on the traditional conceptions, and our procedures on the assumption that the static relations depicted in pictorial stimuli might be easier to perceive, control and understand, than stimulation received by a moving observer, or changing (moving) stimulus relations by a stationary observer. Our procedures thus made exclusive use of pictorial stimuli (slides, photographs, perspective drawings, abstract stimuli), like others before us.

But, despite the partiality of perceptionists to the use of pictorial stimuli in investigating perceptual relations, this may not be the best way or even a good way to begin the study of perception. To do so, as Gibson contends, "is to reduce the chance of understanding the processes of perception, since in a 'frozen' array none of the variant relations are included and only some of the invariant ones in the real world, in particular, only those features in an array that are composed of (the cross-sections of) visual solid angles, or forms".

In spite of this serious disadvantage, the use of pictorial stimuli has something to recommend it. As Gibson admits, pictures, perspective drawings, slides, and so on, can be looked at again and again by the same observer and by many observers, can be "applied" by the experimenter to an adult or to a baby, and in principle to animals too, and responses are relatively easily "scored". But the consequences, which are not negligible, for the interpretation and generalization of one's results should be kept in mind, since many of the ambiguities and misleading inferences taken in perception studies are in part due to the faulty assumptions about the nature of perception underlying the use of severely impoverished stimuli (Gibson, 1979, pp. 268–69).

For us though, at the time, these advantages seemed to outweigh the disadvantages. Also, the spirit of the times in the early seventies was against Gibson's radical approach to perception, and to his stress on surfaces and optical flow as *the* important variables in perception of the environment. Still, and in spite of the cursory dismissal of clinicians of the physical properties of environments as significant sources of danger, and thus of little relevance to phobia except in terms of their symbolic interest, the fact that most phobics seemed unduly preoccupied with these physical characteristics of environments was reason enough to try to find out whether or not this preoccupation was justified. The findings of the studies to be described in the following pages suggest unsuspected relations worthy of further exploration.

As our studies show, relatively few, and clearly circumscribed aspects of environmental structure seem to determine or play a rôle in anxiety and avoidance behaviour of phobic patients; and some of these seem to be quite effective too in eliciting similar reactions in normal persons.

These aspects pertain to the following "invariants" of structure: the relations between the height, breadth, and depth (distance) of spaces; ratios of illumination or relative brightness; heterogeneity of arrangements of elements; occlusion of space by (moving) objects; compactness or dense overlap; and wide, open, unoccluded space. For some phobics too, irregularity of shape or contour is moderately effective.

In later chapters, possible relations between these characteristics of environments (surfaces) and the stability and constancy experienced are explored.

In the *first* study (Bleeker, Velthuizen & McNab, 1972) to be reported on, our aim was unpretentious: to obtain from actual phobic patients, in a systematic way, information about the aspects of environmental structure which seem to trigger or sustain their phobic reactions, and to do so without influencing their perceptions by our preconceived ideas. In the four subjects investigated, the characteristics of the environment (i.e., tunnels) which trigger feelings of displeasure and avoidance tendencies seem to be: those ratios of the height, breadth and depth (H/D and B/D ratios) of these architectural spaces that elicit feelings of being pressed down by the ceiling or sucked through the shaft of the tunnel, in other words, a "funneling" effect associated with feelings of suffocation, unfamiliarity or strangeness. Illumination ratios that elicit feelings of sombreness, dismalness or darkness, and which make such spaces difficult to oversee. In some cases too, the presence or absence of people or vehicles that elicit feelings of busyness or quiet, and which seem to be associated with feelings of unsafety, and loneliness.

In the *second* study (McNab, Batstra & Vrouwe, 1975), these variables are systematically manipulated and controlled in different classes of (pictorial) situations, to ascertain in how far misperception or distortion of the phenomenal characteristics of these spaces is related to ratios of objective stimulation, type of situation, or to the state of anxiety operating in patients suffering from tunnelphobia. The results of this study indicate that the crucial factor in the misperception of these phenomenal characteristics (i.e., compared to a "norm" stimulus) is the ratios of stimulation present in the situations.

In the *third* study (McNab, Nieuwenhuyse, Jansweyer & Kuyper, 1978), two of the above-mentioned variables, namely H/D ratio and B/D ratio, are more extensively explored as variables influencing feelings of enclosure, anhedonic responses, anxiety and avoidance. An increase in H/D ratio proves to be a valid predictor of perceived enclosure of architectural spaces, for phobic as well as normal persons, and is significantly correlated with a decrease in hedonic feelings in phobic and normal persons. A decrease in B/D ratio, though having negligible effect on normal persons, is also a good predictor of perceived enclosure and of strength of anxiety and avoidance responses for phobic patients.

In the *fourth* study (De Leeuw & McNab, 1977) and the *fifth* study (McNab & Hansen, 1978; McNab & Beerthuizen, in McNab, 1981) an exploration of other structural components of situations, namely those relating to the uncertainty-complexity dimensions of space, is undertaken. In the fourth study, in which *abstract stimuli* were shown only to a group of mainly agoraphobic patients, the relevant components for these patients seem to be heterogeneity of elements, irregularity of shape or contour, and irregularity of arrangement of elements. Their anhedonic responses and feelings of arousal were explored but not their responses of anxiety or avoidance. In the fifth study, using *real-life* (pictorial) stimuli of street situations, and normal controls of the phobic patients, the structural components that elicit feelings of unpleasure, arousal, anxiety and avoidance responses, in phobic patients, are high complexity situations characterized by compactness or dense overlap (occlusion of space), the bustle of streets with people (moving occluding forms), heterogeneity of arrangement of elements in space (situations of moderate complexity), and wide, open spaces that elicit strong feelings of loneliness, solitariness or bleakness (situations of low complexity).

The evidence on which these statements are based is systematically reviewed in the following sections.

A Preliminary Exploration of the Characteristics of Some Environmental Structures that Play a Rôle in Phobia (Study I)

As said earlier, the aim of this study was to explore, in a systematic way, characteristics of environmental structures which seem to trigger or sustain phobic reactions to situations; and to do so without influencing the perceptions of the phobic patients by our preconceived ideas. In this preliminary study, in order not to multiply the problems, we limited ourselves to one class of structures that phobic persons fear, namely tunnels, because we expected the characteristics of these structures to be more easily represented, and more easily controlled (than, for example, in street situations).

Method

Subjects

From the patients in treatment at our departmental clinic, we obtained the voluntary participation of four female phobics whose main complaint included a phobia for tunnels. Their ages varied from 34 to 39 years. Two of these patients had been undergoing therapy for a few months, one had been in therapy for a year, and the fourth had been in therapy for several years. The first patient (S 1) suffered from claustrophobia in tunnels, elevators, cinemas and large shops; the second patient (S 2) from agoraphobia, tunnelphobia, and fear of being looked at; the third patient (S 3) from agoraphobia, being far from home, social phobia, and claustrophobia in tunnels, cinemas and large shops; and the fourth patient (S 4) from a phobia for driving a car, tunnel- and tram phobia, and being far from home.

Stimuli

Twenty black-and-white photographs of tunnels in and around Amsterdam, sized 12×17.5 cm, mounted on cardboard. Ten depicted pedestrian subways, and ten traffic tunnels. This collection formed a fair sample of the types of tunnels that the patients might encounter in daily life. Table 5.1 describes them.

Selection of Stimuli

Before selecting the stimuli for the study, 18 black-and-white photographs of pedestrian subways were shown to 15 normal persons (students), who varied in age and sex. They were asked to describe the characteristics of each tunnel stimulus in order to gain an idea of the number of relevant concepts such stimuli might elicit, and also to try out the feasibility of the description task for patients. A large number of concepts was elicited, relating to the *objective* dimensions of structure such as length, breadth, depth, curvature, illumination, state of the construction and kind of materials used, time of day and weather conditions. Also, concepts relating to more *subjective* dimensions and experiences, such as the aesthetic and hedonic feelings that tunnels evoke, attractiveness, familiarity, crowdedness, lugubriousness, and so forth. Ten of the pedestrian subway stimuli included in the try-out were then used in the main study. The ten stimuli selected elicited highest agreement in concepts. No tunnels for vehicles had been included in this try-out, but since we expected (from the dossiers of the patients) that heavy traffic tunnels can also elicit anxiety and avoidance, ten of these were included in the study.

Table 5.1 Brief descriptions of the tunnel elements (black-and-white photographs) used in the investigation

Pedestrian subways:	
E1	J.D. Meyerplein: entrance to subway, brightly lit, empty of people.
E3	Prins Hendrikkade: entrance to subway, dark, empty of people.
E4	Central Station: underpass giving entrance to platforms, brightly lit, people, *affiches*.
E5	J.D. Meyerplein: exit, two persons at exit, raining.
E6	Central Station: freight tunnel, very dark, long and empty of freight or people.
E8	J.D. Meyerplein: inside the subway, one man in foreground, brightly lit.
E9	Central Station: same as E4 but empty of people.
E10	Prins Hendrikkade: exit, dark, empty of people.
E11	Miranda pool: pedestrian-bicycle subway, brightly lit, a few people half-hidden by pillars on one side.
E20	Same as E11: inside the subway, dark, empty, exit clearly visible.
Traffic tunnels:	
E2	Schiphol: 2-lanes, brightly lit, one car, exit visible.
E7	Schiphol: 3-lanes, entrance, very dark, one bumper of a car visible.
E12	Schiphol: 3-lanes with wide emergency lane visible, brightly lit, cars and speeding lorry in the foreground.
E13	Schiphol: the same as E12 but half-lit, middle tunnel, long, two cars and lorry in the distance.
E14	Schiphol: the same as E13, half-lit, long and empty, except for car lights in the distance.
E15	Coen-tunnel: 2-lanes, brightly lit, 5 cars in middle of tunnel, exit not visible.
E16	Ij-tunnel: 2-lanes, half-lit, a few cars, exit visible.
E17	Coen-tunnel: the same as E15, brightly lit, a few cars, exit barely visible.
E18	Schiphol: the same as E2 but empty of traffic.
E19	Schiphol: 3-lanes, dark, two lorries visible near the exit.

Technique of Eliciting Relevant Personal Constructs

To elicit information about the dimensions of the tunnel situations that evoke feelings of unpleasure, anxiety or avoidance, we made use of a personality technique specifically designed to elicit relevant personal constructs from individuals, namely, the Repertory Grid technique (Kelly, 1955; Bonarius, 1965; Bannister, 1968).

In this technique three elements or figures (i.e., tunnel stimuli) are presented to each subject and he or she is asked to say in which way two of these are similar and differ from the third. That is, the person is asked to name the *construct* dimension which separates two of the three elements. The pole of difference is called the *contrast* dimension. This is called the "triad" method. All elements are presented in triads until these no longer elicit new constructs, or up to a previously determined maximum number of trials, depending on the design. When this stage is completed, the person is then asked to rate each element on the extent to which it contains each of the elicited constructs or contrasts. This method ensures the general applicability of the construct dimension to all other elements not appearing in a given triad. When the test is completed, the experimenter has available a list of personal constructs as they have been formulated in the triads, plus a score for each construct which represents the extent to which the construct (or contrast) is present in or absent from a given element.

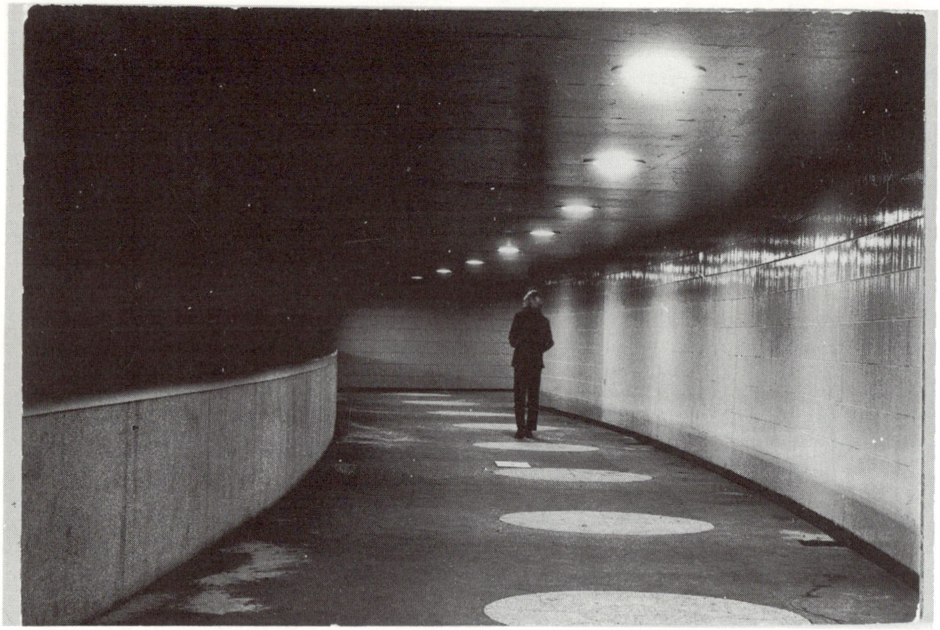

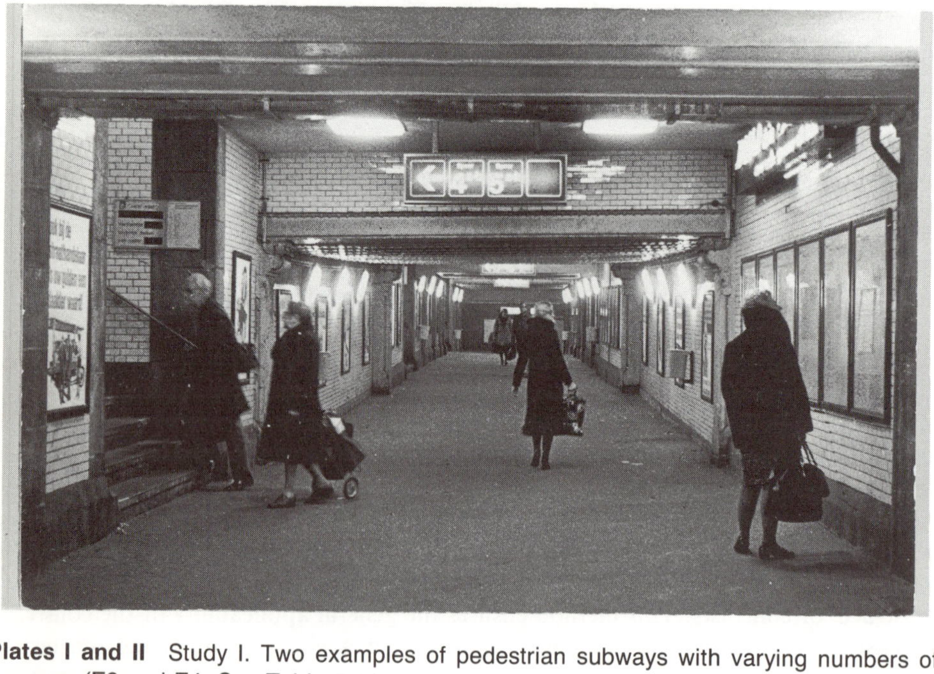

Plates I and II Study I. Two examples of pedestrian subways with varying numbers of persons. (E8 and E4. See Table 5.1.)

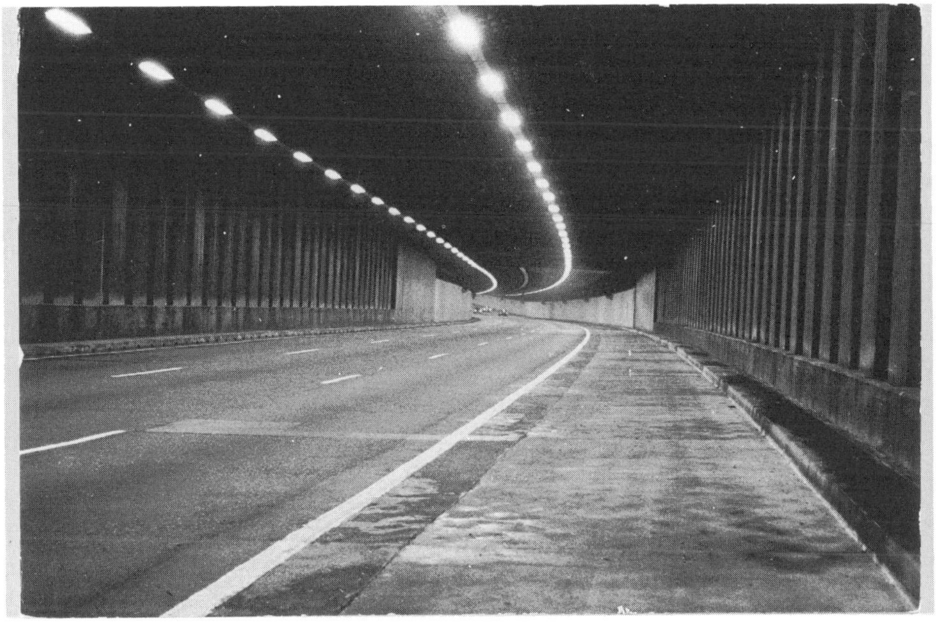

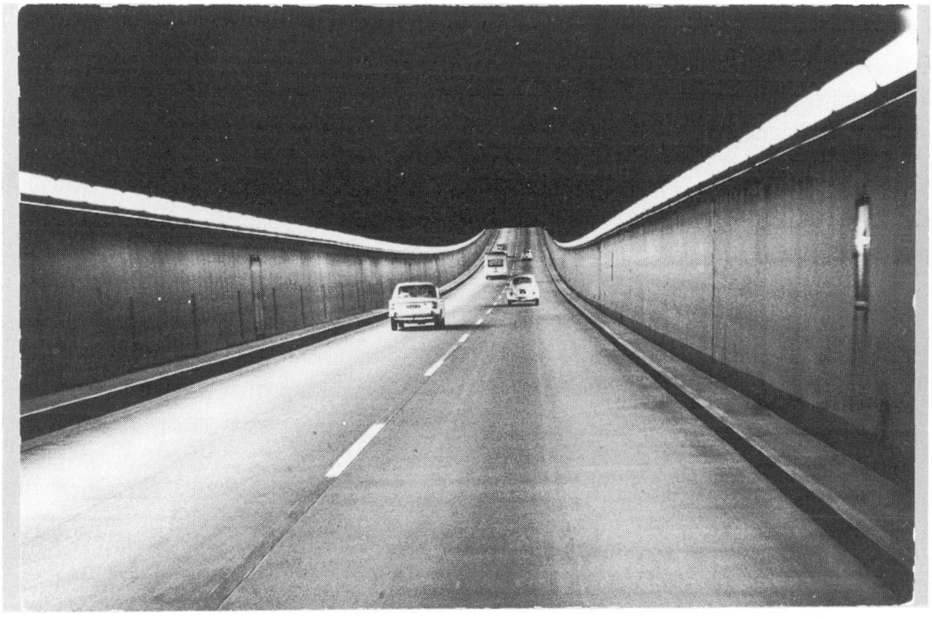

Plates III and IV Study I. Two examples of traffic tunnels with varying numbers of cars. (E14 and E17. See Table 5.1.)

Procedure

In this study each patient was tested individually, in two separate sessions, on separate days. In the first session each subject was given 40 triads in a previously randomized order. Each triad was viewed for 5 seconds and then removed, after which the construct (and contrasting concept) was elicited. The experimenter then made a note of these, and of any observations spontaneously given by the subject. In the second session, and in order to determine the relevance of each tunnel stimulus to feelings of unpleasure or anxiety, the patient was first asked to rank order the tunnel stimuli on the basis of feelings of unpleasure (*onprettigheid*) that the tunnels, as depicted, give rise to. Using a variant of Stephenson's Q-technique, the experimenter asked the patient first to pick out from the unsorted pile of photos on the table the one judged to be most displeasing and the one judged least displeasing. These formed the extreme poles of the hierarchy. Other photos were placed in one or other pile, according to the feelings of unpleasure elicited by the stimulus. The patient was asked to place in a third pile those tunnels which could not be sorted into either pile. When this task was completed, each pile was again rank ordered from "most displeasing" to "least displeasing". The patient was allowed as much time as necessary to do so. At completion of this task, the experimenter noted down the rankings of stimuli given by the patient. Each tunnel stimulus was then separately rated on bipolar, seven-point scales on the degree in which the construct or contrast was present. The scale ran from +3 (the construct) to −3 (the contrast in the depicted tunnel situation). To the list of constructs (and contrasting concepts) obtained from the patient, we added a few constructs of apparent relevance to the phobia of the person, which were taken from the dossier of the patient, or from spontaneous asides made by the patients during the sessions, and they were asked to rate these as well on the basis of presence or absence in a given tunnel. These constructs were: "low ceiling"; "narrow" tunnel; "apparent dead end"; "slant of (road) surface"; "busyness"; and, in one case, "displeasingness" (see Tables 5.1 a–d, where the added concepts are indicated by an asterisk).

Data Analysis

Originally a cluster analysis (according to Bonarius, 1965) was carried out on the Repertory grid data for each subject, and correlations between the construct ratings and the ratings of displeasingness of the tunnels determined (Bleeker & Velthuizen, 1972). Characteristic of the cluster analysis is the making of a classification of the constructs or of the elements by a repeating process of trying to group the constructs or the elements by similarity between patterns of the grid.

In this way constructs within a group are aligned to achieve higher agreement than between constructs that are placed in another group, thereby yielding the so-called *probeerfactoren* (trial factors). At a later date, when a computer program for analysing Repgrid data became available, using principal component analysis (PCA), the data were re-analysed by this method. The analysis of the Repgrid applied PCA is based, however, not on the correlation matrix (as in cluster analysis), but on the matrix of deviation scores (the scores in each row are expressed as deviations of the mean score of that row in the original matrix). Since the PCA method yields similar but more detailed information about the constructcomponents and their vector loadings (the PCA is a factor analytic approach), the results from this analysis are given here instead of the rougher trial factors of the original cluster analysis (see Bonarius, 1980).

Summary of the Results of the Principal Component Analyses for Eeach of the Four Subjects Separately

S 1: *Claustrophobic Patient* in Tunnels, Elevators, Cinemas, and Large Shops

Sixteen constructs (and contrasting concepts) were obtained. To these four were added by the experimenters, because of their apparent relevance, and these 20 constructs (contrasts) were rated by her (see Table 5.1a, in which these are described, with the added constructs indicated by an asterisk). PCA results show 16 constructcomponents of the tunnels. Of these, the first three account for 77.16% of the total variance. Since the other 13 constructcomponents contribute little more of interest, these will not be described here. In Table 5.1a, vector loadings on the constructs are given, but vector loadings smaller than 4.00 are omitted, to facilitate a quick grasp of the constructs (contrasts) that are most relevant to the component (i.e., according to the Repertory grid PCA).

The first constructcomponent (*Eigenvalue*, i.e., the sum of squared vector loadings: 1070.88) accounts for 43.36% of the total variance, and is thus the most important of the three. This component relates to *traffic tunnels*, which are most displeasing to this patient (Vector loading: 6.09). Highly significant, positive relations between displeasingness of these tunnels and the following characteristics are found: "pressure from above", "long tunnel", "dismalness", "funneling effect", "narrow opening", "low ceiling", "exit far off"; "darkness", "difficulty to oversee the tunnel", "unfamiliarity".

All these aspects correlate very highly with displeasingness ($.75 \leqslant r \leqslant .90$) and are also highly intercorrelated ($.53 \leqslant r \leqslant .95$). "Exit not visible", "bend in tunnel", and "apparent dead end", though loading relatively highly on the component, are not highly correlated with displeasingness (respectively $r = .46$; .41; .24). [See Appendix A, Table 5.1e, for an overview of the intercorrelations.] The second constructcomponent (*Eigenvalue*: 448.96) accounts for 19.44% of the total variance. This component relates to *pedestrian subways*, which are neither displeasing nor pleasing to this patient (VL: −.765). The constructs with high vector loadings on this component are: "no traffic", "don't know where you are", "seems a dead end", "narrow", and "no funneling effect". However, only the constructs "dead end", "don't know where you are", and "narrow tunnel" are fairly highly intercorrelated ($.62 \leqslant r \leqslant .65$). [See Table 5.1e in Appendix A.] The third constructcomponent (*Eigenvalue*: 262.36) accounts for 11.36% of the total variance. This component describes a relation between: "apparent dead end", "traffic", "roomy opening", "exit not visible", and a lack of feelings of displeasure in *pedestrian subways* (VL: −1.039). Only "exit not visible,", and "apparent dead end" are highly intercorrelated ($r = .72$) [see Table 5.1e, Appendix A.] None correlate highly with displeasingness.

From these results we may assume that for this claustrophobic patient traffic tunnels are most displeasing, particularly those in which the height is low and length long, and

Table 5.1a Composition of the first three constructcomponents for S 1

Construct	Contrast	I	II	III
displeasing (*onprettig*)	pleasing	6.090	(−.765)	(−1.039)
pressure from above	no pressure	10.336		
exit far off	exit nearby	10.296		
difficult to oversee	easy to oversee	9.911		
unfamiliar	familiar	9.311		
long tunnel	short tunnel	9.298		
funneling effect	no funneling	9.243	−5.390	
exit not visible	exit visible	9.101		4.833
low ceiling	high ceiling	8.436		
narrow opening	roomy opening	8.097		−5.541
dark	lighted	7.937		
traffic tunnel (cars)	pedestrian subway	7.813	−6.812	(−3.467)
bend in tunnel	no bend	6.154		
seems a dead end*	no dead end	5.675	6.672	6.149
dismal (*triest*)	cheerful	5.118		
don't know where you are	know where you are		9.195	
narrow*	broad		6.139	
quiet*	noisy			
no people	people			
traffic	no traffic		−9.450	5.009

N.B. Columns I, II and III give the vector loadings, according to the Repertory Grid PCA.
* Construct not elicited during test but taken from dossier.

the width narrow compared to length, which dimensions seem to elicit feelings of pressure from above, and a strong funneling effect. Also, in these tunnels those illumination ratios (i.c., darkness) which make the tunnels difficult to oversee, appear dismal, and unfamiliar. Pedestrian subways, with or without traffic (people, bicycles) are not displeasing, when no funneling effect is present and the opening roomy, even though the patient feels disoriented (doesn't know where she is), and the subway seems to look like a dead end, with the exit not visible.

S 2: *Agoraphobic- and Tunnelphobic Patient* with a Fear of Being Looked At

Nineteen constructs (and contrasting concepts) were obtained. To these three were added (see Table 5.1b, where these are indicated by an asterisk). PCA results show 17 constructcomponents. Of these, the first three account for 64.38% of the total variance. The other 14 components contribute little more to these, and are not described. Table 5.1b describes these three components of tunnels, with the highest vector loadings.

The first constructcomponent (*Eigenvalue*: 930.548) accounts for 34.14% of the total variance. This component relates to *pedestrian subways*, which are highly displeasing (Vector loading: 7.306). This component has high vector loadings on the following characteristics: "no traffic", "short tunnel", "no bend", "exit nearby", "no people", "other people accessible", "strange", "unsafe", "not a real tunnel"; "old", "uncompleted", "rough walls", "ugly"; "difficult to oversee", "dark". Except for the second group of constructs, and the contrasts: "short tunnel", "no bend", "exit

Table 5.1b Composition of the first three constructcomponents for S 2

Construct	Contrast	I	II	III
displeasing	pleasing	7.306	5.760	(– 1.724)
traffic	no traffic	– 10.155	4.236	
strange	familiar	10.036		
long tunnel	short tunnel	– 9.313	5.778	
old	new	9.125		
uncompleted	completed	8.266		
ugly	fine	7.914		
traffic tunnel	pedestrian subway	– 7.883	8.191	4.118
bend in tunnel	no bend	– 6.737		
smooth walls	rough walls	– 6.283	– 4.133	
real tunnel	not a real tunnel	– 5.938	4.896	– 5.395
difficult to oversee	easy to oversee	5.746	6.353	
no people	people	5.555		
unsafe*	safe	5.247	6.496	
exit far off	exit nearby	– 5.187	5.451	
other people inaccessible	others accessible	– 5.063	– 4.108	
dark	lighted	4.294	7.472	
narrow*	broad			9.291
road slanted down	slanted up			
low ceiling*	high ceiling		– 6.351	9.005
no daylight	daylight		6.658	
seems a dead end	not a dead end			4.220

N.B. A positive loading signifies that the constructpole relates positively to the component and the contrastpole negatively. A negative loading signifies that the constrastpole relates positively to the component and the constructpole negatively.

nearby", "not a real tunnel", these constructs are moderately to highly correlated with displeasingness (.50 ⩽ r ⩽ .66) and moderately to highly intercorrelated (.51 ⩽ r ⩽ .87). [See Appendix A, Table 5.1f for an overview of the intercorrelations.] The second constructcomponent (*Eigenvalue*: 497.476) accounts for 18.25% of the total variance. This component relates to *traffic tunnels*, which are displeasing (VL: 5.760). Fairly high vector loadings are found on: "dark", "no daylight", "difficult to oversee", "unsafe"; "high ceiling", "long tunnel", "exit far off", "real tunnel", "rough walls"; "traffic", "other people accessible". High intercorrelations are found between constructs on this component (.52 ⩽ r ⩽ .79). [See Table 5.1f in Appendix A.] The third constructcomponent (*Eigenvalue*: 326.671) accounts for 11.99% of the total variance. This component relates to *traffic tunnels* which are fairly pleasing (VL: – 1.724). This loads highly on the constructs: "narrow tunnel", "low ceiling", "not a real tunnel", "apparent dead end"; but have low or negative correlations with displeasingness (.05 ⩽ r ⩽ – .21). The only constructs which are highly intercorrelated are: "Real tunnel", "narrow tunnel", "low ceiling" (.55 ⩽ r ⩽ .65). [See Appendix A, Table 5.1f.]

For this agoraphobic patient, pedestrian subways and, to a lesser extent, traffic tunnels are most displeasing when these are dark, difficult to oversee, without people but with people accessible, strange and unsafe. High to moderately high ceilings in long (car) tunnels and in short tunnels are also displeasing; and aesthetically displeasing are old, uncompleted tunnels with rough walls, which are experienced as ugly. When traffic tunnels do not appear to this patient to be "real ones", they are not found to be displeasing, whether or not these tunnels are narrow, have low ceilings, or seem to culminate in a dead end.

S 3: *Agoraphobic- Social Phobic- Claustrophobic Patient*, with a Fear of Being Far from Home

Sixteen constructs (and contrasting concepts) were obtained. To these four were added (see Table 5.1c, in which these are indicated by an asterisk). PCA results show 17 constructcomponents. Of these, the first three constructcomponents account for 71.47% of the total variance. The other 14 components contribute little more to these, and are not described. Table 5.1c describes the first three constructcomponents of tunnels with the highest vector loadings.

The first constructcomponent (*Eigenvalue*: 788.931) accounts for 39.15% of the total variance. This is related to *pedestrian subways*, which are most displeasing (Vector loading: 7.901). This component has high vector loadings on the following characteristics, but only the first group is highly correlated with displeasingness: "sombre", "dark", "strange", "other people accessible", "no people present", "difficult to oversee", "unsafe"; "low ceiling", "narrow tunnel", "short tunnel", "exit nearby", "no bend in tunnel". Table 5.1g shows that the first group of constructs correlates highly with displeasingness ($.71 \leqslant r \leqslant .91$) and the constructs are highly intercorrelated ($.54 \leqslant r \leqslant .94$); but the second group, although moderately to highly intercorrelated ($.51 \leqslant r \leqslant .71$), are not correlated significantly with displeasingness ($-.01 \leqslant r \leqslant .44$). [See Appendix A, table 5.1g for an overview of the intercorrelations.] The second constructcomponent (*Eigenvalue*: 476.528) accounts for 23.86% of the total variance. This is related to those *pedestrian subways* which are highly pleasing (VL: −5.025). These subways are those with the following characteristics: "lighted", "cheerful", "familiar", "people" and "other people inaccessible", "low ceiling", "exit nearby", "short tunnel", "modern tunnel". [The constructs (and contrasts) that are significantly intercorrelated are shown in the r-values in Table 5.1g Appendix A.] The third constructcomponent (*Eigenvalue*: 161.825) accounts for only 8.10% of the total variance. This component is only slightly related to pleasingness (VL: −1.325), and has high vector loadings only on the constructs: "old", and "uncompleted". None of the constructs on this component are significantly intercorrelated. [See Table 5.1g in Appendix A.]

For this patient, then, only those pedestrian subways that are sombre, dark, strange, difficult to oversee, with no people present but people accessible, are found to be highly displeasing and judged unsafe. These subways are generally short and straight, narrow and with low ceilings.

S 4: *Travel Phobic- and Tunnel Phobic Patient*, with a Fear of Being Far from Home

Eighteen constructs (and contrasting concepts) were obtained. To these three were added (see Table 5.1d, in which these are indicated by an asterisk). PCA results show 17 constructcomponents. Of these, the first three account for 73.01% of the total variance. The other 14 components are not described. Table 5.1d shows the first three components with the highest vector loadings.

Table 5.1c Composition of the first three constructcomponents for S 3

Construct	Contrast	I	II	III
displeasing*	pleasing	7.901	−5.025	(−1.325)
dark	lighted	9.762	−5.086	
sombre	cheerful	9.165	−4.399	
low ceiling*	high ceiling	9.118	6.401	
bend in tunnel	no bend	−8.479		
narrow	broad	7.742		
traffic tunnel	pedestrian subway	−7.379	−9.160	
strange	familiar	6.656	−4.970	
other people inaccessible	others accessible	−6.512	4.670	
unsafe*	safe	6.387		
exit far off	exit nearby	−5.597	−7.323	
long	short	−5.413	−8.031	
no people	people	5.281	−4.114	
difficult to oversee	easy to oversee	5.230		
real tunnel	not a real tunnel			
silence	noise			
uncompleted	completed			6.086
slanted surface*	not slanted surface			
quiet	busy			
old	modern		−8.676	6.919

The first constructcomponent (*Eigenvalue*: 936.160) accounts for 41.09% of the total variance. This component is related to *traffic tunnels*, which are highly displeasing (Vector loading: 7.567). This component has high vector loadings on the following characteristics: "long, real tunnel", "cars", "exit far off", "narrow opening", "exit not visible", "no possibility to turn away"; "suffocating", "sombre", "lonely", "difficult to oversee". The constructs "exit not visible" and "no possibility to turn away" are not significantly correlated with displeasingness; but all the other constructs are highly correlated ($.58 \leqslant r \leqslant .85$), and are also highly intercorrelated ($.50 \leqslant r \leqslant .97$). [These intercorrelations are shown in Table 5.1h in Appendix A.] The second constructcomponent (*Eigenvalue*: 482.146) accounts for 21.16% of the total variance. This is related to *pedestrian subways*, which are fairly displeasing (VL: 3.192). This component has fairly high vector loadings on the following characteristics: "no people", "quiet", "lonely", "no vehicles"; "narrow, with narrow opening", "don't know where you are"; "dark", "difficult to oversee". Of these constructs, only "narrow opening" "difficult to oversee" and (feelings of) "loneliness" are significantly correlated with displeasingness ($.65 \leqslant r \leqslant .73$). Intercorrelations between constructs are fairly high ($.51 \leqslant r \leqslant .71$). [See Table 5.1h Appendix A.] The third constructcomponent (*Eigenvalue*: 245.248) accounts for 10.76% of the total variance. This component relates to tunnels characterized by: "exit nearby and visible", "end of tunnel", "busyness".

This patient seems to find traffic tunnels which are narrow and long (exit far off or not visible), cars (traffic) present, highly displeasing, suffocating, sombre, lonely and difficult to oversee. Pedestrian subways without people or vehicles, which are dark, quiet, difficult to oversee and narrow, with a narrow opening are also fairly displeasing. As the exit approaches, and the busyness of the outside world becomes visible, their displeasingness seems to become less.

Table 5.1d Composition of the first three constructcomponents for S 4

Construct	Contrast	I	II	III
displeasing	pleasing	7.567	(3.192)	(2.328)
cars	no cars	11.543	−4.353	
traffic tunnel	pedestrian subway	11.304	−5.627	
long tunnel	short tunnel	11.028		
real tunnel	not a real tunnel	10.733		
exit far off	exit nearby	8.859		−4.513
suffocating	feel relieved	8.373		
exit not visible	exit visible	8.235		−8.975
lonely	not lonely	5.554	4.392	
difficult to oversee	easy to oversee	5.531	5.481	
no possibility to turn away	possibility	4.787		
sombre	cheerful	4.606		
narrow opening	roomy opening	4.302	5.747	
don't know where you are	know where you are		7.000	
no people	people		9.372	
end of tunnel	begin tunnel			8.706
low ceiling*	high ceiling			
narrow	broad		7.854	
dark	lighted		7.546	
quiet*	busy		6.784	−4.345
seems a dead end	not a dead end			

Other Observations

When we compared the actual tunnel stimuli with the constructs and contrasts these elicited in the different patients, some striking omissions or reversals of "objective" structural components present in the stimuli were noted. For instance, S 1 (claustrophobic patient) rated three car tunnels (E2, E13, E19) and one pedestrian subway (E11) "without people or cars", although these were clearly present.

S 2 (agoraphobic patient) rated one car tunnel "extremely light" when, in fact, all that she could see of it was a black hole (E7). Actually, this patient rated all car tunnels "well-lighted", and new, pedestrian subways "dark" and "old", whether or not this was the case. The same patient rated three pedestrian subways (E9, E10, E20) and two car tunnels (E14, E18) as "full of people or vehicles," whereas three were totally empty, and two contained people who were hardly visible to the naked eye. S 3 (agoraphobic + social phobic + claustrophobic patient) and S 4 (travel phobic patient) rated two tunnels in which no clues at all about their length could be seen, as respectively "short" and "long", apparently because of the connotation "short" with pedestrian subway and "long" with car tunnel (E3, E7).

Comments

These misperceptions were difficult to interpret. It was not clear if these were linked to the nature of the phobic complaint (e.g., the claustrophobic patient's phobia had started after a fight with a close friend during a drive in a car tunnel, which had led to a regretted break in the relationship; the agoraphobic patient complained that people in the street stared at her as if they knew she was mad, and saw eyes everywhere; and so on), or to the phenomenal aspects of these architectural spaces, or to learned associations or anxiety state. The fairly high to high intercorrelations between different characteristics of these tunnels, for all the patients, suggested that the different variables might interact, and their combined effects give rise to or intensify feelings of unpleasure and other negative experiences (e.g., suffocation) in the situations; for instance, the funneling effect might well be increased when the tunnel was dark.

Because of the careful procedure we had followed in this study, without knowing it we had obtained from these four patients, with different complaints, one of the keys to the possible resolution of the problem of perceptual dysfunction in phobia, as will become clear in later chapters, namely, the linkage of quite specific (though not idiosyncratic) experiences of these spaces to the structural relations present in them. Instead of following through this association, which might have led us earlier out of the woods, we focused instead on the striking misperceptions of the objectively present stimulus relations, as the clue we were looking for. With hindsight, it is easy to see that this was probably due to our bias then towards thinking of the problem in terms of faulty coding of stimulus inputs, or of meanings of situations. This led us off at a tangent; but, as it turned out, a turning off which did not prove to be an entirely unfruitful one. The next study (Study II) describes this (ad)venture.

A Second Attempt to Explore some of the Characteristics of Environmental Structure that Play a Rôle in Phobia (Study II)

Redefining the Problem

From study I we had learned that what all four patients had in common was the linking of feelings of unpleasure, and other negative feelings such as suffocation, dismalness, sombreness, loneliness to structural components or relations of tunnel situations. For instance, the ratios between the height of the tunnel and the distance (depth) and between the breadth and the depth seemed to elicit feelings of enclosure, of being thrust through the shaft of the tunnel or pressed down by the roof which was described as a sort of "funneling", and which gave rise to feelings of suffocation. The luminance levels or illumination ratios (especially dark) seemed to give rise to feelings of darkness, sombreness or dismalness ("*triestheid*"), making these spaces also difficult to oversee. The presence or absence of people, or vehicles gave rise in some to feelings of unsafety, busyness or quiet, or loneliness. All four patients appeared to misperceive some aspect(s) of these structures or objects, in different tunnels. Also, the kind of tunnel and/or the nature of the phobic complaint seemed to be important in determining misperception, or feelings of displeasure, etc.

Besides this, the high intercorrelations for all four subjects between structural components (physical dimensions) and phenomenological experience suggested that different components of these tunnels might interact to strengthen (or weaken) their anhedonic experiences. Having ascertained this much, several questions loomed large. First of all, what weight might we give to these findings? Although we had followed a careful procedure and abstained from influencing the patients in their conceptions, we had after all only investigated four patients. And we had used stimuli to do so whose variables had not been systematically manipulated, even though we had taken care to achieve as fair a sample as possible of the kinds of tunnels the tunnelphobics would come across in daily life. We had also made use of rating scales, which might mean that the results were an artefact of the procedure employed, because of the tendency of neurotic patients to make use of extreme scoring categories on rating scales. The results could also be due to chance factors, since no controls were used, neither for the subjects nor the stimulus conditions. A second question was whether these structural components of tunnel situations, which are present in other kinds of spaces, might have similar effect on these patients. In other words, are feelings of anxiety or unpleasure a function of ratios of stimulation present in the situation, that are not specific to tunnels alone? Or are these feelings a function of idiosyncratic meanings that are only marginally related to ratios of stimulation? A third point concerned the locus of misperception. Are the physical aspects of situations misperceived, or the relations between physical variables? Or are the phenomenal aspects misperceived (that is, the appearances of these relations)?

In order to improve the chances of obtaining answers to at least some of these questions, we decided to make use of a design in which the independent variables could be systematically manipulated and controlled in different classes of situations, that is, situations structurally similar to tunnels but with different connotations. To resolve the question whether misperception is due to ratios of stimulation in the situation, or to anxiety-level of the phobic patient, we decided to make use of control groups varying in anxiety-level, and in kind of phobia (in case misperceptions had to do with the relevance of the situation to the phobia); and also to vary different characteristics (holding others constant), in different types of situations. To exclude as much as possible the operating of chance factors or response bias, a method was chosen where these are minimized (Method of constant stimulus differences; see Procedure). Having settled on these improvements, we had to make a choice on the problem to attack first, given the context for such exploration (i.e., experiments to be carried out by students). We chose to focus on the misperceptions because, as said earlier, at the time our theoretical orientation biased us towards a conception of perceptual malfunction in phobia in terms of miscoding of stimulative effects. The misperceptions in the previous study seemed to be the key to much of the distress felt in these situations by phobic patients.

Expectations and Hypotheses

We reasoned that if the anxiety of tunnel phobics is linked to some specific, idiosyncratic meaning that tunnel situations have for these patients, then one might expect their perceptual behaviour in these situations to differ from other phobic persons, who have no “vested interest” in such situations; and also to differ from normal persons, who feel no fear at all in tunnels, or in other tunnel-like situations. One might also expect to find a difference between their perceptual behaviour in tunnel situations, compared to other situations that do not usually give rise to anxiety. These expectations are formulated in the first hypothesis. If, however, the findings of the first study are not artefactual, one might expect different characteristics of tunnels to have different relevance for phobic patients of different complaints, compared to their normal controls. These expectations are formulated in the second hypothesis. Of course, if the ratios of stimulation and/or the phenomenological aspects of these determine misperception, then we ought to find few differences between the groups, although the responses of the phobics might be "stronger" (i.e., show more misperception) than the normal subjects.

Given the choice of procedure, misperception is operationalized in terms of the frequency with which the subject gives an incorrect judgment on the amount of stimulation or ratios of the characteristic present, whether or not this pertains to objective ratios or phenomenological characteristics of the situation.

Hypotheses

H1: Persons who feel high anxiety in specific situations (i.c., tunnels) will significantly more frequently misperceive the characteristics of these situations, compared to (a) persons who are relatively free from anxiety in the same situations; and (b) compared to their own perceptual responses to neutral situations.

H2: In "phobogenic" situations (i.c., tunnels), certain levels, intensities, or ratios of stimulation are more effective than others in inducing misperception. Specifically, high levels, intensities, or ratios of stimulation yield more misperception of these than low levels, intensities or ratios. Furthermore, these (high) stimulative effects combine or interact to intensify or strengthen negative feelings to these situations.

H0: Perceptual effects are nil (or misperception equal) whether or not differences exist in anxiety level of the person, or in characteristics of the situation.

Pilot Studies

Having made a choice to investigate eventual differences between phobics and normals on the accuracy of their perception of variables of architectural spaces (i.c., tunnels), we started with those characteristics which had been found in the first study to have significant effect in eliciting feelings of unpleasure, namely, height-distance and breadth-distance ratios associated with feelings of (strong) funneling, presence or absence of people or vehicles associated with busyness or quiet, and illumination ratios associated with darkness, dismalness or sombreness. Three pilot studies were carried out to resolve problems of instruction, and construction of stimuli. Two of these, because of their relevance to the main study, are briefly described.

In the first study we wished to determine whether the judgments of people differ greatly when they are asked to judge the objective relations in a situation (e.g., estimate the ratios between height, breadth and depth of a space) and when asked to judge phenomenological or perceptual experiences of these objective relations. We were of course aware of the work of Thurstone (1959) and others in this field; but for our purposes (investigation of phobic perception) we needed to know just how much these might deviate, and to try out the task and the instructions for use with phobic patients.

Although we did not expect phobics, compared to normals, to misperceive the objective ratios of stimulation more than normals, we expected that their phenomenological experiences of these might well differ from normals. Also, we wished to ascertain how reliable their estimates of objective ratios and judgments of subjective experiences of these ratios might be; and how they might relate.

Eighteen psychology students compared different examples of two types of tunnels (namely pedestrian and bicycle tunnels) on a paired comparison task. Judgments were elicited several weeks apart under the different instruction conditions. In the first session they were told what would be expected of them, about the different ways of perceiving (judging) aspects of a situation (i.e., focusing on the objective or on the phenomenal characteristics of situations), and asked to judge the stimuli according to which had more of a given characteristic. The phenomenological aspect was first judged, and a week later estimates were made of the objective characteristics (by paired comparison).

In the phenomenological-instruction the subject was asked to judge the stimuli on the basis of "the feeling or impression of being sucked through the shaft of the tunnel, pressed down by the roof or ceiling, and/or feeling or impression of being enclosed in the spaces". This was dubbed the "funneling effect". In the physical-instruction condition the subject was ask to attend exclusively to the physical parameters of the tunnel, namely the length, height, breadth (or narrowing) of the tunnel, and estimate which of the two tunnels had higher/lower ratios of height to distance (H/D) and breadth to distance (B/D).

In both conditions the subject was asked only to respond with the indication: (the one on the) "left" or "right". The standard (level 3) and the comparison stimulus were viewed *simultaneously*, *side-by-side*. The stimuli were presented in random and counterbalanced order, to minimize order and location effects. Each subject was given eight trials for each comparison of the different levels of "funneling" or H/B/D ratios. Four levels were distinguished, so that six comparisons were made by each subject. In all 864 comparisons were made for each type of tunnel and for each instruction condition (or a total of 144 judgments per type tunnel, per type instruction, per comparison).

Since the breadths of pedestrian and bicycle tunnels do not differ as much as in car tunnels, in order to obtain noticeable differences of "funneling", this variable was manipulated by photographing the tunnel with different camera lens sizes. Using the lens sizes 135 mm, 105 mm, 50 mm and 35 mm, the funneling effect was manipulated. No or little funneling corresponded to lens size 135, moderate funneling to lens size 105, much funneling to lens size 50, and very much funneling to lens size 35 mm. Photographing the tunnel with a lens size of 135 mm gave the impression of a "high, broad, short tunnel" (little or no funneling effect); and a lens size of 35 mm gave the impression of a "low, narrow, long tunnel" (very much effect). Table 5.2.1 shows the mean percentages and z-scores for each paired comparison on the measures "funneling effect" (phenomenological instruction), and estimates of H/B/D ratios (physical dimension instruction) for bicycle and pedestrian tunnels. Figure 5.1 shows the relation between height-breadth-distance ratios, "funneling" and discrimination ("hits"), H/B/D ratio (and funneling) as a function of lens size.

The results show that estimates of objective ratios and judgments of phenomenal experience of these (i.e., "funneling effect" of H/B/D ratios) are functionally and linearly related ($rxy = .90$ for bicycle tunnels and $rxy = .91$ for pedestrian subways).

Table 5.2.1 shows that on all comparisons the physical-dimension-instruction yielded slightly higher percentages correctly than the phenomenological-instruction.

Table 5.2.1 Mean percentages and z-scores for each paired comparison on the measures "funneling effect" (phenomenological instruction) and estimation of H/B/D ratios (physical dimension instruction) for bicycle and pedestrian tunnels. (Each comparison is based on 144 observations)

Mean values

		phenomenological instruction				physical dimension instruction			
stimulus pair	lens size in mm.	% hits bicycle	z-score	% hits pedestrian	z-score	% hits bicycle	z-score	% hits pedestrian	z-score
1–2	35–135	87.4	1.15	84.7	1.02	91.0	1.34	92.6	1.45
1–3	35–105	78.4	.78	90.0	1.29	88.2	1.19	91.2	1.35
1–4	35–50	50.6	.01	77.0	.74	41.9	–.21	77.0	.74
2–3	135–105	60.4	.26	36.8	–.34	79.5	.82	60.0	.26
2–4	135–50	85.4	1.05	61.1	.28	94.9	1.64	86.0	1.08
3–4	105–50	88.1	1.18	87.5	1.15	95.6	1.71	90.0	1.29

Overall means: Bicycle tunnels					Pedestrian tunnels			
stimulus	s1	s2	(s3)	s4	s1	s2	(s3)	s4
phenom. instr.:	.65	1.18	–	.65	–.03	1.15	–	.99
physical instr.:	1.23	1.71	–	.77	.67	1.29	–	1.18

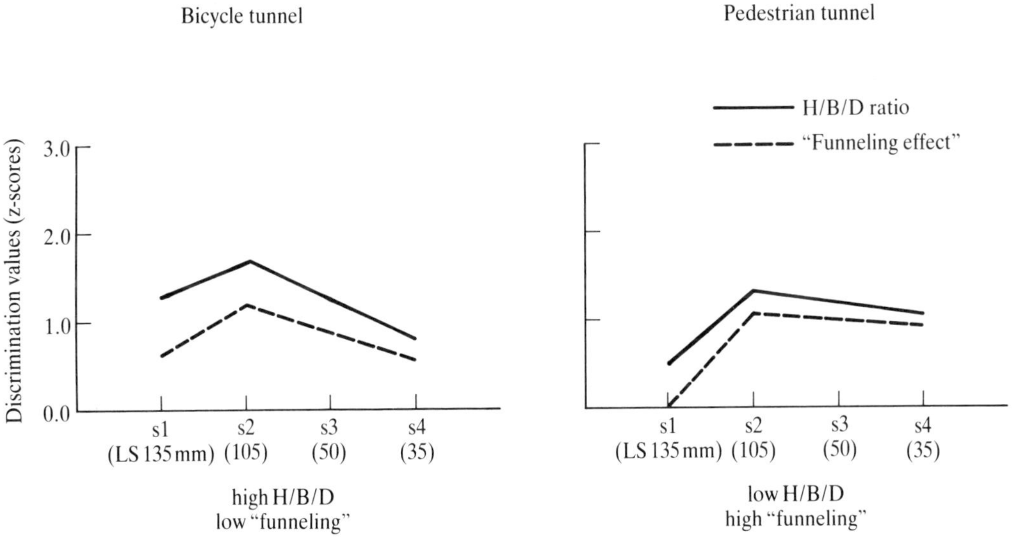

Figure 5.1 Relation between H/B/D ratio, "funneling effect" and discrimination (normal subjects)

The high correlations between responses under both conditions suggest that subjects are indeed basing their responses on certain structural components common to both perceptual responses. Figure 5.1 shows that for these normal subjects H/B/D ratios and the "funneling effect" are better discriminated when the H/B/D ratios are neither low nor high, but moderately high, and the levels of funneling also moderately high.

The next problem was to find a satisfactory criterion for judging whether responses to varying illumination ratios were "correct" or not, or even possible on the basis of "feelings of sombreness, dismalness or darkness" that these elicit.

In this pilot study we presented two groups of 18 and 26 psychology students with tunnel stimuli in which the overall luminance levels had been manipulated by the photographer and ranked by him from "dark" to "light". It concerned eight examples of the same bicycle tunnel. In individual sessions, the students were asked to rank order these stimuli on the basis of the feelings of "sombreness, dismalness or darkness" which these stimuli elicited. This was done by paired comparison, each pair being judged by each individual eight times. In the second group, and to facilitate the task, which proved not at all easy to do, the stimuli were presented in overlapping subsets (log.lux units 1.5; 2; 2.5). Even these results deviated so much from the ranking of the photographer ($r = .12$), highly differing pairs not always yielding better discrimination of this experiential variable, as related to luminance levels, that we could not assume a linear relationship with the phenomenal experience of these. These were puzzling results, for it was not clear whether they were task-dependent or stimulus-dependent. (Of course, before projecting the stimuli onto a screen, the subject had been given time to dark-adapt.) Before giving up on this variable, we decided to make one more attempt, by asking the experimental and control groups in the main experiment to discriminate between the stimuli on the same basis (i.e., "Which gives rise to stronger feelings of sombreness, dismalness, or darkness"?). Here, too, each subject was given the paired-comparison task after the eyes were dark-adapted.

A much higher agreement was found between their rankings of the stimuli on this basis, and the ranking of the photographer on the basis of overall luminance levels (tunnelphobics: $r = .90$; other phobics: $r = .62$; normals: $r = .86$). The concordance between the groups was also high ($W = .82$). Since the task proved possible for these subjects, once again we tried to obtain a criterion for measuring "accuracy of response" to the variable, by asking a new, but smaller group of normal subjects ($n = 5$) to rank the stimuli on the same basis, and by the same procedure. These rankings accorded well with that of the photographer, ranked on the basis of overall luminance levels, and so were used in the main study as a criterion. These normals did not take part in the experiment.

In the third pilot study it proved an easy task to relate feelings of "busyness or crowdedness" to the number of persons or vehicles in a tunnel, so we will leave these findings unreported, and turn now to the main study.

Aims of the Main Study

As one may recall, our aim was to find out if (tunnel)phobics misperceive phenomenal characteristics of feared situations more than normals do, and more than they misperceive phenomenal characteristics of neutral situations. Also, to determine whether this misperception is a function of levels or ratios of stimulation of structural components in the situations with which certain phenomenal experiences are associated; or whether this is due to anxiety level and/or specific meaning that a feared situation may have for the phobic.

To investigate this perceptual behaviour, a design was used in which responses in different classes of situations (tunnels, and tunnel-like situations), to the different experiential variables could be compared. As a control of the effect of anxiety level on this perceptual behaviour, a normal control group was included, as well as a phobic control group, for the relevance of the complaint to their eventual (mis)perceptions of these variables.

The investigation was carried out in two stages. In the first stage anxiety hierarchies for tunnels were obtained individually from all those participating in the experiment, using a paired-comparison task. In the second stage, a few weeks later, subjects judged phenomenal aspects of the stimuli in different classes of situations, using the method of constant stimulus differences. Except on "darkness", the standard was always at level 3 within a series.

Subjects

The *experimental* group consisted of five tunnelphobic patients, all women between the ages of 28–50 years (mean age: 37 yrs). Two of these women suffered from tunnelphobia as main complaint, and three others as a subsidiary complaint, their main complaints being claustrophobia, phobia for swallowing, and phobia for water. The *control* groups consisted of one group of five phobic patients who had no fear of tunnel situations, and one group of five normal women who had no known phobias. The phobic control group, four women and one man, was a little younger than the tunnelphobic group, aged 25–28 years (mean age: 25.8 yrs.). Two women suffered from social phobia as their main complaint, one woman from a fear of death or disease, another woman from phobia for snakes, and the man from a fear of injections.

The normal control group consisted of five women between the ages of 24–50 years (mean age: 32.4 yrs). Four women were departmental secretaries at the laboratory, and the fifth was a housewife (the mother of one of the experimenters).

To avoid the knotty problem of finding an objective criterion for measuring anxiety, the groups were chosen on the basis of the available clinical information. However, we decided to check the anxiety levels for the relevant tunnel stimuli by asking all participants to rate the tunnel stimuli on the basis of anxiety felt in those situations.

Stimuli

Forty-eight stimuli were used, specially prepared slides of three different classes of situations: 16 tunnel stimuli, 8 of car tunnels, 4 of bicycle tunnels and 4 of pedestrian subways; 16 stimuli of corridors (in the laboratory); and 16 stimuli of street lanes lined with trees on both sides, with overhanging boughs. In each of these situations three objective characteristics, that is, the height-breadth-distance (depth) ratios, illumination ratios (overall luminance levels), and numbers of people or vehicles, were varied at four levels, which corresponded to low, moderate, high and extremely high levels.

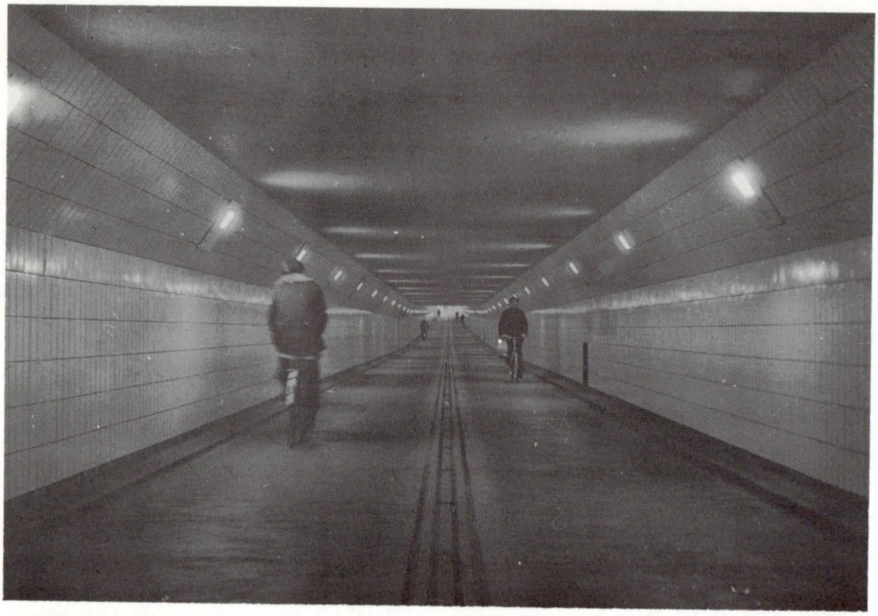

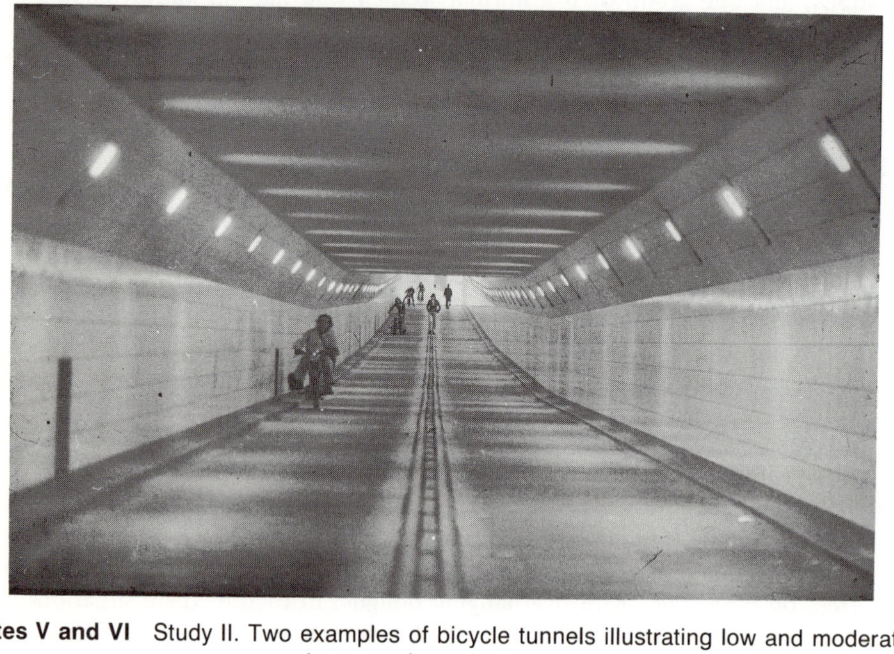

Plates V and VI Study II. Two examples of bicycle tunnels illustrating low and moderate busyness/crowdedness.

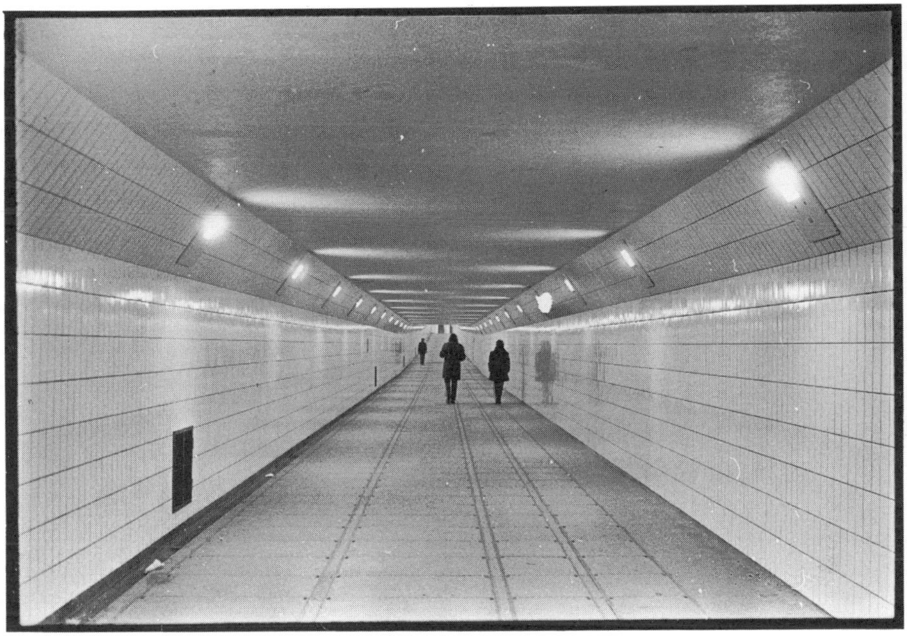

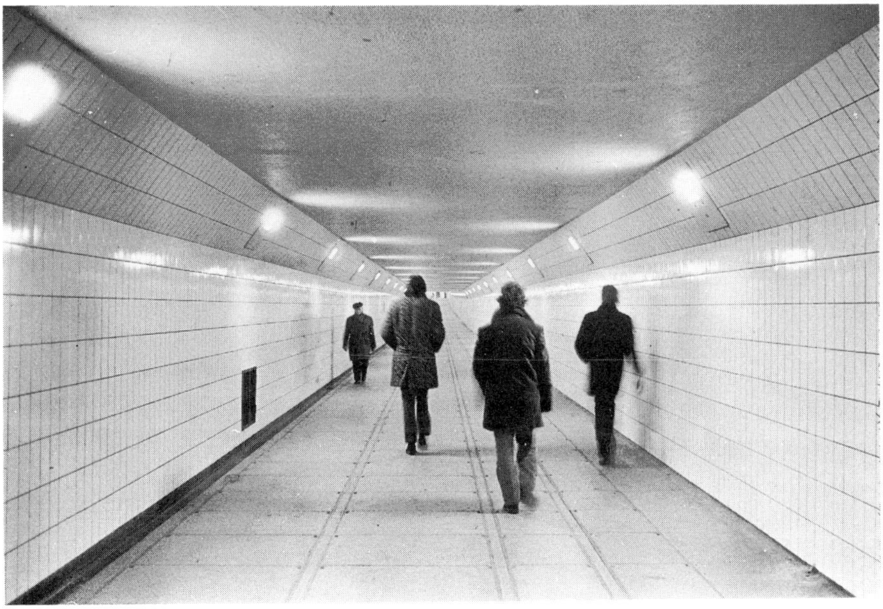

Plates VII and VIII Study II. Two examples of pedestrian tunnels illustrating high (standard stimulus) and very high busyness/crowdedness.

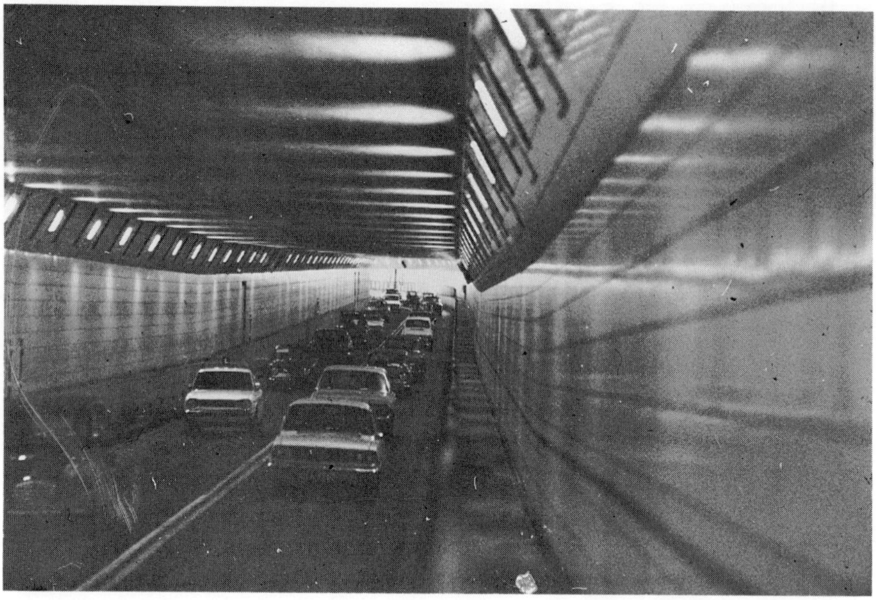

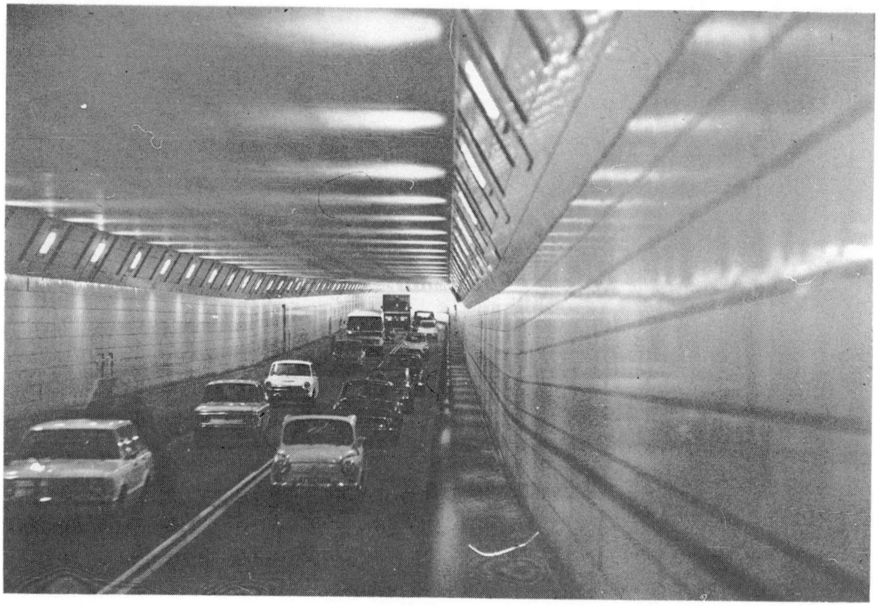

Plates IX and X Study II. Two examples of car tunnels illustrating low and moderate funneling effect.

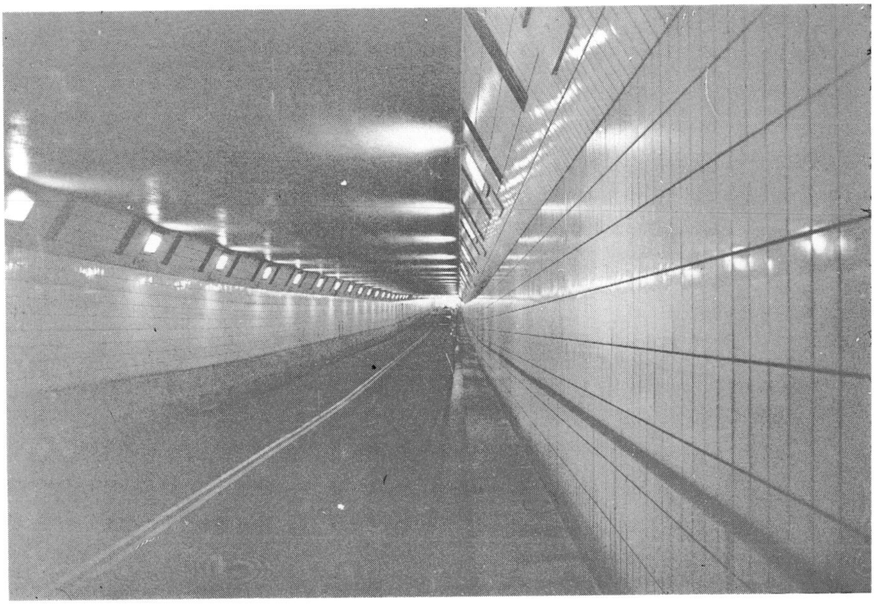

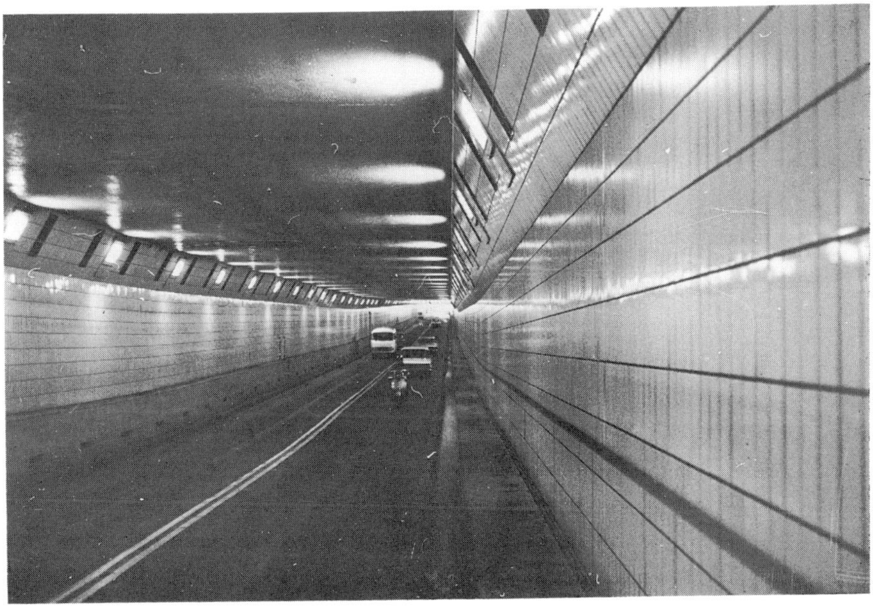

Plates XI and XII Study II. Two examples of car tunnels illustrating high (standard stimulus) and very high funneling effect.

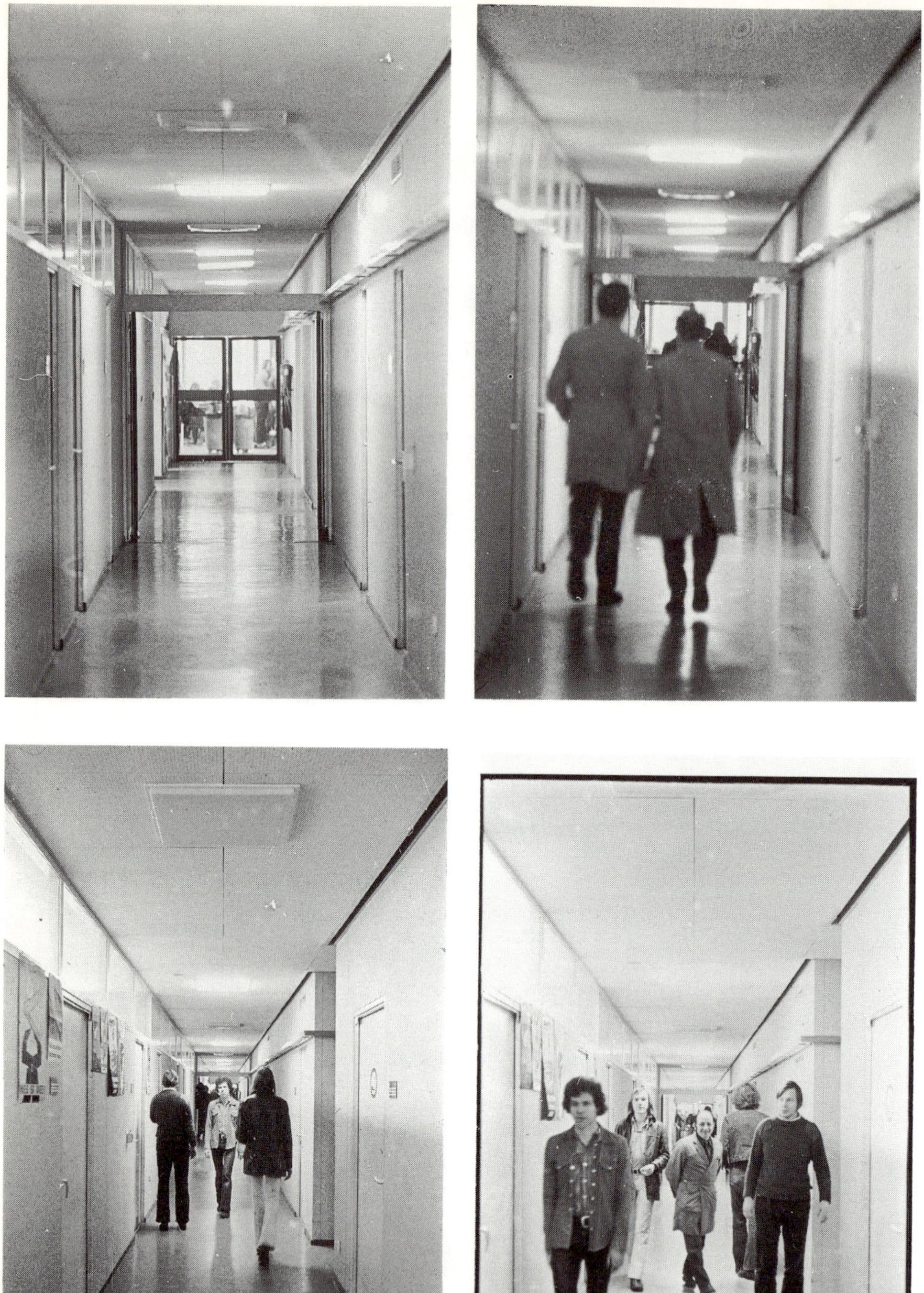

Plates XIII Study II. Four examples of corridors illustrating low, moderate, high and very high busyness/crowdedness. Bottom left (high) is standard stimulus.

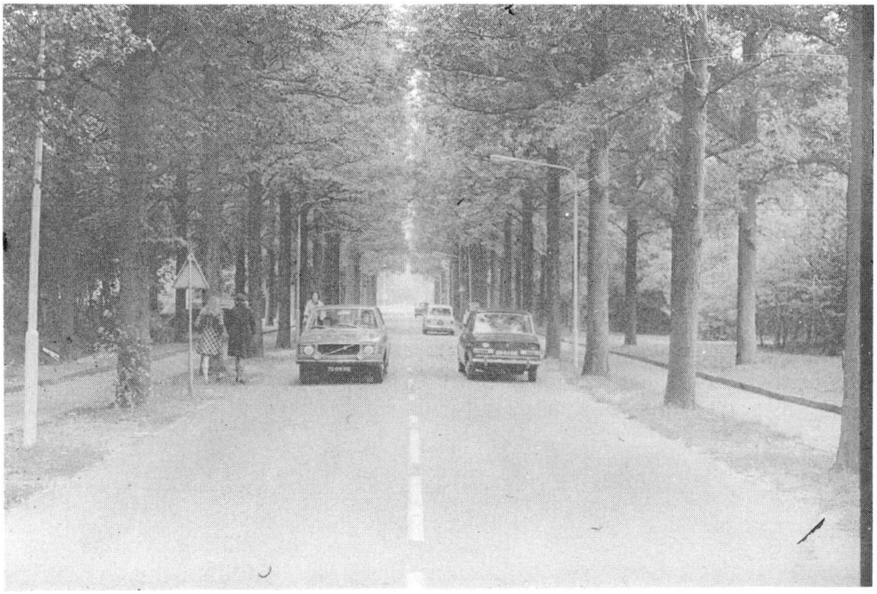

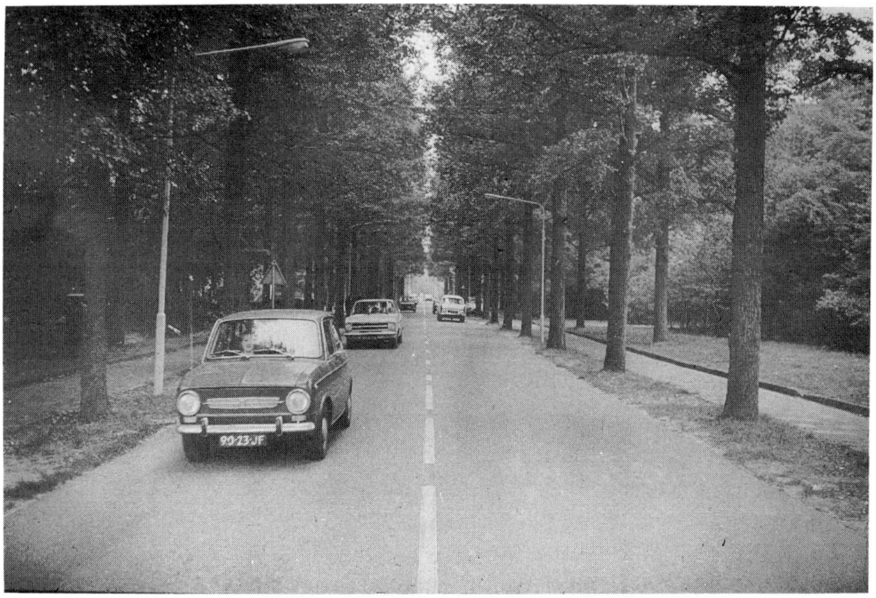

Plates XIV and XV Study II. Two examples of street lanes illustrating low (top) and moderate darkness/dismalness/sombreness.

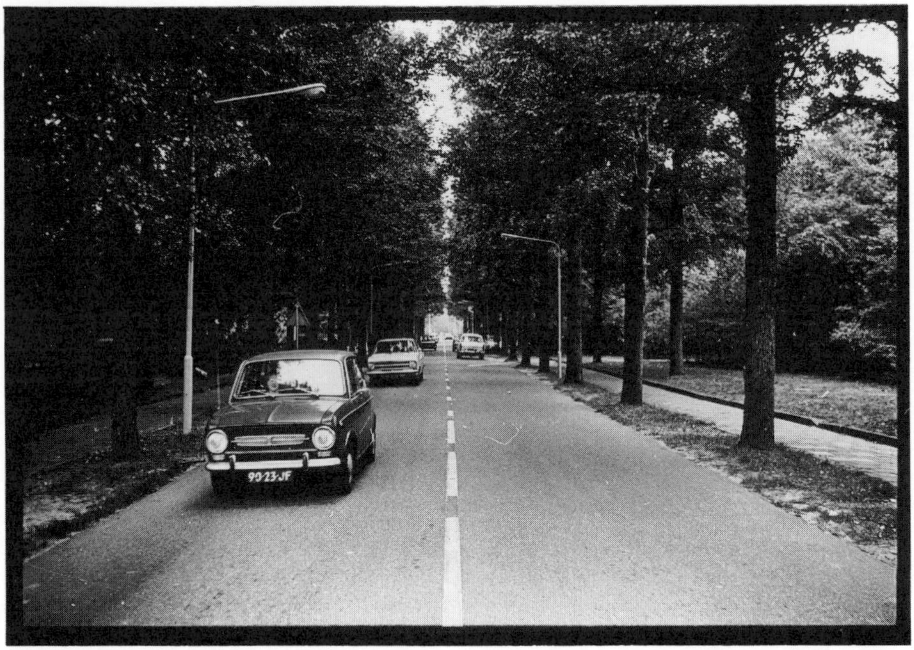

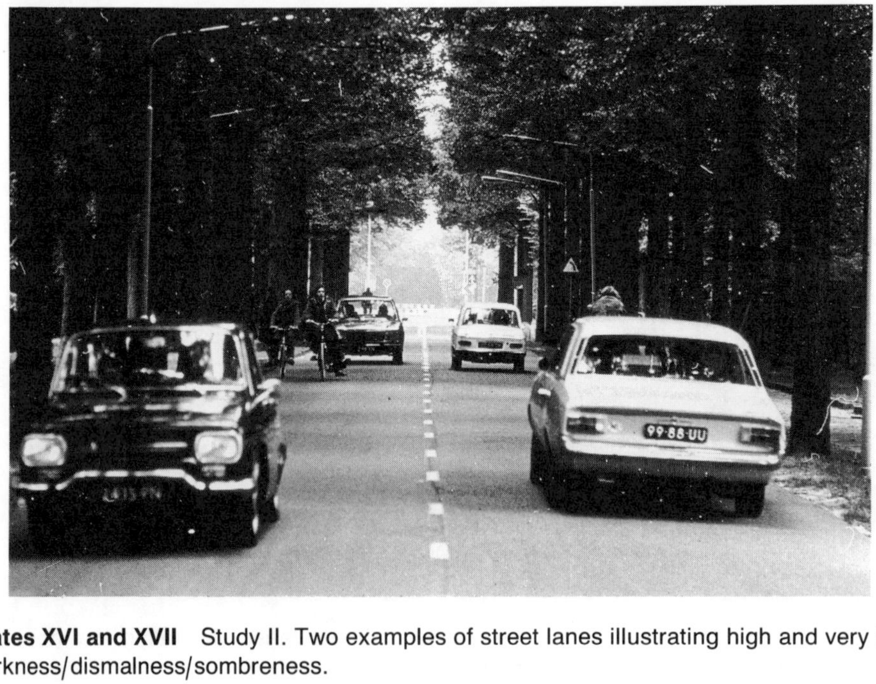

Plates XVI and XVII Study II. Two examples of street lanes illustrating high and very high darkness/dismalness/sombreness.

In real-life situations, for example in tunnels, it is difficult to separate B/D ratios and H/D ratios and manipulate these independently (of the type of tunnel) since the type of tunnel determines the relation of B/D ratio to H/D ratio. For instance, pedestrian subways are generally narrower and shorter than bicycle or car tunnels. Because of the difficulties in manipulating these ratios so as to control the "funneling effect", we decided to do this by photographing the different scenes at different points (i.e., at the beginning, middle and end of the tunnel), using four different camera lenses (i.e., of 135, 105, 50 and 35 mm). See the first pilot study for the procedure and results of this manipulation.

Overall luminance levels were determined by the photographer, and the stimuli were selected on his instructions and classified accordingly in four levels of illumination, ranging from dark to light. The number of persons and vehicles was varied at four levels: none or one; two to three; four to six; and eight or more. The function of this pilot study was to determine these levels and relate them to feelings of busyness or crowdedness in these situations. Within each series, one variable was manipulated while keeping the other two constant (that is, varying the number of people while holding H/B/D ratios and overall luminance levels constant); but between series the levels of the variables held constant within series, were varied. This necessarily yielded incomplete series. The comparison tasks, for patients, would not have been feasible (that is, would have been an extremely onerous task) if, having systematically varied all levels of all the variables in these stimuli while keeping the other variables constant, all of the stimuli were then compared. The tunnel stimuli used in the ratings of anxiety, in the first stage, consisted of 16 stimuli, 8 car tunnels and 8 bicycle and pedestrian tunnels (four of each kind). The levels of "funneling", "darkness" and "busyness/crowdedness" present were varied, but not in any systematic way, since this would not have made the ranking task feasible.

Apparatus and Procedure

The subject was seated at about two metres from an opaque screen, in a dark, soundproof room. Placed on a table behind the subject were two slide projectors, with a timing device set at 5 seconds (for simultaneous projection of two stimuli). In each session the subject was given sufficient time to ensure dark-adaptation of the eyes before the task began. Oral instructions were always followed by five practice trials. Stimuli were presented in blocks of trials, randomized and counterbalanced to minimize order and location effects, and with short breaks between blocks of trials to lessen fatigue or boredom with the task. Each level of a given variable was judged eight times by each subject, by means of paired comparisons in stage One (to determine the anxiety hierarchy), and by the method of constant stimulus differences in stage Two (namely, the discrimination tasks). Instructions were kept simple. The person was asked to choose between the two projected stimuli, designating her choice by saying only "left" or "right", to indicate which stimulus induced a stronger impression or feeling. In this way we hoped to eradicate bias in response. In stage One, the subject was simply asked: "Which of the two scenes before you induces stronger feelings of anxiety"? In stage Two, and according to the characteristic being judged, the instructions were: "Which of the two scenes before you induces stronger feelings of: being sucked through the shaft of the space or pressed down by the ceiling, or a combination of these feelings (the so-called funneling effect); or: feelings of busyness or crowdedness; or: feelings of sombreness, dismalness or darkness, or a combination of these?". Since the pilot study had shown that the phenomenal experiences that are associated with objective characteristics could be judged as reliably as estimations of objective ratios of stimulation, and since we expected the phenomenal experiences to be more relevant to the phobic complaint, and thus more susceptible to distortion or misperception, only judgments of phenomenal characteristics were made.

Data Analyses

The raw data from the discrimination tasks were first converted into z-scores.Then three-factor analyses of variance with repeated measures (subjects nested under the factor group; see Winer, 1970) were carried out on these data for all classes of situations, and for the three variables in each class. Anxiety ratings were determined by transforming the cumulative frequencies per group into z-scores. Intercorrelations between discrimination of the three experiential characteristics of tunnels and anxiety ratings were calculated.

Results

Three-factor analyses of variance (with repeated measures) show no difference in perceptual behaviour between groups, neither for the different types of tunnels nor for the neutral (control) situations, that is, corridors and street lanes. A nearly significant *main effect* for groups is found only for the variable related to the "funneling effect" in car tunnels and corridors (F: 3.60, df.: 2/12, $p = .06$; F: 3.66, df.: 2/12, $p = .06$).

A glance at Figure 5.2, plotted on the basis of these data, shows that, in contrast to normals, tunnelphobics and other phobics tend to discriminate better between subjective funneling characteristics of the ratios of stimulation present; but since this does not reach significance, the related null hypothesis may not be rejected.

In *all classes of situations significant main effects* are found for the three variables. For the variable relating to the "funneling effect" by H/B/D ratios, significant main effects are found (pedestrian subways and bicycle tunnels: F: 18.37, df: 2/24, $p = .01$; car tunnels: F: 29.07, df: 2/24, $p < .01$; corridors: F: 36.76, df.: 2/24, $p = .01$; street lanes: F: 26.70, df.: 2/24, $p = .01$).

For the variable relating to "busyness or crowdedness" induced by the presence of people or vehicles, significant *main effects* are found (pedestrian subways and bicycle tunnels: F: 5.71, df.: 2/24, $p = .01$; car tunnels: F: 22.29, df: 2/24, $p < .01$; corridors: F: 32.14, df: 2/24, $p < .01$; street lanes: F: 40.82, df: 2/24, $p < .01$).

For the variable relating to "sombreness, dismalness or darkness" induced by illumination ratios, significant *main effects* are also found (pedestrian and bicycle tunnels: F: 5.49, df: 3/36, $p < .01$; car tunnels: F: 9.01, df: 3/36, $p < .01$; corridors: F: 6.11, df: 3/36, $p < .01$; street lanes: F: 5.96, df: 3/36, $p < .01$).

Significant *interactions* are found between the three variables in two classes of situations, pedestrian tunnels and bicycle tunnels, and in corridors. Only in car tunnels and in street lanes does the variable "busyness or crowdedness" not interact with other variables. A significant interaction is found between the variable "busyness or

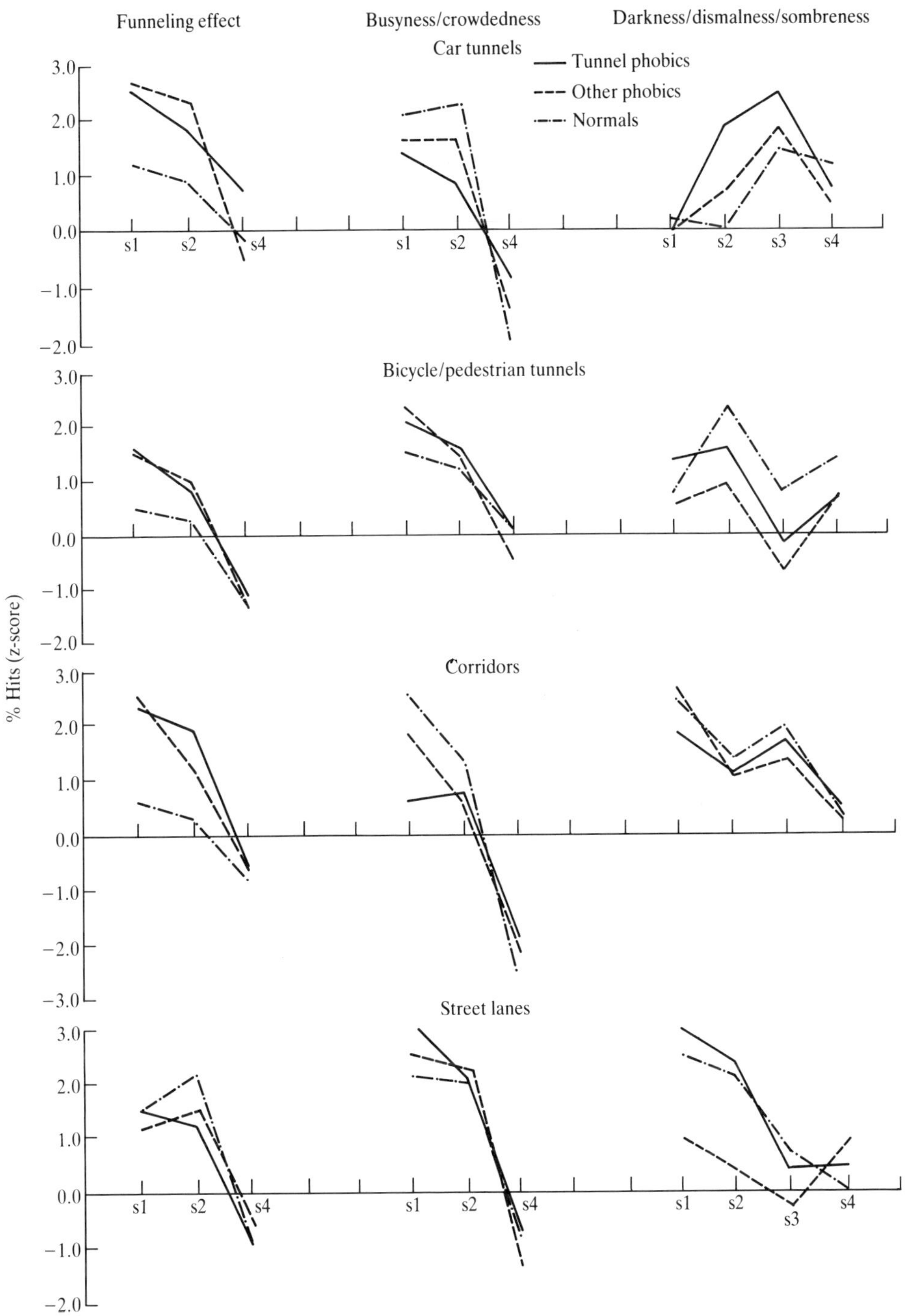

Figure 5.2 Relations between experiential variables and discrimination (Study II)

crowdedness" and groups in corridors, and between "funneling effect" and groups in car tunnels (F: 2.06, df: 6/72, p = .03; F: 2.18, df: 6/72, p = .02, respectively).

Figure 5.2 depicts these relations. For all these classes of situations and for all groups, discrimination of the phenomenal experiences associated with H/B/D ratios, and with number of people or vehicles, depends on the levels or ratios of stimulation present in the situations. Trend analyses show that for the "funneling effect" in all classes of situations the relation is mainly linear, with a small but significant quadratic component (Car tunnels: Flin.R: 126.08, df.: 1/176, p = .001; Fquad.: 15.05, df.: 1/176, p = .001; Pedestrian-bicycle tunnels: Flin.: 99.05; Fquad.: 12.12, df.: 1/176, p = .001; Corridors: Flin.: 103.71; Fquad.: 15.05, df.: 1/176, p = .001; Street lanes: Flin: 137.41; Fquad.: 71.73, df.: 1/176, p = .001). Trend analyses show a similar relation for the variable "busyness", a mainly linear one with a small but significant quadratic component (Car tunnels: Flin.: 217.76; Fquad.: F 65.25, df.: 1/176, p = .001; P/B tunnels: Flin.: 73.20; Fquad.: 7.07, df.: 1/176, p = .001; Corridors: Flin.: 338.09; Fquad.: 37.94, df.: 1/176, p = .001; Street lanes: F: 279.05; Fquad.: 53.78, df.: 1/176, p = .001).

For the variable "darkness etc.", trend analyses show that the relation is quadratic and linear in car tunnels (Fquad.: 16.22; Flin.: 11.11, df.: 1/176, p = .001); in pedestrian subways and bicycle tunnels, the relation is non-linear (quartic) (F: 11.95, df. 1/176, p = .001). All other relations are not significant (F < 1). But in corridors and street lanes the relation between "darkness, etc.," and discrimination is only linear (Corridors: F: 29.75, df.: 1/176, p < .001; street lanes: F 36.41, df.: 1/176, p < .001). All other relations are not significant (F < 1).

On the basis of these results there appears to be some support for the part of the hypothesis that relates misperception, as defined, to ratios of stimulation (of the experiential variables), but these errors are not tied in to the phobic complaint.

All groups, regardless of anxiety level or nature of phobic complaint, show the same trends. As a rule, high levels of these experiential variables are more often misperceived (show error in judgment) than lower levels. Also, the effects of these variables do seem to combine or interact in such a way as to intensify their effects. "Busyness" in car tunnels, and in street lanes forms the only exception.

Anxiety Ratings of Tunnels and Discrimination

Because we wished to make sure that the (tunnel) stimuli were indeed anxiety-evoking for the tunnelphobic subjects, we asked both the experimental group and the control groups to rank these sixteen tunnel stimuli (by paired comparisons) on the basis of the degree of anxiety or unpleasure felt in these situations. The stimuli were the same that were used in the main study. All tunnelphobics, in their protocols, professed to feel high anxiety in some of these situations. The other phobics and the normal subjects expressed feelings of apprehension in some tunnels, but said that no anxiety was felt in these situations; although some were more displeasing than others. But, as the coefficients of concordance within the groups illustrate, the different individual rankings deviated much (tunnelphobics: W = .334; other phobics: W = .315; normals: W = .185). The concordance between groups was also not high (W = .376).

Examining the individual profiles of "anxiety", it appeared that between groups certain individuals showed more similarity in their negative preferences than within the groups. That is, certain individuals rated pedestrian subways as highest in the hierarchy of anxiety, others rated car tunnels as highest, and still others bicycle tunnels as highest. On the basis of these preferences, we rearranged the groups.

Group I (Pedestrian subways: highest rating on anxiety) consisted of three tunnelphobics, one social phobic, and two normal persons.

Group II (Bicycle tunnels: highest rating on anxiety) consisted of one tunnelphobic, one snake-phobic, one phobic with a fear of injections, and one normal person.

Group III (Car tunnels: highest rating on anxiety) consisted of one tunnelphobic, one social phobic, one phobic with a fear of death and disease, and two normals.

Their concordances are now of course higher (WI: .631; WII: .769; WIII: .614). The intercorrelations between anxiety ratings of these tunnels and the mean (z-)scores for the groups, per experiential variable in these tunnels on the discrimination tasks show that there is either little relation between discrimination of their effects and anxiety or, if there is, the relation is not linear (see Table 5.2.2).

Discussion and Interim Conclusion

While pondering these results which, in spite of our efforts, had yielded mainly the assurance that phobics do not differ from normals in their perception of the experiential variables of objective ratios of stimulation, that is, in the degree to which they misperceive these, the unhappy thought occurred to me that all these results might be explained by Weber's law; in which case the time and effort spent had only gone into "re-inventing the wheel". But there is one argument against. The proportionality law (Weber's constant) is only valid when stimuli (comparison and standard) are presented *non-simultaneously* as was reported by Weber (1849). The variability of judgments, a very old psychophysical problem, was first attacked by Weber, who determined the just-noticeable-difference (jnd) in size between a standard and a comparison line of various absolute length. Weber summarized his results by his famous law, which states that the jnd is a constant proportion of the stimulus

Table 5.2.2 Intercorrelations between discrimination of three experiential characteristics of tunnels and anxiety

experiential variable	TP	OP	N	I	II	III**	type of tunnel
	anxiety			anxiety			
anxiety	1.00	1.00	1.00	1.00	1.00	1.00	
"funneling"	.23	.10	−.03	.22	.46	−.12	Pedestrian/
"busyness"	.04	.10	.06	−.79	.96*	−.13	Bicycle tunnel
"darkness"	−.01	.04	−.15	.10	−.33	−.10	
anxiety	1.00	1.00	1.00	1.00	1.00	1.00	
"funneling"	−.45	.24	−.08	−.73	−.23	.13	Car tunnel
"busyness"	−.002	−.11	−.04	.37	.36	−.02	
"darkness"	−.37	−.56	−.08	−.55	.01	−.36	

* significant at $p < .02$
** I, II and III = rearranged groups
TP = tunnelphobics; OP = other phobics; N = normals

magnitude. In size and length estimation tasks, the jnd for simultaneous viewing was extremely small (about 2% of the standard size). Baird (1970), in noting this, points out that other researchers (e.g., Miller, 1947) have confirmed this, in showing that under simultaneous viewing the error (jnd) was in most cases less than 5% of the standard (size).

In most cases in our experiments, error in judgment on "funneling effect", and "busyness/crowdedness" was much higher than 5% for the highest level represented (level 4) in the different situations. The error is most striking on the variable "busyness/crowdedness" (see Figure 5.2). Especially in the latter case, Weber's law would not seem to be the appropriate explanation for the sharp drop in discrimination, for all groups. Of course, when ratios of stimulation are high, any added constant has much less effect than when ratios of stimulation are low. And this might explain the drop in discrimination on the variables "funneling effect", and "darkness": an added constant, especially when small, will not be discerned. In this case, judges might switch to a strategy of guessing. But chance guessing would yield a score of zero in this case (z-score for the chance probability of 0.50). But, for the variable "busyness or crowdedness" in car tunnels, corridors and street lanes, the error in judgment of level 4 ranges between 70% and 95%. In other words, the subjects are in fact saying that when these situations contain four to six persons or vehicles, they elicit a stronger feeling of "busyness or crowdedness" than when these contain eight or more persons or vehicles! (The range lay between "none, to eight or more"). The explanation for this behaviour must, I think, be sought elsewhere. Part of this "elsewhere" forms the subject of the next investigation, part will become clear when we look more closely at individual perceptual strategies in chapter VI. So, for the moment, we leave things a bit "up in the air", and move on to the next link in the chain.

Height/Distance Ratio as a Predictor of Perceived Openness-enclosure of Space and Emotional Responses in Normal and Phobic Subjects (Study III)

Before we undertook this study, we consulted the psychological literature on space perception to find out what is known about responses of normal and clinical groups to physical dimensions of architectural spaces. In the rising discipline of environmental psychology, the work of Spreiregen (1965), Gärling (1969), Hesselgren (1971) and Hayward & Franklin (1974) seemed particularly relevant. These researchers consider the variable of perceived openness-enclosure of space to be a crucial one in the experiences of normals to architectural spaces. But they disagree on which physical variables are the best predictors of perceived openness-enclosure. Gärling's hypothesis (for which he found support) is that this variable is best predicted by size (area) of space, and in such a way that the smaller the size, the stronger the experience of enclosure. Spreiregen, as also Hayward & Franklin, hypothesized that perceived enclosure is best predicted by the ratio of boundary wall height to wall distance (H/D ratio), and they too found support for their hypothesis.

In our previous explorations with phobic patients (and a few normals) spatial variables had not been satisfactorily manipulated, in our view, because of the difficulties involved in doing so by means of photographs or slides made from photos of these environmental spaces. Although it seemed that the ratio of breadth to distance (B/D ratio) was as significant as H/D ratio in eliciting feelings of anxiety, unpleasure, funneling, suffocation, and so on, neither these ratios, nor size of the spaces, had been systematically varied. Hayward & Franklin's approach seemed to be a better way of clarifying the relations between physical and experiential variables of space.

Using perspective drawings of outdoor architectural spaces viewed under monocular conditions by university undergraduate students, they found that the ratio of boundary wall to wall distance (H/D ratio) was the main determinant of perceived openness-enclosure. Though size of space had a slight effect on perceived openness-enclosure, the effect was not powerful enough to produce statistical significance. Other variables such as the retinal angle subtended by the back wall, and the inclusive retinal angle of the back wall and floor, were also highly correlated with the ratings of openness-enclosure (resp., $r = .96$ and $.95$). They reasoned that since the H/D ratio expresses a relation of object (back wall) size and distance, and is therefore also positively related to retinal angle size, these correlates and the H/D ratio are but different indices of the same variable. We agree with this. The H/D ratio is a physical variable closely related to other physical variables and the choice of H/D ratio is therefore somewhat arbitrary. The size of the retinal angle subtended by an object is determined by the relation of the object's size and its physical distance. Therefore the first covariable of H/D ratio (height of back wall) is a determinant of a second covariable (retinal angle subtended by back wall), the latter being a part of a third covariable (inclusive retinal angle). It is only for reasons of technical convenience that we decided to use the H/D ratio as our independent variable instead of, for instance, retinal angle size with which the H/D ratio is closely related. If the confounding of descriptive variables indicating the same spatial phenomenon is not damaging to the purpose of our investigation, a source of confounding of another kind might be more serious. To illustrate what we have in mind: Hayward & Franklin varied the H/D ratio as well as the size of the area of space by enlarging the scale of the perspective drawings that represents these spaces, for every (given) level of the variable, H/D ratio. The scale of a perspective drawing of a given space can be varied by manipulating the texture gradient of the drawing (see Figures 5.3.1a and b for examples of this), thereby allowing the experimenter to change the perceived size of the area of space while holding the H/D ratio constant. When one manipulates scale in this way it not only leads to variation of perceived size of space but *also* to variation of perceived spatial volume; which implies that perceived size (area) and perceived volume cannot be experimentally isolated if one decides to hold H/D ratio constant. This is in this context not an urgent problem, since we will not try to manipulate size *and* volume; but it does mean that one should bear this in mind in the interpretation of the effect of perceived size of space on perceived openness-enclosure and other criterion variables. We turn now to our experiments with normal subjects and phobic patients.

Experiment 1 (Normal Subjects)

In this experiment we wished to test not only Hayward & Franklin's (1974) hypothesis that perceived openness-enclosure of architectural space is best predicted by the ratio of boundary wall height to wall distance (H/D ratio), but also the alternative hypothesis of Gärling (1969) that perceived openness-enclosure is best predicted by size (area) of space, and in such a way that the smaller the size, the stronger the experience of enclosure. We decided to do so under modified conditions. Instead of monocular viewing of perspective drawings of architectural spaces, binocular viewing of slides of perspective drawings of these spaces was introduced. Since Gärling (1970) found that such representations of space yielded similar judgments to those obtained from in situ stimuli, this method was chosen. Because we were unable to determine whether or not the subjects in Hayward & Franklin's experiment had actually been able to discriminate between the differences in size of spaces, a matter which might have influenced their results adversely, we decided to vary the size of space in two ways, that is, by varying the width (breadth) of the space as well as the scale. Magnitude estimates of the sizes of these spaces were then obtained in a procedure identical to the one used by Gärling.

Since we not only wished to test these hypotheses, but also with an eye to comparing the responses of normals to those of phobic patients on this variable and on other experiential variables, to ascertain if, and to what extent perceived openness-enclosure is related to hedonic feelings, ratings of a number of experiential variables that reflect the hedonic quality of space were also obtained.

Method

Subjects

Twenty-two undergraduates, psychology students, served as subjects. All participated in the experiment in fulfilment of part of a psychology course. Another group of 33 students also estimated the size of these spaces, in the same context, but their data are not included because of a slight deviation in the material used (objects were placed in the spaces).

Apparatus and Materials

Stimulus items consisted of two sets of 12 slides of perspective drawings of architectural spaces, each set depicting one of two breadths ($B/D = 1/2$; $B/D = 1$) related to distance (B/D: ratio of breadth of back wall to distance). Within each set, four slides depicted spaces which were 5 metres deep, four depicted spaces which were 10 metres deep, and four depicted spaces which were 20 metres deep (respectively, the five, ten, and twenty metre scales). The H/D ratio was varied in each scale at four levels, namely, $H/D = 1/4$; $2/4$; $3/4$ and $4/4$. A standard texture element was chosen (a square), which size became proportionally smaller as scale increased. All pictures were drawn as projections of real spaces from a normal observation height (1.75 m). To provide sufficient cues to depth and size, the floors and walls of all depicted spaces were gridded with perspective lines running parallel and perpendicular to surface edges. The resulting grid pattern covered all wall and floor surfaces with adjoining square texture elements. Figures 5.3.1a and b show examples of the perspective drawings that were used.

A slide projector attached to a tachistoscope that was adjusted to 10 seconds was used to project the stimuli onto a screen placed at a distance of 3.3 metres in front of

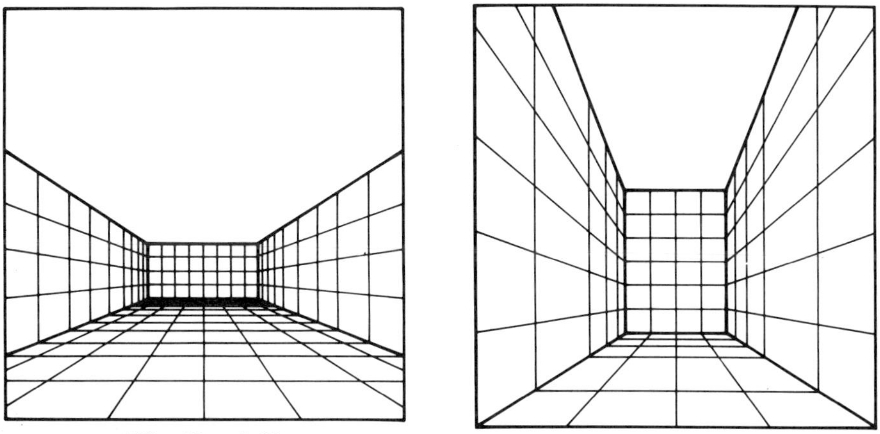

(a) H/D = .25; scale 20; B/D = .50

(b) H/D = 1.00; scale 10; B/D = .50

Figure 5.3.1 Two examples of the stimulus material

the seated subject. Five-point bipolar scales were used to obtain judgments of openness-enclosure and hedonic feelings.

Procedure

The subjects were randomly distributed over two groups of eleven persons, each group viewing one set of 12 slides, each slide within a set depicting one of two breadths. Each subject was allowed time to acquaint himself with the task in one trial session, using a slide of a perspective drawing of space that was not included in the experimental series. The subject was not shown all the depicted spaces beforehand.

The subject was first told in general terms of the reasons for our interest in the phenomenon, relating these to the needs of architects and psychologists to know more about human experiences in spatial environments. Then he was instructed how to use the bipolar rating scales to rate his responses to the following five variables: openness-enclosure, safety-unsafety, pleasure-unpleasure, suffocation-lack of suffocation, protectedness-unprotectedness. Each slide was projected for 10 seconds, the size of the projection being 1.1×1.1 metres. After each projection of a slide (in random order) the subject was given sufficient time to rate his responses on the rating scales. When all the ratings had been obtained, each slide was again presented and the subject was now asked to make magnitude estimations of the size of the area of each space using as standard point of comparison a slide representing 30 units, which did not appear in the series. The method (ratio scaling) and the instruction were similar to the ones used by Gärling (1969). The method is a very simple one to use. The subject is asked to say 60 if the size of a space appears to be twice as large as that of the standard with which it is compared, to say 15 if it appears to be half as large, etc. The experimenter writes down each number as it is given in the appropriate space on his chart. When all 12 slides had been judged, the experiment was concluded.

Results

The data were analysed by means of a three-factor analysis of variance with an error term which consisted of a pooled average of the highest order interaction and the interactions with subjects within groups (see Winer, 1962, p. 319). The level of significance was 5% for all tests. This analysis revealed a significant main effect of H/D ratio (F: 6.97; df.: 3/226) on perceived enclosure. A trend analysis showed that only the linear component of the systematic variance accounted for by the H/D ratio was significant (F = 103; df.: 1/226) and explained 98% of it. These results are depicted in figure 5.3.2. The variables B/D ratio and scale had no significant main effects (both F's: < 1).

A significant effect of the interaction between B/D ratio and scale was found but the size of this effect was very small, and tests of the simple effects of B/D ratio revealed that only the difference between the criterion means for the smallest scale was significant (tobs. for resp., scale 5, 10 and 20: 2.8, 1.2 and 1.1; tcrit.: 1.65). Paradoxically, the effect shows that the spaces of a smaller breadth are perceived as slightly less enclosed than those of a larger breadth, although only in the case of scale 5 m.

The effect of the interaction between H/D ratio and B/D ratio was also significant (F: 2.68; df.: 3/226), but its size was hardly dramatic. Only the simple B/D effect for H/D = .50 was significant (tobs. for resp., H/D = .25, .50, .75 and 1.0: 1.2, 2.2, 0.0 and 1.6; tcrit.: 1.65) showing that for this value, spaces of a smaller breadth were perceived as slightly more enclosed than spaces of a larger breadth (see Figure 5.3.3). However, the above-mentioned significant interaction effects are, in a quantitative sense, almost negligible if we compare their ω^2 effects (% of the total variance explained by a factor) with that for the H/D ratio (29.2, 2.3 and 1.2% for the H/D ratio effect, the effect of the interaction between B/D ratio and scale, and the effect of the interaction between H/D ratio and B/D ratio, respectively).

Finally, a significant effect was found for the interaction between scale and H/D ratio. Figure 5.3.2. shows that the data for the smallest scale are responsible for this

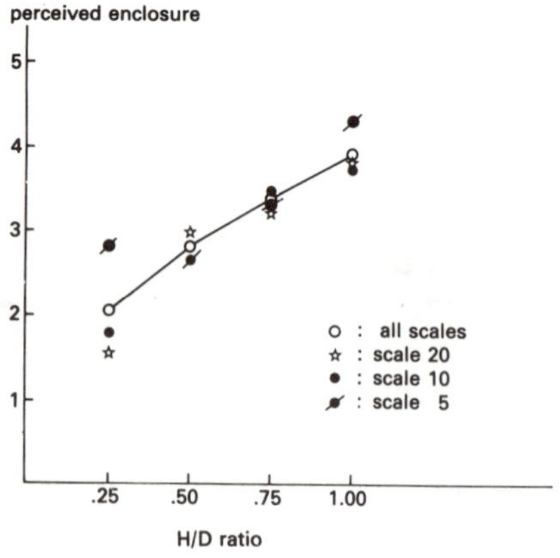

Figure 5.3.2 Relations between H/D ratio, scale and perceived enclosure

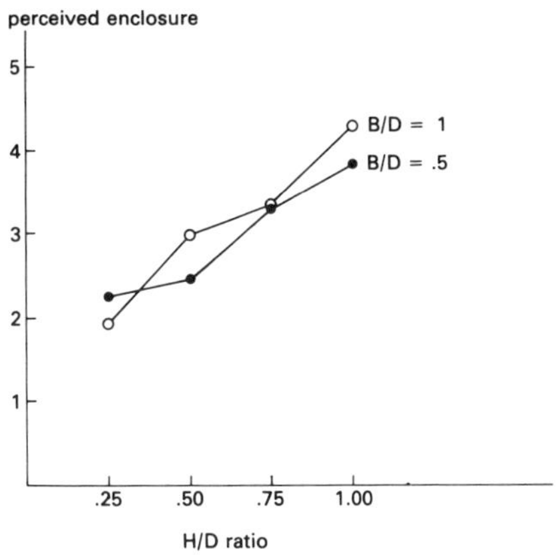

Figure 5.3.3 Relations between H/D ratio, B/D ratio and perceived enclosure

effect. Notice, however, that even for this scale perceived enclosure increases as the H/D ratio increases. Tests of the simple effects of scale on H/D ratio revealed that only the criterion scores for H/D = .25 and H/D = 1.0 differed significantly (F: = 9.71; < 1; < 1 and 3.30 for H/D = .25; .50; .75 and 1.0 respectively; df.: 2/226).

Since it is not wise to capitalize on significance only, we computed the ω^2 effect for the interaction between H/D ratio and scale. As can be seen from an inspection of Figure 5.3.2, the effect is quite small; only 1.88% of the estimated total true variance is accounted for by this interaction effect. Comparing the ω^2 effects for several variables which had significant criterion effects, we have to conclude that, for normal subjects, only the H/D ratio appears to be a substantial predictor of perceived openness-enclosure. It is of course also the only factor which has a consistent and straightforward relation with the dependent variable. Two methods were used to vary the size of space, namely, variation in scale and in the B/D ratio. The physical size of each area of space, as depicted to the subjects by means of perspective drawings, was known to us. Figure 5.3.4 shows the judged size of spaces plotted as a function of logarithmic physical size (base 10). The curve shows a remarkable similarity to other curves generally obtained for such judgmental procedures (see Gärling, 1969), and suggests that the subjects did indeed perceive differences in size of the spaces. [Note: In the group of 33 normals (students) not reported on here, three persons (9.12%) perceived no differences in size of the spaces.] Perceived size increased significantly as physical size increased by manipulation of B/D (t = 1.85; df.: 20), and varied significantly as physical size was varied by manipulation of scale (F: 56.9; df.: 2/40). The independence of perceived enclosure and size of space is seen from the variation in perceived enclosure across conditions of varying size of spatial area (illustrated in Figure 5.3.4).

Finally all intercorrelations between experiential scales used in this study were computed and are shown in Table 5.3.1.

Table 5.3.1 shows that the hedonic quality of the experience of spaces decreases as level of perceived enclosure increases, that is, feelings of unpleasure, suffocation and unsafety increase as spaces are perceived as more enclosed. An unexpected result was the lack of correlation between the variables protectedness-unprotectedness and

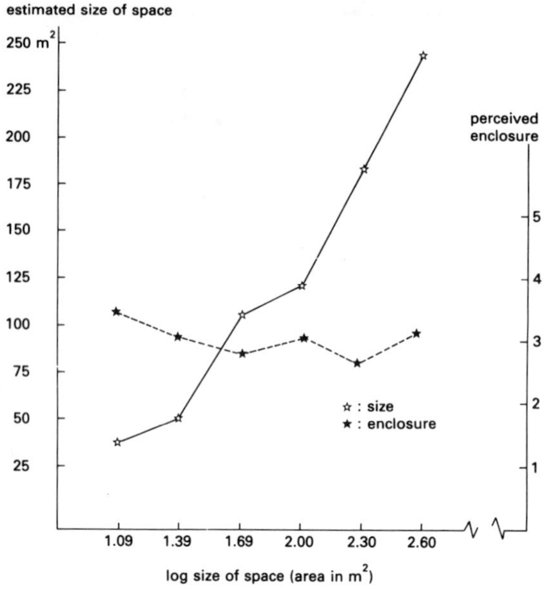

Figure 5.3.4 Relations between physical and estimated size of space and perceived enclosure

Table 5.3.1 Intercorrelations between experiential variables (normal subjects)

	suffocation	unsafety	enclosure	unprotectedness	unpleasure
suffocation	1.00				
unsafety	.36*	1.00			
enclosure	.92	.42	1.00		
unprotectedness	−.46	.47	−.31*	1.00	
unpleasure	.79	.62	.79	−.02*	1.00

* not significant

pleasure-unpleasure. Also, although normals tend to feel more protected in spaces that are more enclosed, this tendency is very weak and the correlation between both variables is not significant. We have to conclude therefore that, for normal subjects, the variable "protectedness" is unrelated to perceived enclosure and did not contribute to the determination of hedonic quality of perceived openness-enclosure of space.

Discussion

Substantial support is found in this experiment for the hypothesis of Hayward & Franklin (1974) that perceived openness-enclosure of space is closely related to the ratio of boundary wall height and wall distance (H/D ratio), and little support for the rival hypothesis (Gärling, 1969) that perceived openness-enclosure is closely related to size of space. However, at this stage of our investigations our conclusions are necessarily tentative. No causal relation is assumed between H/D ratio and perceived openness-enclosure of space, but the assumption that it is a good predictor of perceived openness-enclosure now seems highly plausible. Our reasons for expressing these conclusions in terms of plausibility statements are because of the two points made earlier. First, there may be equally valid indicators of these spatial dimensions (e.g., retinal angle size) which are highly correlated with H/D ratio. Secondly, the fact that different aspects of space are practically impossible to isolate by experimental manipulation. If we hold the size of space (area) constant and vary the H/D ratio, while keeping the form of space constant, then H/D ratio is confounded with volume. If, on the other hand, we allow the size of space to vary (as we did in varying the scale in this experiment) while holding H/D ratio constant, then size of space is confounded with volume. If H/D ratio is held constant while breadth (B/D ratio) is varied, then size of space and volume are again confounded.

However, assuming that a relation exists between size or volume of space and perceived enclosure, we would then expect an increase in volume to have the same effect as an increase in size on perceived enclosure; certainly not to have opposed effects. Since both factors were allowed an equal chance of manifesting this (hypothetical) effect on perceived enclosure, that is, by the introduction of a substantial scale variation, and since, with one exception, neither resulted in a significant variation of the criterion variable, we may plausibly conclude that these variables are not related to perceived openness-enclosure. The same reasoning applies to variation of breadth (B/D ratio). Furthermore, although the size of space was held constant under different conditions (i.e., within each scale manipulation), a substantial criterion variance was effected. H/D ratio, and not size or volume of space, must then be assumed to be the effective variable accounting best for the criterion variance, at least for normal persons.

Of course, this does not mean that further investigation of the problem will preclude other spatial variables as possible indicators of perceived openness-enclosure. Only open, empty spaces were involved in this experiment and innumerable other form variables might possibly be introduced in further exploration. All that we may say at this point is that the conclusion seems justified that, for normal persons, the hedonic quality of the experience of space decreases as the level of perceived enclosure increases.

But does this apply too to phobic persons? If the findings of the studies I and II are not completely artefactual, we should expect B/D ratio (and thus size or volume) to be as effective an indicator of perceived openness-enclosure; and thus too of (decrease in) hedonic quality of experience of space. The next experiment provides answers to these expectations.

Experiment 2 (Phobic Subjects)

Subjects

Thirty-two, mainly agoraphobic patients participated voluntarily in the experiment. Six of these patients had no agoraphobic complaints (two claustrophobics, three claustro- and social phobics, and one social phobic), but the others all had agoraphobic complaints, sometimes mixed with claustro- and social phobia, or with fear of death and disease, etc. These patients were diagnosed by members of the staff of the Department of Personality and Clinical Psychology, and were currently undergoing treatment for their complaints there. Their ages ranged from 16 to 50 years of age.

In deciding to replicate the experiment with phobic subjects, we hoped to find more solid ground for the findings in the first two experiments which suggested that there might be a systematic relation between the relations of H/D ratio and B/D ratio and perceptual effects (perceived enclosure) as well as other experiential effects of these spaces (e.g., suffocation, unprotectedness, unsafety, etc.) which trigger feelings of displeasure, anxiety or avoidance of environmental situations in which these variables predominate (e.g., buildings, squares, streets).

The assumption was made that phobic persons, who are generally classified in the neurotic category, would show similar responses to normals in these situations, although these responses might be more extreme, and that their anxiety and avoidance behaviour would be positively correlated with perceived enclosure, H/D ratio, and possibly B/D ratio too.

We decided to replicate the first experiment as exactly as possible. The method was therefore quite identical to that in the preceding experiment, except for the addition of two rating scales for anxiety and avoidance, and the omission of the magnitude estimation of the spaces from the procedure. The reason for the latter decision was a pragmatic one. In view of the previous results, and the stress imposed on phobic patients, the gain from a shortened version of the experiment seemed to outweigh the loss of these data. Also, instead of 22 subjects, 32 phobic subjects were employed, randomly divided in two groups of 16 persons.

Results

A three-factor analysis of variance of exactly the same type as the one used in experiment 1 revealed a significant main effect of H/D ratio on perceived enclosure (F: 7.5; df.: 3/366), and a significant main effect of B/D ratio on perceived enclosure (F: 39.5; df.: 1/30). All tests had a level of significance of 5%.

No significant effect was found for scale on perceived enclosure (F: 1.05; df.: 2/366); nor were any of the interactions (between B/D ratio and scale, B/D ratio and H/D ratio and between scale and H/D ratio) significant (all F's: <1). H/D ratio and B/D ratio both had significant effects on feelings of anxiety (F: 6.15; df.: 3/366 and F: 16.9; df.: 1/30) and the effects of all other factors (scale and all first order interactions) were not significant (all F's <1). The B/D ratio influenced avoidance behaviour significantly (F: 59.5; df.: 1/30) but the main effect of H/D ratio on avoidance was not significant (F: 2.3; df.: 3/366). No other main factors or interactions had significant effects on this criterion variable (all F's: <1).

[Note: 12.5% of these phobic patients showed no variation in their responses, either to ratios of H/D and B/D or to scale (size) differences; and 18.8% showed only slight variation in their responses to perceived enclosure.]

Trend analyses on the data relating the H/D ratio to perceived enclosure, anxiety and avoidance showed these relations to be mainly linear. In all three cases the non-linear component was not significant (all F's: <1), but the linear component was significant (for enclosure, anxiety and avoidance, resp., F: 22.0; F: 19.4 and F: 6.9; df.: 1/366).

In all cases (all three criterion variables) the linear component explained at least 94% of the systematic variance due to the H/D ratio. This implies that the linear correlation of the type rbetween is almost perfect in all cases. Such a type of correlation is quite adequate to describe the associative strength between variables in terms of more stable group means but it overestimates correlational strength under conditions of more individual variability. Therefore, correlations of the type rwithin were also computed. As is generally the case, these correlations are much lower (r = .42, .46 and .41 respectively for enclosure, anxiety and avoidance). Nevertheless, H/D ratio is an accurate predictor of mean criterion values (see Figure 5.3.5a and b); the inter-criterion correlations being: r = .98, .98 and .94 for the correlation between avoidance and anxiety, enclosure and anxiety, and avoidance and enclosure respectively.

To obtain an indication of the relevancy of the two systematic sources of variation which had significant effects (B/D ratio and H/D ratio) the ω^2 – effects for these factors and for experimental error were computed: these were 12.6 and 16.3 and 71.1% for the criterion variable, perceived openness-enclosure. H/D ratio is still a more important source of variation (but less convincingly so than in the case of normal subjects), in the sense that it contributes more of that part of the estimated total true variance that can be explained by (significant) systematic variation of independent variables.

The correlation between perceived enclosure and decrease in hedonic value is even higher for this sample of persons than for normals (see Table 5.3.2). In contrast to the negative correlations found between enclosure and unprotectedness when using normal subjects (see Table 5.3.1), this variable shows a high positive correlation with other variables (enclosure, suffocation, unsafety, unpleasure) for phobic subjects.

Discussion

The results of both experiments lead us to assume that H/D ratio is a good and useful

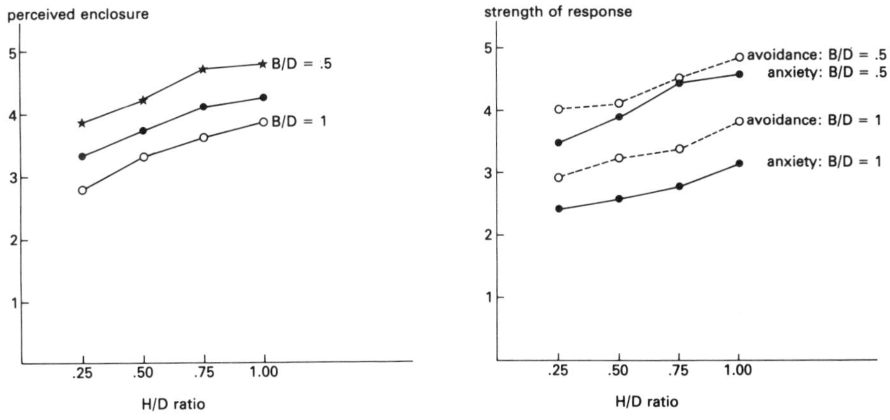

Figure 5.3.5 Relations between H/D ratio, B/D ratio and (a) perceived enclosure (b) anxiety and avoidance responses

Table 5.3.2 Intercorrelations between experiential variables (phobic patients)

	enclosure	unsafety	unpleasure	suffocation	unprotectedness
enclosure	1.00				
unsafety	.84	1.00			
unpleasure	.93	.93	1.00		
suffocation	.93	.94	.96	1.00	
unprotectedness	.76	.91	.86	.87	1.00

predictor of perceived openness-enclosure of space for normal and phobic subjects. Clearly though, for the phobic group, the H/D ratio is not the sole predictor, for the B/D ratio has to be taken into account. We will come back to this in a moment.

The hedonic quality of perceived enclosure has been determined: the stronger the feelings of enclosure, the stronger are the feelings of unpleasure, suffocation, unsafety. These relations apply equally well to normal as to phobic persons. The groups differ, however, on the degree in which feelings of unprotectedness are correlated with perceived enclosure: positively in the case of phobic patients, negatively for normals. Although there is a tendency for normals to feel more protected in spaces that are more enclosed, this tendency is weak. More unexpected is the strong relation between unprotectedness and enclosure for phobic patients. There may be several reasons for this, one of them being the composition of this group of patients, several of whom, although with a main complaint of agoraphobia, suffered also from claustrophobic, and (in some cases) social phobic complaints as well. Before we can reach any sound conclusion on this matter, more systematic investigation of these relations needs to be undertaken. The most intriguing difference between the experimental groups is the one found on the variable B/D ratio: no effect in the normal group, but a significant one in the phobic group, on perceived enclosure, and on anxiety and avoidance measures. Although this finding was reason for surprise for one of the investigators (see McNab, Nieuwenhuyse, Kuyper & Jansweyer, 1978), for me it was a particularly gratifying result. For though unintended, it seemed to vindicate the findings of the tunnel experiments with phobics (Studies I & II), which in comparison suffered from lack of inadequate controls; and, in spite of our efforts, a comparably unsystematic manipulation of the independent variables. What, to us, was even more surprising was the fact that, though a small B/D ratio had considerable effect on mean anxiety level and on mean level of perceived enclosure, in phobics (in contrast to normals), no significant scale effects were found. Since we assumed that a B/D ratio effect, if significant, would support Gärling's hypothesis (1969) that size of space (and/or volume as a confounded variable) explains the criterion variance, it was puzzling to find that, in all cases (on all criterion variables) scale effects were not only nonsignificant but, quantitatively speaking, nil. It is then not unlikely that this group of phobic patients have responded to those spatial properties that are most directly and validly measured by B/D ratio, namely, the *relation* between breadth and distance. It is unlikely that they responded to one of the covariables with which it is confounded. Only such an hypothesis can explain the invariance of the criterion variables across scale conditions. In general, then, one may conclude that architectural variables, such as the ratios of physical dimensions, are important predictors of perceived enclosure and other experiential variables, for normal persons and for phobic patients.

Perceptual and Emotional Responses of Phobic Patients to Structural Components of Complexity, in Abstract Stimuli (Study IV)

From the previous studies we had obtained a fair idea of the physical variables in architectural spaces (tunnels, rooms) which trigger and/or help to maintain phobic responses to these situations. Because many of our patients are also afraid of streets, and some of wide, open spaces as well as of enclosed ones, we asked ourselves whether other variables than those investigated by us might be present in these environments, and be as good predictors of debilitating emotional responses (anxiety, arousal, displeasure) as are H/D and B/D ratios, illumination ratios, etc.

Before attacking the problem of streets, with their many-facetted structures, we consulted the psychological literature on informational uncertainty, because we thought that this parameter might prove to be an important predictor of anhedonic responses too. Berlyne's work over a quarter of a century (1957–1974) seemed a suitable starting-point. He found that certain structural characteristics of environments, such as variations in the dimensions novelty, uncertainty, complexity, ambiguity, and so on, are determinants of attention, exploratory activity, aesthetic preference, interest, and optimal level of arousal. These structural qualities he called *collative variables* since these are dependent on comparison between stimulus elements that are simultaneously or successively present in situations. Berlyne argued that it is the subjective uncertainty arising from informational uncertainty which calls for "structuring," "organization," or "interpretation" of stimulus pattern; and presumably makes demands on cortical information-processing, rather than vegetative functions that facilitate motor activity. He showed that in normal people, subjective uncertainty or perceived complexity of environments is a linear, monotonic function of objective uncertainty of information. Preference ratings and ratings of interestingness, however, relate differentially to stimulus complexity or uncertainty. As the latter increases, feelings of interestingness increase, but are finally sustained at a plateau, with further increase in complexity. Preference, on the other hand, is an inverted-U function of complexity; and so is arousal.

This difference in the relation of preference, interest and arousal led Berlyne to postulate a differentiation between two kinds of exploratory behaviour. One, specific exploration, is primarily aimed at securing information for the individual and is implicated in measures of amount of exploratory activity, or interestingness ratings; while the other, diversive exploration, has an affective, emotion-arousing basis, and is involved in preferential-choice measures, or ratings of pleasingness, liking, etc. In this view, perceptual curiosity is conceived as a condition of heightened arousal whose alleviation through incoming information is rewarding. Perceptual curiosity is held to result from subjective uncertainty, which is regarded as a form of conflict (competition among responses corresponding to alternative hypotheses). The bulk of this research shows a high consistency in the judgments of normal subjects. Berlyne concluded from this that processes of some generality are reflected herein.

Other researchers (e.g., Wohlwill, 1966–1970; Francès, 1976) found that these relations also apply in real-life situations. Francès, who investigated normal subjects of different educational levels (students and manual workers), found a striking difference between these groups in terms of preference (for abstract stimuli, as well as for paintings), but no difference in terms of interest. Where students as a whole preferred complex abstract stimuli (and abstract art) over simple stimuli (and representational art), the manual workers showed the opposite preference. This difference between groups was highly significant.

Because at this point in time the significance of our findings was far from clear, at least to me, I hoped that if I could establish that uncertainty of information was *the* predictor variable into which all the other structural components feed, as Berlyne's work leads one to assume, I might obtain a better understanding of the problem of perception in phobia. Alas, it was not to be; but neither were these explorations "a wild goose chase". The next two investigations describe these attempts to achieve more insight.

In the first of these, the effects of stimulus complexity on perceived (judged) complexity, preference, interest and arousal are investigated, in a group of mainly agoraphobic patients. The paradigm used is one in which artificial, mainly geometric stimuli are dichotomized into low versus high complexity, in six different categories of complexity. In his earlier work on visual complexity, Berlyne showed that the complexity dimension is not one-dimensional but includes several different properties. These are distinct classes:

1. number of elements or independent units in an array (i.e., amount of material)
2. heterogeneity of elements
3. irregularity of shape or contour
4. irregularity of arrangement of the elements in an array (i.e., asymmetry or random distribution)
5. incongruity of elements, and
6. incongruous juxtaposition of elements.

To investigate these, he made use of patterns which fall into the above six classes, and which enable the effects of these distinct properties to be examined both separately and collectively. As dependent variables he made use of (a) verbal ratings, (b) psychophysiological measures, and (c) behavioural measures, such as exploration time, and exploratory choice. In verbal ratings he found that responses to the complexity dimension could be adequately subsumed under twelve dimensions, that comprise three classes of responses. These classes of responses are: (1) Subjective or perceived complexity; (2) Hedonic tone; and (3) Internal state or arousal.

The twelve dimensions can be represented by three scales in the first class, five in the second and four in the third. The first three describe (i) informational content (the principal complexity dimension: Simple-complex); (ii) ease of perceptual organization (Clear-indefinite); and (iii) degree of redundancy present in the information (Disorderly-orderly).

The second class of responses describes the evaluative factor (or hedonic tone) which includes preference and interest. This "hedonic value or tone" is adequately denoted by the five scales: ugly-beautiful; displeasing-pleasing; dislike-like; uninteresting-interesting; and weak-powerful.

The third class of responses describes the internal state of the person, that is, autonomic and cortical arousal, and is denoted by four scales: no pleasure-extreme pleasure; no discomfort-extreme discomfort; relaxed-tense; and drowsy-alert.

Expectations and Hypotheses

The first four of our hypotheses are in line with the relations found by Berlyne, and others, for normal subjects. In the previous studies we had seen that phobics do not differ significantly from normals in the perception of relations between stimuli, so there was little reason to expect them to differ here on perceived complexity. As to preference, interest and arousal, we expected their behaviour on these variables to describe similar functions to normals, although these might be more extreme, one way or the other. If, as some clinical findings (Marks, 1970; Van Zuuren, 1976) imply, there is a relationship between lower educational level, socio-economic status and agoraphobia, and bearing in mind the findings of Francès (1976) with students and manual workers, we expected agoraphobics to show higher preference and lower arousal for simple stimuli, compared to complex ones; but not necessarily lower interest for complex stimuli. But if, as Berlyne suggests, perceptual curiosity is a condition of heightened arousal whose alleviation through incoming information is rewarding, we might expect stimuli that generate more conflict to elicit heightened arousal and lower preference. These expectations are formulated in hypotheses 5 and 6.

In the former study (H/D ratio and perceived enclosure), the individual data showed that 12.5% of the phobic patients (though none of the normal subjects) did not change their responses regarding perceived enclosure at all, either as a function of H/D or B/D ratio, or of scale (size). If disturbances in information-processing as uncertainty of information increases is an indication of defense against increasing anxiety and feelings of unpleasure, we might expect to find among these phobic patients that those who are poor discriminators of complexity will show heightened arousal and lowered preference as the stimuli become more complex. These expectations are formulated in hypotheses 7 and 8.

Hypotheses

The effect of complexity of stimuli, regardless of kind of collative variables

H1: Subjective (judged) complexity increases monotonically as uncertainty of information (stimulus complexity) increases.
H2: Preference increases and then decreases as judged complexity increases. That is, preference describes an inverted-U shaped function of judged complexity.
H3: Interestingness increases monotonically as judged complexity increases.
H4: Arousal levels increase and then decrease as judged complexity increases.
H0: Main effects are nil, regardless of uncertainty of information or judged complexity.

The effect of kind of collative variables, regardless of the level of complexity

H5: As stimuli become more irregular and/or incongruous, preference for these will diminish.
H6: As stimuli become more irregular and/or incongruous, arousal level will increase.
H0: Main effects are nil, regardless of irregularity or incongruity of stimuli.

The effect of poor discrimination of complexity on preference and arousal

H7: Poor discriminators will show significantly lower preference for complex stimuli than good discriminators.
H8: Poor discriminators will show significantly higher levels of arousal for complex stimuli than good discriminators.
H0: Effects of discrimination on preference and arousal are nil.

Method

Subjects

Twenty-four phobic patients, 6 men and 18 women, varying in age from 21–56 years (mean age: 35.5 yrs). At the time of the investigation, all were being treated for their complaints in our clinical department. None had participated in earlier perceptual studies. Sixteen of the patients suffered from agoraphobia as main complaint, with additional fears of death and disease and being alone. Six patients had mixed complaints of agoraphobia and/or claustrophobia and social phobia. One patient was mainly claustrophobic, with fear of blushing and obsessive compulsive complaints, but had subsidiary agoraphobic and animal phobic complaints, and one suffered from neurotic depression and aggression, without the phobic extension.

Apparatus and Materials

The stimulus items consisted of two sets of six slides representing the six classes of collative variables that define the complexity dimension, each set depicting a Simple and a Complex version. These figures (see Figures 5.4.1 and 5.4.2) are variants of those used by Berlyne, which were constructed by Francès (1976). They were chosen instead of the Berlyne figures because they seemed more meaningful for phobic patients.

A slide projector attached to a tachistoscope, adjusted to 5 seconds, was used to project the stimuli onto an opaque screen at a distance of 3.2 m in front of the seated subject. Each stimulus projected a visual image of size 145 × 96 cm.

Rating Scales

Twelve 7-point bipolar scales (Berlyne scales) were translated into Dutch and used to obtain judgments of perceived complexity, preference and interest (hedonic value), and arousal. The first three describe the complexity-uncertainty factor: 1. simple-complex, 2. clear-indefinite, 3. disorderly-orderly. The next five describe the evaluative factor (hedonic value): 4. ugly-beautiful, 5. displeasing-pleasing (*onaangenaam-aangenaam*), 6. dislike-like (*onaantrekkelijk-aantrekkelijk*), 7. uninteresting-interesting, 8. weak-powerful. The last four scales describe the arousal factor: 9. no pleasure-extreme pleasure (*onplezierig-plezierig*), 10. no discomfort-extreme discomfort, 11. relaxed-tense, 12. drowsy-alert (*slaperig-waakzaam*).

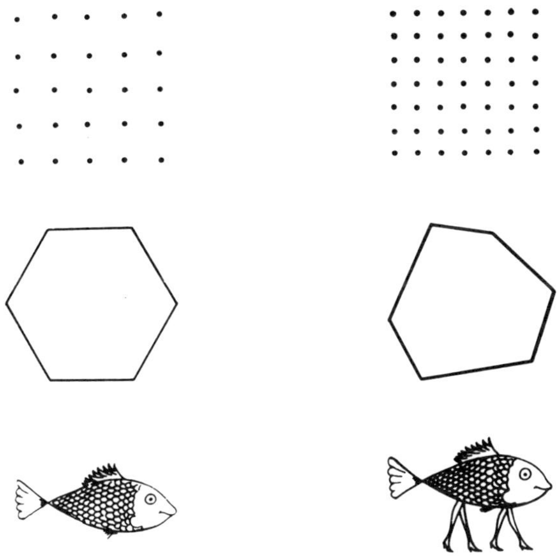

Figure 5.4.1 Examples of pairs of designs in Study IV showing three of the collative variables. (Top to bottom: I. number of elements; III. regularity of figure; and V. incongruity) [taken from Francès, 1975]

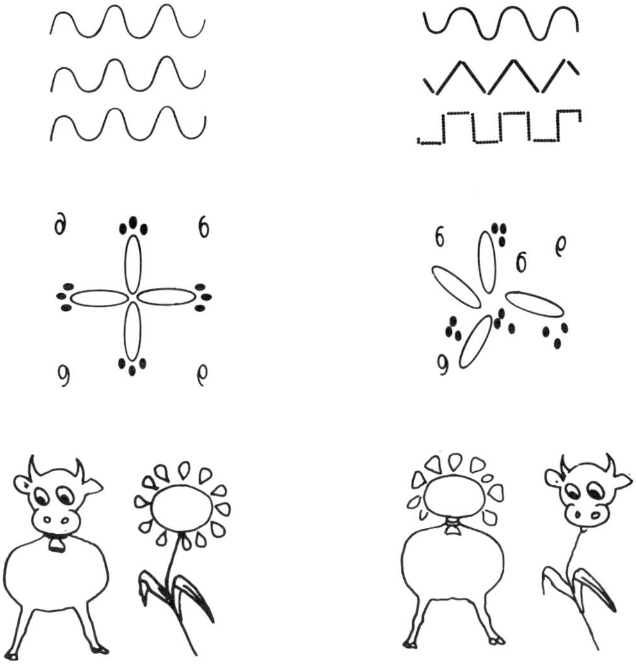

Figure 5.4.2 Examples of pairs of designs in Study IV showing three of the collative variables. (Top to bottom: II. heterogeneity of elements; IV. regularity of disposition; and VI. incongruous juxtaposition) [taken from Francès, 1975]

Procedure

Before projecting the series of stimuli, each subject was given some time for the eyes to become dark-adapted. He or she was then shown three examples of the stimuli, depicting the range to be viewed. This precaution was taken to help the subject to adapt rating behaviour to the distribution of the stimuli. Each subject was also given one practice trial to ensure a proper use of the rating scales.

The 12 figures were then presented in a randomized order, the series for each subject beginning with a different example, determined by means of a balanced Latin square design. When all 12 figures had been judged on all the 12 scales, the experiment was concluded.

Data Analyses

The null hypotheses relating to the effects of complexity of stimuli, regardless of kind of collative variables, are tested by means of three-factor analyses of variance with repeated measures, subjects as random factor, and fixed factors I–VI (stimulus categories) and S–C (simple-complex dimension).

The null hypotheses relating to the effect of kind of collative variables are tested by means of four-factor analyses of variance, with the categories nested under factor X–Y, X representing categories I, II, and III and Y representing categories IV, V and VI.

The null hypotheses relating to the effects of discrimination of complexity are tested by means of analysis of variance with repeated measures, subjects nested under the factor Dp–Dg. Dp stands for "poor discriminator of complexity" and Dg stands for "good discriminator". "Good" and "poor" discrimination are measured by difference scores for the Simple and Complex stimuli on the first three scales (the Complexity factor). The level of significance is 1% for all tests.

Results

Perceived Complexity, Preference, Interest, and Arousal in Agoraphobics

Analyses of variance on the data "perceived complexity" (mean values on the scales 1 to 3) show significant *main effects* of categories I to VI (F: 8.67, df: 5/115, $p < .001$); of complexity levels S–C (F: 11.81, df: 1/23, $p < .001$); and an *interaction effect* between categories I–VI and levels S–C (F: 12.80, df: 5/115, $p < .001$). In all categories except category I, the complex is perceived as more complex than the simple stimulus (S–C in category II: F: 11.52; S–C in category III: F: 28.89; S–C in category IV: F: 71.65; S–C in category V: F: 18.47; S–C in category VI: F: 25.38; df.: 1/253, $p < .001$). The first hypothesis finds strong support in these data. [Incidentally, 33% of these patients showed little or no change on perceived complexity for the simple figures across categories of complexity.]

Analyses of variance on the data "preference" or hedonic tone (mean values on the scales 4 to 8) show significant *main effects* of categories I–VI (F: 6.63, df: 5/115, $p < .001$); of complexity level (F: 23.12, df: 1/23 $p < .001$); and an *interaction effect* between I–VI and S–C (F: 3.71, df: 5/115, $p < .001$). For these subjects significant differences exist in preference per category of complexity, but the relation does not describe an inverted-U curve. The subjects prefer the stimuli in categories I and II above those in category III, and the stimuli in category IV and V more than in category VI. On the simple-complex dimension, the simple stimuli in all categories are much preferred to the complex, but the difference is significant for categories III, IV and V but not for those in categories I, II and VI (III: F: 14.31; IV: F: 13.59; V: F: 13.73, df: 1/253, $p < .001$). For categories III to VI there is a tendency for preference to increase and then decrease with perceived complexity, but this does not apply to the lower dimensions of complexity.

These results lend only partial support to the second hypothesis.

Analyses of variance on the data "interestingness" (mean values on the scale 7) show a significant *main effect* of categories I–VI, regardless of complexity level (F: 5.69, df: 5/115, $p < .001$). Contrary to our expectation, no significant differences are found for complexity level, although there is a tendency among subjects to rate the simple stimuli as more interesting than the complex ones. No interaction effect is found between categories I–VI and complexity levels.

No support is found then for the third hypothesis. In this group interest is not a monotonic function of the stimulus categories, nor of complexity level. On the contrary, the results go in the opposite direction.

Analyses of variance on the data "arousal" (mean values of the scales 9 to 12) show significant *main effects* of categories I–VI (F: 4.83, df: 5/115, $p < .001$); and of complexity levels S–C (F: 12.74, df:1/23, $p < .001$); but no interaction effect between categories I–VI and levels S–C. Analysis of variance per category shows a significant difference in arousal between the simple and the complex stimulus in category IV (F: 10.87, df:1/253, $p < .001$), but not in the other categories. In this category only arousal level increases with increase in complexity.

Only partial support, then, for the fourth hypothesis. Across categories, and for category IV there is support for the hypothesis, but not for separate categories I, II, III, V and VI. Figure 5.4.3 describes the functional relations found between the experiential variables perceived (judged) complexity, preference, interest, and arousal to objective complexity.

The effect of kind of collative variables, regardless of level of complexity

Since the total scores of the subjects on the *hedonic factor* with regard to the complex stimuli on variable Y (categories IV, V and VI) are higher (289.8) than the total scores on variable X (categories I, II and III: 243.2), further analysis was unnecessary. Contrary to the formulated expectation, as stimuli become more irregular and/or incongruous, preference for these increases. No support for the fifth hypothesis.

Since the total scores of the subjects on the *arousal factor* with regard to the complex stimuli on variable Y (see above) are lower (247.5) than the total scores on variable X (289.75), further analysis was unnecessary. Contrary to our expectation, as stimuli become more irregular and/or incongruous, arousal level decreases. No support for the sixth hypothesis.

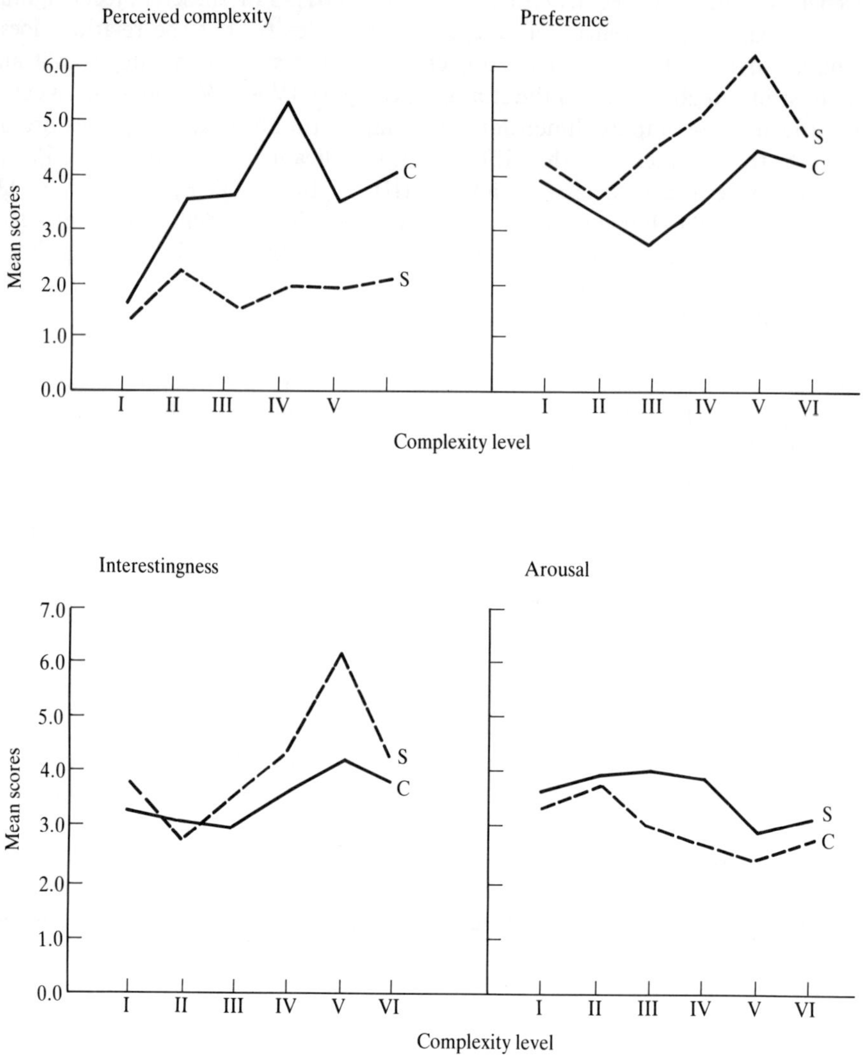

Figure 5.4.3 Relations between four experiential variables of six categories of complexity (abstract stimuli) [Agoraphobics]

The effect of discrimination of complexity on preference and arousal

There is a small, but not significant difference between poor and good discriminators on the *hedonic factor and the arousal factor* for the complex stimuli in categories I, II and III. The poor discriminators show less preference and higher arousal for these stimuli, compared to good discriminators. No support for the seventh hypothesis.

Analyses of variance show that poor and good discriminators of complexity differ significantly on the *arousal factor* with regard to categories I–VI (F: 4.69, df: 5/110, $p < .001$); and with regard to complexity level (F: 12.42, df: 1/22, $p = .005$). But no difference is found in arousal with regard to the complex stimuli across categories. The eighth hypothesis then finds no support.

Of incidental interest are some spontaneous responses of these patients to the stimuli in category III. These undulating lines were greeted with expressions of disgust or apprehension by some, who said that they were reminded of "snakes". The incongruous stimuli in categories V and VI (a sunflower's head interchanged with a cow's head; a fish on a pair of lady's legs) elicited smiles and comments. These emotional responses may have influenced the scoring of these elements and lowered difference scores.

Conclusions

In this first exploration of the relations between stimulus uncertainty, perceived complexity, hedonic tone and arousal in agoraphobic patients our conclusions are necessarily tentative. For these phobic subjects perceived complexity does seem to increase monotonically as a function of objective complexity. The slightly lower, and unexpected, values for the classes of stimuli relating to "incongruity" and "incongruous juxtaposition" may be a result of the kind of stimuli used. These were found to be more meaningful than the other stimuli, in spite of their incongruity, which might have led to a "chunking" of the information into simpler conceptual configurations.

The relation between perceived complexity and preference accords only partially with our expectations or with the work of others. There was a greater preference for the lowest categories of complexity, which was unexpected; and of the complex stimuli, those relating to irregularity of shape or contour, heterogeneity of elements and asymmetry or irregularity of arrangement of elements were the least preferred, found least interesting, and elicited higher arousal.

Interestingness went opposite to our expectations. Although not reaching significance, these subjects tended to find the simpler stimuli in all classes more interesting than the complex ones. Nor was the expectation that preference would decrease and arousal increase with increase in irregularity and incongruity ("conflict") borne out, although this may have been a result of the stimuli used. On the whole, then, these results do not agree with what one would expect from Berlyne's work.

A Second Exploration of Perceptual and Emotional Responses of Phobic Patients and Normal Persons to the Complexity Dimension of Real-life Situations (Streets) (Study V)

Central to Berlyne's theory is the concept of an optimal level of stimulation, according to which positive affect is produced by stimuli, up to a certain value on the scale of complexity; a value that is determined by the individual's optimal level of stimulation (see also Wohlwill's work, 1968 on, which inspired this study).

Berlyne's concept of an optimal level of stimulation, as Wohlwill notes, clearly dictates a research design embodying systematic variation of stimuli along the continuum of complexity. But in the earlier work of Berlyne, and in that of others inspired by him, stimuli are typically dichotomized into high versus low complexity or at most, trichotomized.

In a study in which Wohlwill explored the shape of the function relating stimulus complexity to (a) amount of voluntary exploratory activity, and (b) affective ratings (preference) in 28 normal subjects (students), he made use of two domains of stimuli varying along this dimension. One domain was taken from the physical or geographic environment to which the individual is exposed in his daily life or travels, the other domain from twentieth-century non-representational art. Independent judges were used as "variation-detectors" to obtain seven levels of complexity on the complexity continuum. His main hypothesis was that stimulus complexity would be found to be a monotonically increasing function of number of exposures (viewings) requested by the subjects, and be an inverted-U function of affective ratings. For both the environmental stimuli and for the art stimuli, though more consistently for the latter, the hypothesis was confirmed. Amount of voluntary exploratory activity (measured by number of exposures requested by the subjects) increased monotonically as a function of stimulus complexity, while the preference judgments followed a curvilinear trend, reaching a maximum at an intermediate point of the complexity scale, namely, level 5. The major departure from these general patterns was a dip in both the "number of exposures" and "preference" measures at level 5 of the complexity scale for the environment slides. The basis for these aberrant values was difficult to fathom, especially since the two slides at that level contributed to them about equally, even though they were quite dissimilar in content. Trend analyses confirmed the differences between the shapes of these two functions. Wohlwill thus concluded that his results inspire confidence in the generalizability of findings based on artificially constructed visual (and auditory) patterns to more meaningful or aesthetically relevant ones. We will leave his work, and others who come after him at this point, to take up our own concerns. Wohlwill offered us a paradigm for investigating the complex situations in real-life, particularly streets, which so many of our patients fear and avoid. Still pursuing the elusive idea of informational uncertainty as the key to a better understanding of phobic responses to these environments, we set out to test this hypothesis, using normal controls.

Hypotheses

The first four hypotheses are identical to those postulated for abstract stimuli (see the previous study). Although phobic patients, compared to normals, may show reduced preference and interest, and higher arousal to an increase of uncertainty or complexity in the environment, as yet we have no solid basis to suppose this. But we would expect them to show higher anxiety in and stronger avoidance of situations as complexity increases. For both normals and phobics we postulate then that:

- H1: Subjective or perceived complexity is a linear (monotonic) function of uncertainty of information.
- H2: Preference (hedonic tone) is an inverted-U shaped function of perceived complexity.
- H3: Interestingness is a linear (monotonic) function of perceived complexity.

H4: Arousal is an inverted-U shaped function of perceived complexity.

Furthermore, and only for the phobics patients we expect that:

H5: Anxiety is a linear (monotonic) function of perceived complexity.
H6: Avoidance is a linear (monotonic) function of perceived complexity.
H0: Main effects are nil, regardless of uncertainty of information or perceived complexity.

Method

Complexity Scaling

Because many phobic patients show extreme anxiety in and avoidance of streets, stimuli were selected from the domain of streets in and around Amsterdam.

The use of real-life stimuli poses difficult problems of scaling. In deciding to use different groups of persons as "variation-detectors" à la Wohlwill, we hoped that their rankings might yield values of a lesser order of subjectivity than would be the case from direct ratings of phenomenal complexity.

From the municipal archives of the city of Amsterdam we obtained 66 (black-and-white) photographs of street scenes which showed a wide range of complexity and diversity in the natural and man-made environment. The streets had been photographed in different districts, and at different times of day.

Two groups of 12 normal persons (staff-members of the Department of Personality and Clinical Psychology) were then asked to rate these stimuli on the basis of the amount of variation they contained, that is, on the basis of the number of elements, variety in the elements, irregularity of arrangement or intricateness, and degree of clarity of the scenes. During the relatively informal task, each subject was encouraged to voice the criteria used by him or her to rank the stimuli, as well as criticisms of the stimuli. The first group consisted of 9 men and 3 women; the second group of 6 men and 6 women.

In individual sessions each person was first asked to sort the stimuli into 7–8 piles, according to their apparent complexity. Then each pile was presented separately, and the person was again asked to rank these "from simple to complex". When this task was completed, he or she was shown the rankings of the entire series, and permitted to change the position of any of the stimuli which, when seen in the whole series, no longer appeared in the correct place in the rank ordering. On the basis of variability in rankings and observations of the judges on the suitability of the stimuli, 26 stimuli were removed after group I's rankings were completed, and another 10 stimuli after the rankings of group II.

The remaining 30 stimuli were then ranked by a group of 16 phobic patients, three men and thirteen women, following the same procedure. This was done to explore the possibility that they might differ considerably on perceived complexity, because of the anxiety states of these persons, or because of differences in educational level. But their rankings of the same stimuli showed a very high correlation with those of the normal groups ($r = .84$, corrected for ties, significant at $p < .005$).

Table 5.5.1a Descriptions of street scenes and levels of complexity

Level	General description of class	Specific description of the individual scenes
I	Wide, open spaces (including water); perspective emphasized	1. dyke road near harbour, open space and wide sky, one man on a bicycle 2. quayside, open spaces, wide sky, high office building background, water foreground 3. plain, sombre schoolbuilding (2-storey) in narrow street, a few cars, few people
II	Predominantly greenery (shrubs and trees); openness-enclosure optimal	4. empty street, much greenery, wide pavement, empty cars in parking-lot nearby. 5. nearly empty street, much greenery, modern suburban, wide pavement 6. nearly empty boulevard crossing, wintry, cloudy day, open spaces, wide sky, bare trees
III	Regularity and symmetry of architectural spaces emphasized (street, square, houses)	7. nearly empty street, much greenery, very wide pavement, suburban, regular houses 8. symmetrical blocks of houses (4-storey) enclosing a paved square; young trees, few people, woman with dog on leash; windy day 9. square in front of Central Station; a few people at a bus-stop; old tree trunks visible; in background ornately sculptured facades
IV	Compactness in architectural spaces (occlusion through trees, traffic, housing); few people; dull atmosphere	10. very compact scene; small, straight street flanked on both sides by 3-storey houses, cars chock-a-block in street 11. parallel streets, two rows of large trees, high, large houses, parked cars; cycling group approaching (foreground) 12. very compact scene: broad street with blocks of houses, bombed-out spaces, many cars but few people walking
V	Busyness of streets emphasized: occlusion and overlap by milling crowds of people, heterogeneity of arrangement in structures; stimulating atmosphere	13. Canal Singel: foreground intricate branching of trees in spring, 5-storey houses with varied gables, parked cars aside water; sunny 14. cross-roads (Rokin-Damrak) of broad streets in centre of city, full of traffic, much variety in buildings 15. very busy shopping-street (Regulier Breestraat) rush-hour: jam-packed with cars, people, bicycles, shopping-signs, etcetera

This high agreement allowed us to select 15 of the stimuli for the main investigation, namely, those stimuli which showed highest agreement between judges in all the groups, and which described increasing levels of complexity. These 15 stimuli provided us with a set of five approximately equally spaced points on the complexity continuum, each level of complexity defined by three stimuli. Tables 5.5.1a and b list different rank orderings (with corrected z-values; Guilford, 1954) of both the groups in the scaling study and the three groups in the main experiment, with brief descriptions of the scenes and the classes. Figure 5.5.1 illustrates some striking differences between the normal and phobic subjects in the scaling study on their impressions of aspects that make streets complex. For the phobic patients, compactness of buildings and congestion of streets by traffic, the bustle or busyness of streets (milling crowds), heterogeneity of arrangement of elements, and wide, open spaces that elicit feelings of loneliness, solitariness, or bleakness, seem to be the structural components that determine their rankings of complexity. For the normal persons, though, complexity is more often determined by the amount of information, and by the number of decisions one must make to navigate traffic or the spaces.

Table 5.5.1b Rank ordering of street scenes according to level of complexity showing ranking in the pilot study [r = .84] and the z-values in the main study (normals and phobics) [*W* = .64]

			Rank order pilot study			Rank order main study		
		RO	N1	P	RO	N1	N2	P
level	street stimuli		(n = 24)	(n = 16)		(n = 20)	(n = 30)	(n = 12)
I	dyke road	1	1.32	1.20	2	1.74	2.48	1.94
	empty street greenery	2	.95	.97	7	1.83	2.10	1.32
	school street	3	.93	.81	1	2.31	1.68	2.03
II	empty street green, parking	4	.83	.50	4	2.70	1.69	1.22
	quayside	5	.66	.33	3	1.81	1.84	2.23
	boulevard cross	6	.39	.13	5	2.29	1.95	1.60
III	empty street greenery	7	.24	.01	6	3.14	3.09	1.53
	symmetrical block houses	8	.01	−.41	8	2.09	2.02	1.40
	square C.S.	9	−.08	−.19	9	2.39	2.28	1.47
IV	compact street 3-storey houses	10	−.46	−.26	10	2.61	3.30	2.27
	cycling group	11	−.55	−.70	11	2.52	2.46	2.67
	compact, broad	12	−.59	−.59	12	2.75	2.44	2.38
V	Canal in spring	13	−.75	−.47	13	2.50	2.74	2.21
	Rokin-Damrak	14	−.89	−1.09	14	4.80	3.43	3.29
	rush-hour in Reg. Breestreet	15	−2.14	−2.03	15	5.79	4.00	5.50

N1 = staff members of department; N2 = normal, employed adults (external); P = phobic patients

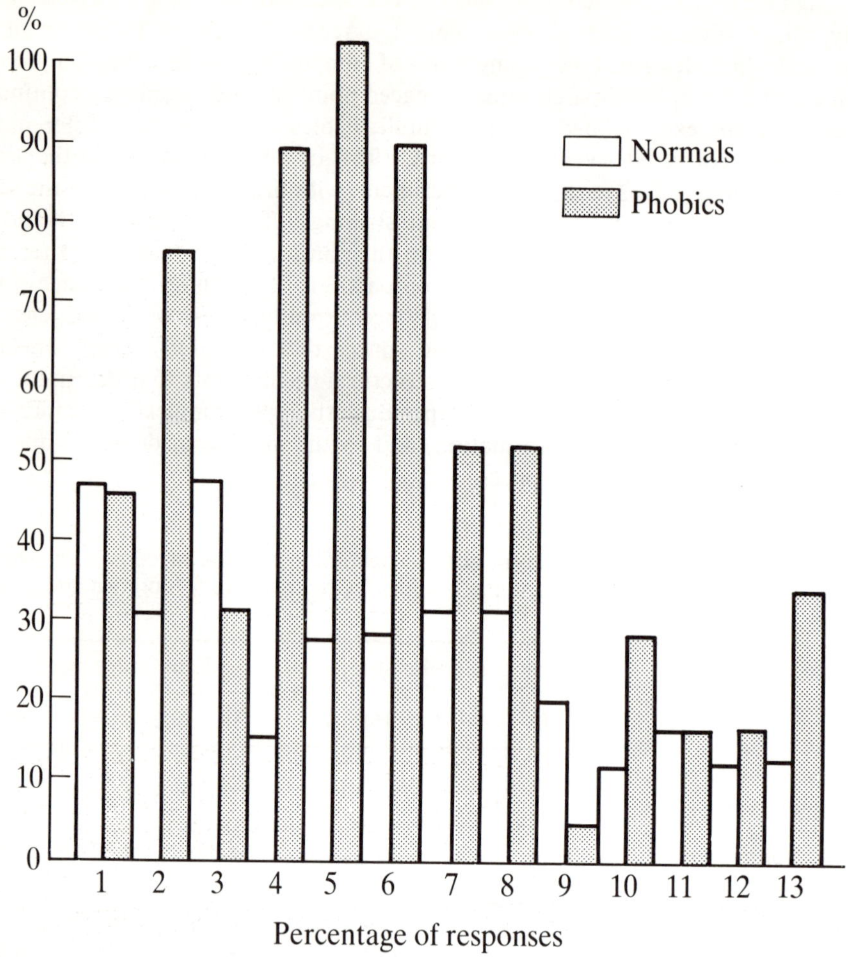

Figure 5.5.1 What makes a street complex? Some striking differences between normal and phobic persons

Complexity of street:
1. amount of information (overload)
2. heterogeneity of arrangement
3. number of decisions to navigate traffic
4. bustle/busyness of street (milling crowds)
5. compactness of buildings/traffic
6. open spaces (N); open, lonely, bleak spaces (P)
7. enclosed spaces, narrow streets
8. speed of traffic
9. gaiety; attractiveness; interestingness
10. sombreness; greyness
11. greenery (shrubs; trees)
12. unfamiliarity
13. rest category

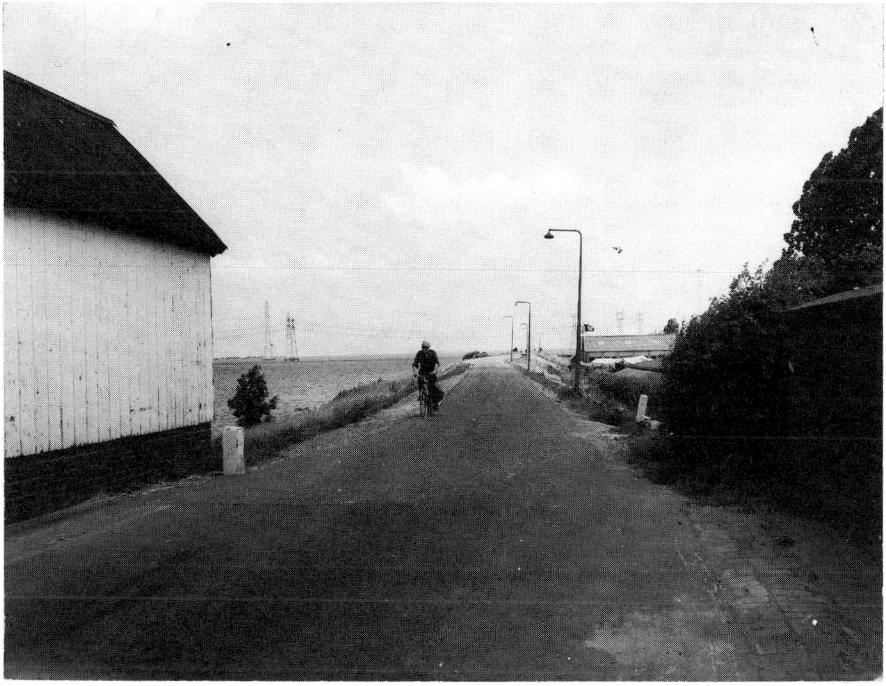

Plate XVIII Study V. Complexity of streets: Level 1. Wide, open spaces (Stimulus scene no. 1, see Table 5.5.1a).

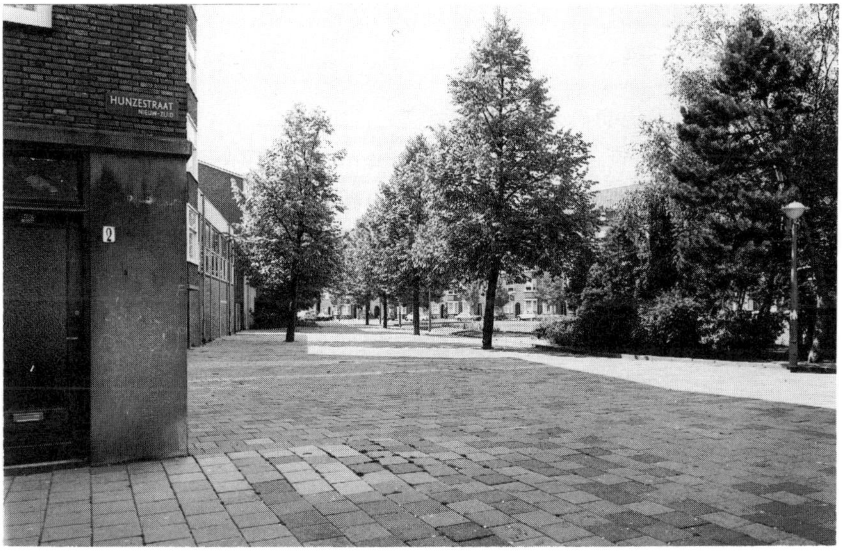

Plate XIX Study V. Complexity of streets: Level II. Predominantly greenery (Stimulus scene no. 5, see Table 5.5.1a).

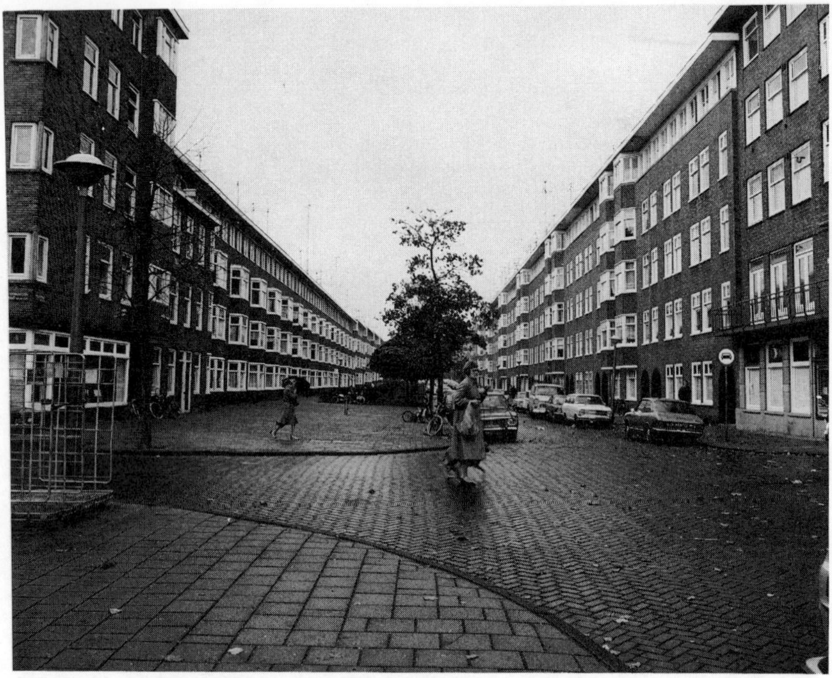

Plate XX Study V. Complexity of streets: Level III. Regularity and symmetry of architectural spaces (Stimulus scene no. 8, see Table 5.5.1a).

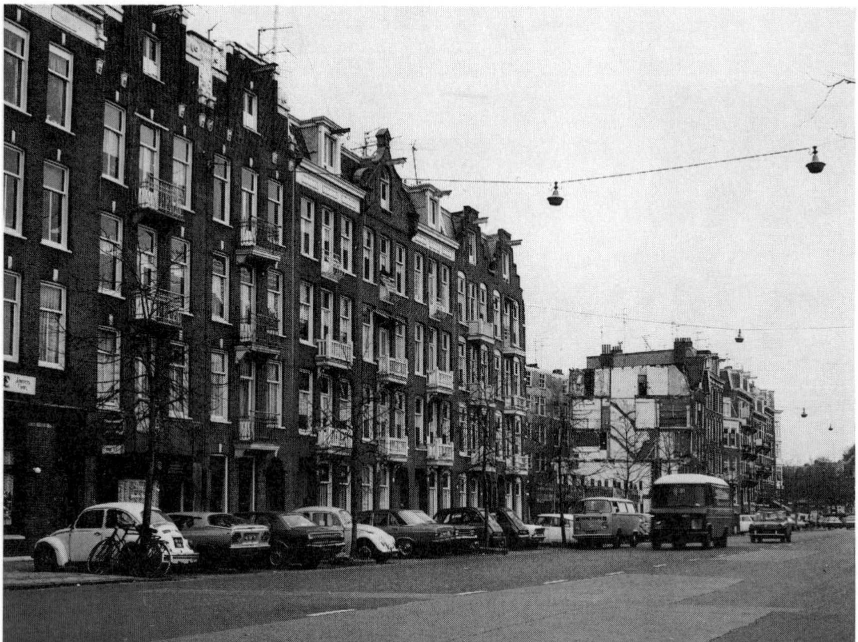

Plate XXI Study V. Complexity of streets: Level IV. Compactness in architectural spaces (Stimulus scene no. 12, see Table 5.5.1a).

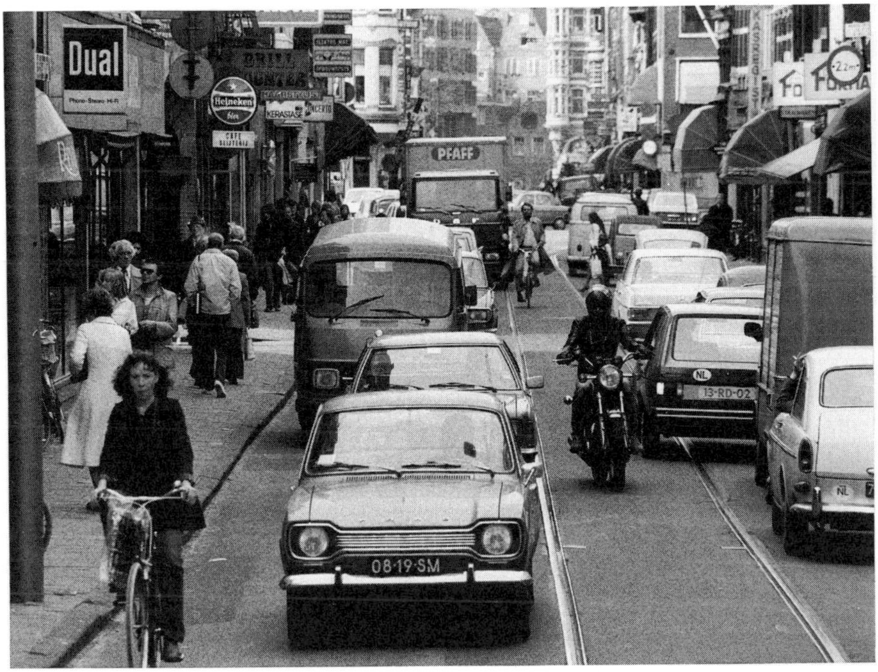

Plate XXII Study V. Complexity of streets: Level V. Busyness; occlusion and overlap (Stimulus scene no. 15, see Table 5.5.1a).

An indication of the reliability of these scaled complexity values is obtained by comparing the rank orderings of the normal group of 20 persons with that of the phobic group (12 persons), on their ratings of perceived complexity of the same streets three months later (test-retest condition). The correlation between rankings and judgments is lower for the normal group than for the phobic patients. For the normal group this is: $r = .66$, for the phobic group: $r = .77$ (significant at $p < .005$).

Three years later, the experiment was replicated with a normal group of 30 persons outside the environs of the laboratory. A moderate correlation between their judgments and those of the phobic and normal control group suggests that the judgments and the choice of stimuli are fairly reliable ($W = .64$).

Subjects

The *experimental* group consisted of twelve of the old group of sixteen phobic patients who had functioned as "variation detectors" in the scaling study, and who were still undergoing treatment in the clinic at the time of the main study (i.e., three months after the scaling of stimuli). These three men and nine women varied in age from 23–44 years (mean age: 32.7 yrs). Their phobic complaints varied: three suffered from agoraphobia, fear of being alone, and other complaints; three from complaints of agoraphobia, claustrophobia and/or social phobia; one from claustrophobia and fear of being alone; one from fear of death and making decisions; one from fear of storms and high wind, with obsessive overtones; one from fear of animals, groups, being alone, and medical instruments; and one from fear of travelling, supermarkets, and fear of a heart attack.

The first *normal control* group consisted of twenty persons, eleven men and nine women who had also participated in the scaling study as "variation detectors". They varied between the ages of 23–60 years (mean age: 42.2 yrs). Twelve of them were members of the scientific subfaculty and staff of the department, two were graduate students, three were administrative staff members, and one an (external) accountant.

The second *normal control* consisted of thirty persons, twelve men and eighteen women, between the ages of 23–62 years (mean age: 34.2 yrs). This group contained housewives, skilled and semi-skilled technical and manual workers, and a sprinkling of academically trained persons. In making use of this group, we wished to control for the sometimes supposed "deviant" behaviour on psychological tests by psychology students and staff.

Materials

The 15 stimuli of street scenes, mounted on cardboard, sized 16 × 24 cm, all black-and-white photographs with a highly polished finish. And fourteen 7-point bipolar scales (that is, the 12 Berlyne scales and 2 scales for measuring ratings of anxiety and avoidance. See scales in study IV).

Procedure

Each subject was individually tested. Prior to the experiment, the phobic subjects and those in both normal control groups were given one practice trial in how to use the fourteen bipolar rating scales.

The instruction on how to fill in the scales, and information on the purpose of the study, was read aloud to the phobic and to the (external) normal control groups; but the (internal) staff-members were permitted to read the instructions themselves before filling in the scales.

Each stimulus was presented in a previously randomized order, and for the different subjects, according to the Latin square principle, to partially control for sequence effects. Each stimulus was placed on a table in front of the subject, and he or she was then asked to look carefully at the scene for 60 seconds, and try to imagine himself (or herself) in the situation. After 60 seconds the stimulus was removed, and the subject was asked to rate his (or her) response on the different scales with respect to: (a) perceived complexity of the situation, (b) hedonic feelings, (c) arousal felt in the situation, (d) anxiety in the situation, and (e) avoidance tendency in the situation.

Data Analysis

To test the null hypotheses three-factor analyses of variance with repeated measures on the second factor (subjects nested under groups; Winer, 1970) were carried out. To determine which levels of stimulation were significant a Newman-Keuls analysis was also done where necessary. The level of significance for all tests is 1%. Also, in the scaling study, rank order coefficients (Kendall's tau) were computed for the rankings of the stimuli by the different groups.

Results

Relations between stimulus complexity/uncertainty and perceived (judged) complexity

Three-factor analysis of variance showed a significant main effect only for levels of complexity (F: 134.30, df: 4/236, p = .001). All three groups, phobics and normals, perceive significant differences in levels of complexity of the stimuli (see Figure 5.5.2). But the groups do not differ in their perception of these ($F < 1$). Nor is the interaction between the groups and complexity significant. Further analysis (Newman-Keuls) showed that, except for level II compared to level I, each level of increasing complexity is perceived as significantly more complex than the previous one. Level II is judged by the internal normal group as significantly less complex than level I, and both groups judge level I to be significantly more complex than the phobic group judges it. Trend analyses on these data showed that the relation between stimulus uncertainty and perceived complexity is mainly linear (F: 474.88, df.: 1/236, $p < .001$) but has also a significant quadratic component (F: 60.505, df.: 1/236, $p < .001$).

This result confirms the expectations formulated in hypothesis 1, and accords with the findings in the literature. As uncertainty of information increases, perceived (judged) complexity increases, for normal and phobic persons.

Relations between hedonic feelings (tone) and perceived complexity

Analysis of variance revealed a significant *main effect* on the factor "groups" (F: 17.38, df: 2/59, p = .001), and a *main effect* on the factor "stimulus levels" (F: 14.94, df: 4/236, p = .001). Significant differences exist between normal and phobic persons in the amount of hedonic feeling experienced in these situations. The interaction between groups and complexity levels though does not reach significance (F: 1.84, df: 8/236, p = .071). Newman-Keuls analysis showed that, for phobics, levels I and IV differ significantly from levels II and III, but the latter two do not differ. Level V differs significantly from all other levels. This means that levels I and IV, compared to levels II and III, elicit less positive hedonic feeling, but level V elicits highest hedonic feeling in this group.

The normal groups also differ significantly from each other on this variable, except for levels I and II where no difference exists. The external group of normal persons judged all other levels of complexity as more pleasing than the internal group (the psychologists); and level V as having highest hedonic tone. At all levels of complexity the phobic patients experience less hedonic feeling than the normals. Figure 5.5.2 shows this difference between normal and phobics. Trend analyses showed that the relation between hedonic tone and stimulus complexity is mainly a linear and quartic one (Flin.: 20.989; Fquartic: 20.336, df.: 1/236, $p < .001$). Other non-linear relations are not significant. The hypothesis thus finds no support in these data.

Relations between interestingness and perceived complexity

Analysis of variance revealed a significant *main effect* on the factor "groups" (F: 12.87, df.: 2/59, p = .001) and on "stimulus levels" (F: 31.24, df: 4/236, p = .001), but again no significant interaction between groups and levels (F: 1.80, df: 8/236, p = .078). Newman-Keuls analysis showed further that, except for level II, normals and phobics differ significantly on the amount of interest (experienced). The phobic patients find all other stimulus levels less interesting than the normal subjects. Levels I, II, III and IV do not differ significantly for the phobic patients, but interest rises significantly for level V. The normal groups also differ significantly from each other, except on levels I and II. Level IV yields in both groups significantly lower interest than levels III and V. The normal externals score highest. Trend analyses showed that the relations between interest and perceived complexity have linear (F: 80.98), quadratic (F: 13.42) and quartic (F: 15.07, df.: 1/236, p < .001) components. The linear relation accounts for most of the variance (82.7%) and the non-linear for 15.9%. On the basis of these analyses therefore, support is found for the hypothesis that interestingness is a linear function of perceived complexity. However, differences do exist between phobic and normal persons in the amount of interest they have towards these scenes (see Figure 5.5.2).

Relations between arousal and perceived complexity

Analysis of variance revealed significant *main effects* on the factors "groups" (F: 4.59, df: 2/59, p = .01) and on "stimulus levels" (F: 8.61, df: 8/236, p = .001), but no significant interaction between them (F: 1.80, df: 8/236, p = .08). Newman-Keuls analysis showed that the normal groups differ significantly only at level V, but the phobic group differs from both normal groups significantly at all levels. As one might expect, their arousal levels are higher than the normal controls, and highest for levels I, IV and V. Trend analyses showed that the relations between arousal and perceived complexity are quadratic (F: 14.84), linear (F: 11.32, df.: 1/236, p < .001) and a small part quartic (F: 3.421, df.: 1/236, p = .05). The quadratic relation explains 51.6% of the variance and the linear component 47.8%. (See Figure 5.5.2.)

These relations then take the form of a U-curve rather than an inverted U-curve as Berlyne predicts, and in the case of the normal subjects this is even a flattened curve. The hypothesis therefore finds no support in these data.

Relations between anxiety and perceived complexity

Analysis of variance revealed significant *main effects* on the factors "groups" (F: 16.03, df: 2/59, p = .001) and on "stimulus levels" (F: 5.95, df.: 4/236, p = .001), as well as a signficant *interaction effect* between them (F: 3.45, df.: 8/236, p = .001). Newman-Keuls analysis showed that all three groups differ significantly from each other, with the phobic group showing highest levels of anxiety to the stimuli. At level I and at level V, anxiety is higher in the phobic group than at other levels.

Trend analyses showed the relations between anxiety and perceived complexity to be quadratic (F: 13.54) and linear (F: 6.784, df.: 1/236, p < .001), the quadratic component explaining most of the variance (98.8%) (see Figure 5.5.2). The hypothesis finds little support in these data.

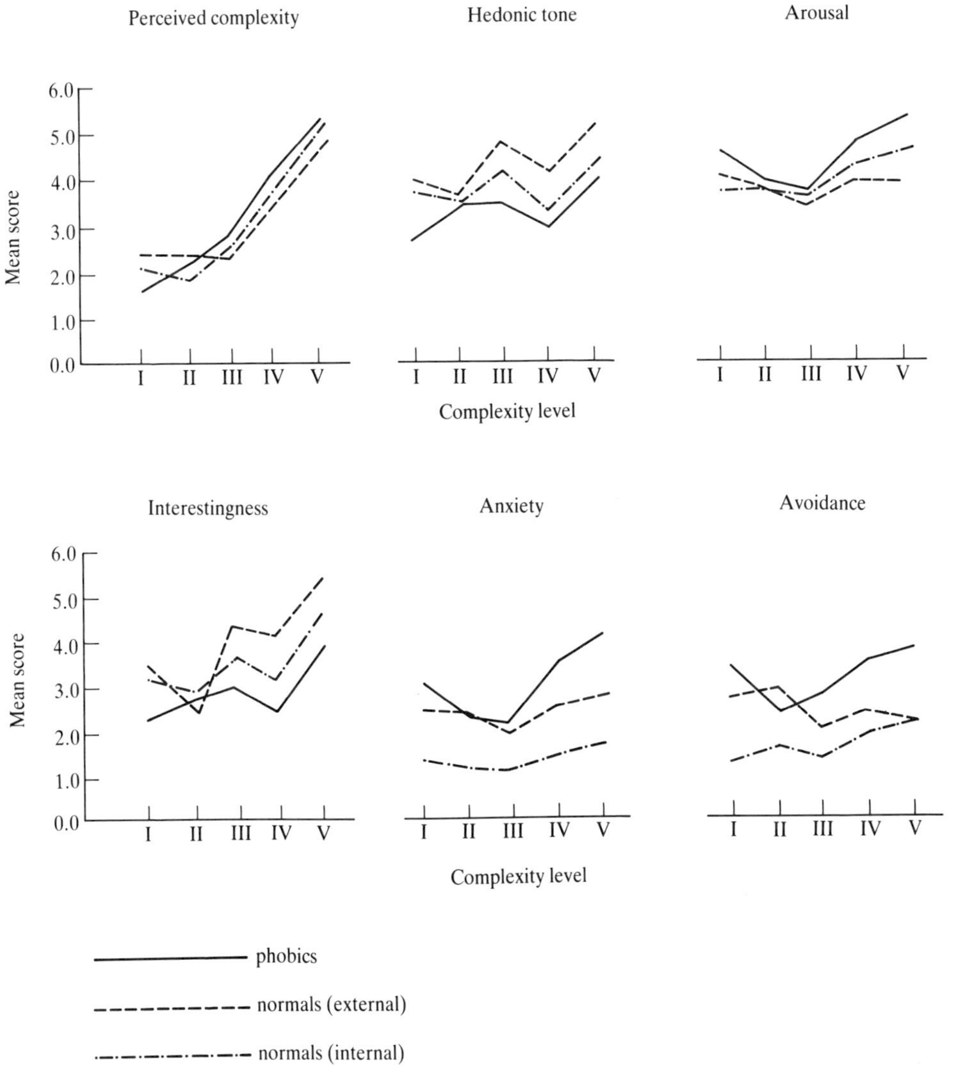

Figure 5.5.2 Relations between stimulus complexity and six experiential variables in streets (normal and phobic subjects)

Relations between avoidance tendency and perceived complexity

Here too analysis of variance and Newman-Keuls analysis revealed similar relations between avoidance tendency and perceived complexity. Significant *main effects* were found on the factors "groups" and "stimulus levels" (respectively, F: 7.85, df: 2/59, p = .001; and F: 5.05, df: 4/236, p = .001), as well as a significant *interaction effect* between them (F: 4.00, df: 8/236, p = .001). Again, all three groups differ significantly, the phobic group showing highest avoidance at all levels excepting level II. The normal groups do not differ significantly in avoidance tendency at level V, but at all other levels the external normal group shows significantly more avoidance tendency than the internal group, and even higher avoidance than the phobic group at level II. In fact, they tend to avoid the lower complexity level situations more than the higher. In contrast, the internal normal group shows little avoidance tendency to the lower three complexity levels, but increasing avoidance tendency at levels IV and V (Figure 5.5.2).

Trend analyses showed that the relation between avoidance tendency and perceived complexity is quadratic F: 15.19, df.: 1/236, $p < .001$). This relation explains 98.7% of the estimated total variance. Neither linear nor other nonlinear relations are significant ($F < 1$). The hypothesis is not supported by these data.

Discussion and Conclusion

In this study the only relations that support Berlyne's, and conform with our expectations as formulated in the hypotheses, are those relating perceived complexity to (objective) uncertainty, and, to some extent, between interestingness and perceived complexity. For all groups, normals and phobics, perceived complexity is mainly a linear, monotonic function of uncertainty. The interestingness of these stimuli is mainly a linear function of perceived complexity, although having significant non-linear components too. On the whole, and for all levels of complexity, these street situations arouse in the phobics significantly less interest than in the normal groups. For phobics, interest increases only for the highest level of complexity, which describe the busyness or bustle of streets. These situations also elicit the highest feelings of pleasure. In contrast to normals, this is one of the characteristics that phobics say makes a street complex (see pilot study, Table 5.5.1). But these situations also elicit the highest feelings of arousal, anxiety and avoidance. To a lesser degree, this applies also to the normal subjects. I will come back to this.

Another interesting finding is that streets characterized by wide, open spaces (and expanses of water) are judged to be more complex by normals than by phobics; but phobics show more subjective arousal, more anxiety, and more avoidance in regard to these situations, as well as less interest. It follows that their hedonic feelings are also less positive in these situations.

Hedonic tone, in this study, is not an inverted-U function of perceived complexity, but a more complex one, with linear and quartic components. Levels I and IV (wide, open spaces and compactness in streets, see Table 5.5.1a) elicit less pleasurable feeling than other levels of complexity in phobics. For both normal and phobic persons, but to a lesser degree in phobics, the street situations that elicit higher hedonic tone are those characterized by symmetry and regularity, and, as said, by busyness and bustle.

Another important difference found in this study, for both phobics and normals, is the relation between arousal and perceived complexity; between anxiety and perceived complexity; and avoidance tendency and perceived complexity. Arousal is not an inverted-U function of perceived complexity but a more complex one, having quadratic and linear components. Anxiety is partly a linear, and partly a quadratic function of perceived complexity. Avoidance is mainly a quadratic function of perceived complexity. This means that subjective arousal, anxiety, and avoidance tendency are higher at lower levels of complexity than at moderate ones and high at high levels. Lowest arousal is felt in moderately complex street situations in which, not surprisingly, greenery, or regularity and symmetry of spaces predominate. Why the difference then? In Berlyne's work and that of others (e.g., Wohlwill; Francès) pictorial stimuli were also used to vary complexity in real-life situations, so the reason for the difference cannot lie in this. Nor does it seem to lie in the fact that the range of stimuli used was too narrow (see table 5.5.1a., where these are described).

A possible explanation for the deviating findings may lie in the nature of the stimuli, in different classes of complexity. Level I is best characterized by open spaces with wide expanses of sky or water, and few occluding or distracting objects. Perspective and distance are emphasized. Level II is mainly characterized by streets that are empty of people (or nearly so), but high in greenery (shrubs, trees, flower beds, grass and shade), that may give an optimal feeling of protected enclosure. This is the only level at which no differences are found between phobics and normals on any of the experiential variables. Level III is more difficult to categorize, but seems to be best described by symmetry, moderate amounts of variety and heterogeneity of arrangement of elements. Level IV is predominantly characterized by compactness of structure (high buildings occluding the spaces, cars chock-a-block in the streets, and so on). Finally, level V is best characterized by the busyness or bustle of streets, people milling around (moving and occluding forms) and traffic. Even the view of a canal, that was generally rated as more pleasing and more interesting than the other city streets, the complexity of the trees' branches budding in spring and occluding the view over the water, the ornate gables, high houses and parked cars give a similar feeling of man and nature cluttering up space.

It is not surprising that quiet streets with lots of foliage and ordinary, everyday scenes (e.g., in a suburban area) will elicit feelings of calm, even sleepy content; hence less interest, less arousal, and little or no anxiety (level II). Nor is it surprising that streets with greater compactness of structure, or with wide, open spaces, and few people present are experienced by these phobic patients and also by normals as to be more disturbing (that is, less pleasurable, more anxiety-evoking, inducing higher arousal, and avoidance tendency). Phobics react to these more extremely, but the difference would seem to be a quantitative, rather than a qualitative one. What is a little more surprising is the finding that the busier the streets are, the more pleasant they seem, the higher interest they seem to elicit, but also the higher is the arousal, anxiety, and avoidance tendency, felt! This is the case not only for phobics but also for normal persons. Do we have here an indication of how conflict may arise, even in normals, by what the environment supplies? Busyness ("*drukte*") is exciting, stimulating, attractive. But it has another side too. It can turn one off: elicit a feeling of being hemmed in, crowded out, overpowered, trodden underfoot by an amorphous mass of people, who are inviting and indifferent to one, at one and the same time.

What these results, taken overall, suggest is that in streets informational uncertainty is probably not the predictor variable we are looking for, to understand phobic responses to such environments. To understand fully why situations of this kind, differing greatly in complexity, can arouse feelings of unpleasure, anxiety and avoidance responses, we may need to take into account the differential effectivity of structural components of another kind than formulated by Berlyne in the six dimensions. That is, in rather more dynamic terms of their optical effects and visual events to which they give rise. Even thinking back to the puzzling results that Wohlwill's study showed, the discrepancy (and dip) found at level 5 in his study, using seven levels of complexity, might be better explained by this differential effectivity on exploration and preference.

As one may recall, the two stimuli differed widely in content at this level, although they contributed equally to judgment of complexity of the level. Of these two environmental stimuli, one depicted a farmstead with ploughed fields, and the other (the one responsible for the dip in preference and exploratory behaviour) depicted a factory in a downtown area of a small town. Judging from the responses in our study to buildings of this kind, and to compactness in streets, as well as to wider, more open spaces, Wohlwill's finding might be better understood in terms of the differential effect of structural components.

In the next chapter we will consider another side of the coin, in looking at individual response patterns which may determine these effects.

VI

The Enemy Within: Strategies of Perceptual Control?

Nonlinearity in Perceptual Response Strategies and Bipolarity of Experience

In the preceding chapter the data presented in the five studies concerned the different response functions of *groups* of phobic and normal persons to some relevant physical parameters of the environment. In this chapter we take a closer look at *individual* variability in the subjects' responses to perceptual variables in these investigated situations.

The idea that an important aspect of phobic perceptual functioning might be concealed by the group analyses of the data (and thus easily overlooked) occurred to me when I noticed that, in general, the normal individuals changed their perceptual responses as the stimulation varied (only 9.1% of normal students in the experiment on depth estimation of H/D ratios showed no variation in response to H/D ratio as a function of scale (size) of the spaces, though they discriminated the different ratios of H/D). In contrast, some of the phobic patients varied their perceptual responses to varying stimulation hardly or not at all. For example, 12.5% of the patients in the H/D ratio experiment showed no variation whatever in response, either to ratios of H/D and B/D, or to scale (size) differences, and 18.8% showed only slight variation in responses to change in stimulation. In the experiment on "collative variables of complexity in abstract stimuli", 33% of the patients showed no or little change in response to the simple figures across categories of complexity. In the experiment on the complexity of streets, one patient showed no variation at all in response to 14 of the 15 stimuli, rating them all as extremely simple and the 15th stimulus as only slightly less simple than the rest. Most patients thus responded maximally or minimally. Others (and some normals) responded extremely to low and high levels of stimulative effects, swinging from minimum to maximum response (or vice versa). This tendency of neurotic persons to respond extremely to stimulus situations has been noticed before (e.g., Van Haasen, 1972; Schaper, 1974), and it is often attributed to a tendency to complain about their suffering. Others have shrugged it off as an artefact of the measurement techniques often employed in clinical studies (i.e., rating scales). I could not do so, since the tendency was also found in the experiment on tunnels and tunnel-like situations (study II), where we made use of the method of constant stimulus differences. In many psychological studies, and certainly in perception work, such extremely deviating responses are usually expunged from the data before analysis, the argument being that these subjects behave as if they do not understand the instruction, and are therefore not responding to stimulus variables as defined. But in our case we could not justifiably say this for it was clear that the patients understood the instructions (which were generally very simple indeed). Also, the different investigators in the different studies remarked on the care, even conscientiousness, with which the individual patients approached, and carried out the task, even when its purpose appeared absurd to them, undoubtedly thinking of the possible importance of these studies for clinical intervention. Normals, on the whole, tended to be more cavalier about their responses; yet, given the results (in Chapter V), were apparently paying more attention to the tasks than may have seemed to be the case.

Yet we found that in not one or two of the experiments, but in all the studies, over a period of roughly eight years, using different patients and different investigators, some individuals would deviate so much in their responses from the group, or from the stimulation presented (some responses remaining the same throughout all changes in stimulation, some going contrary to what one might expect given the task), that stimulus and response did not seem to have a related function for these individuals. We were brought up a little short by this; and intrigued. After examining the data carefully, these apparent fluctuations in response seemed to have a certain consistency in pattern, and yet differ in pattern of response for different individuals. This observation brought to mind Helson's work (1964), and Schneirla's work (1959, 1965). Helson showed that these behaviours are not random but are lawfully determined. Schneirla argued that one's responses are directly related to the nature of environmental stimulation. In brief, Schneirla found that animals and neonates tend to approach weak energies of stimulation, and withdraw from intense sources of stimulation. What is effectively weak or strong though depends on the adaptive state of the organism. Approach and withdrawal, in his view, are not all-or-nothing responses, but manifest varying degrees of acceptance or rejection. This is so at least for normal, non-neurotic behaviour.

Less striking, but equally pervasive, is the tendency to adapt to stimulation in systematic ways. Helson noted that one-to-one correspondence between stimuli and perception, judgment, cognition or memory responses occurs only in special cases. Nonlinearity between stimuli and response is the rule rather than the exception, and is found in all behavioural responses, not only in simple perceptual judgments. That is, responses tend to deviate in an orderly and definite pattern from linearity. Most of these departures from linearity, according to Helson, concern overestimation and underestimation of magnitudes, intensities, qualities and spatial properties of stimuli. They represent ways in which organisms have adapted to their conditions of life (1964, p. 94). Because in this study on perceptual control I assume that this tendency to nonlinearity of response, that is, overestimation and underestimation of magnitudes and ratios of stimulation, may be the linchpin on which perceptual distortion revolves, let us follow Helson's exposé a little further

> "One of the most striking departures from linearity of responses to stimulation is found in overestimation of small magnitudes and underestimation of large magnitudes, with an intermediate range where 'error' is minimal or absent. This double deviation from linearity of response usually takes the form of a negatively accelerated curve in which the lower part of the curve lies above the straight line of unit slope and the upper part of the curve lies below [see Figure 6.1.1] Hollingworth (1910) made this discovery in a study of motor behaviour and referred to it as the 'central tendency' effect ...(.) Later research showed that over-estimation judgments for small values and underestimation judgments for large

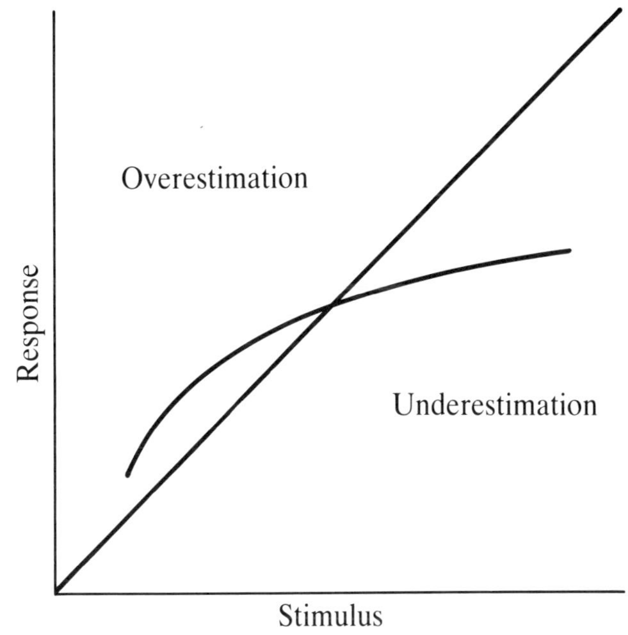

Figure 6.1.1 Departures from linearity of stimulus-response functions tend to result in overestimation of small quantities and underestimation of large quantities as shown in this negatively accelerated curve (taken from Helson, 1964)

> values of stimuli are found only when the adaptation level lies within, and usually near the center of the series being judged. Central tendency is thus a special case of O and U departures from linearity (p. 96).
>
> Cases where small magnitudes are underestimated and large magnitudes are overestimated have been found to occur, but are much less frequent. Occasionally, all stimuli in a group are underestimated or overestimated, deviations from linearity occurring in one direction only. This is the case, for instance, when anchor stimuli at the high end of the continuum lower the judgments by raising adaptation level, or those at the low end raise the judgments by lowering adaptation level" (1964, p. 100).

When no anchor stimuli are present in a series, stimuli are judged with respect to internal norms that represent the pooled effects of past and present stimulation. Adaptation level is a function of past and present stimulation, and is generally defined as "the weighted geometric mean of focal, background and residual stimuli". Adaptation level can be understood as the neutral level that a perceiver reaches as a function of all the stimuli (internal and external) operating at a given moment in his or her perceptual activity. It is comparable to the point of subjective equality in psychophysics theory. Although this neutral level of adaptation determines behaviour, in Helson's view, it is not the same as a cognitive style or trait. It is a function of changing levels of stimulation. Adaptation level theory takes into account that a person to a large extent can determine the nature and degree of stimulation that is received by selective processes (e.g., by "gating" of stimulation, walking around in the environment, and so on).

The processes involved in this behaviour have sometimes been described in the clinical and social psychology literature in terms of the concepts *contrast* and *assimilation*. When differences in judgments of scale items are enhanced, or displaced away from the judgments of the anchor stimulus, contrast is said to be operative. When differences in judgment are reduced, or displaced towards the judgments of the anchor stimulus, assimilation is said to be operative. Contrast denotes difference, repulsion, complementarism and movement away from the attributes or position of an object, whereas assimilation denotes likeness, attraction and movement towards these attributes or position. But, as Helson stresses, these processes are complementary, not independent as is sometimes thought. They go together, and are not independent of the situations in which they are manifested (Helson, 1964, p. 225).

In Helson's book, in which he is mainly concerned with demonstrating the empirical bases for his theory of adaptation-level, these patterns of overestimation and underestimation are defined in terms of the adaptation level of the individual. But the experiments from which the data to be discussed are derived were not planned with an eye to determining the adaptation level of the individual; so no measurements of the actual point of adaptation to the series of stimuli can be made, since neither the focal, background or residual stimuli impinging on the person can be exactly determined. But I did find one study in which he illustrated overestimations and underestimations in a perceptual or cognitive task (judgments of attributes) by taking the means for the stimuli in the sample as approximations of the true values for the stimuli, and expressing overestimations and underestimations in terms of deviations from the means relative to the distribution of scores per stimulus. These values may have been based on larger groups than the ones on which I shall try to demonstrate similar patterns of response. At least, I could not ascertain how large these groups were from the text and table illustrating this, since no further data were given.

This brings me to one difficulty concerning the problem of measurement. In the literature on perception, the problem of intra-individual variability is given little attention. Most textbooks are concerned with establishing perceptual functions and relations between functions, and are thus concerned with data for large groups, or inter-individual variability which is expressed in terms of relative error, or in terms of, for example, per cent frequency of a given exponent for different attributes (e.g., length, area, volume). So our choice of analysis is somewhat arbitrary, and subject to criticism. Another difficulty about the data used to illustrate the point I wish to make lies in its *ad hoc* character. Since the data were obtained for a different purpose, these can only indicate the possible operation of perceptual control mechanisms, not prove this in any way. To do so, proper experiments designed for such purpose must be carried out. Still, given the consistency in patterns of response across the years, in patients in different categories of complaint, my hunch is that we are on to something more real than fluctuations due to chance factors. And it is this hunch that makes me feel it will not be entirely a waste of time to consider, and ponder, the implications of these data, in spite of the *ad hoc* analysis.

In discussing the differences between normal and phobic persons in the following pages, I will refer to the departures from linearity in their perceptual responses to the stimuli as *strategies* of perceptual control. I do this for two reasons. Mainly because the term carries the connotation of *active* participation of the person in the process, whereas a more neutral term, such as pattern, does not. But active participation does not imply conscious manipulation of levels of stimulation; more often than not this manipulatory activity is unconscious. Secondarily, to remind the reader that what we are concerned with is not a cognitive style, in the sense that, for instance, Witkin (1965) uses the term, as a personality trait; but with perceptual behaviour that changes and adapts, or should change and adapt, as the situation changes.

Although 110 normal persons and 82 phobic patients participated altogether in the studies mentioned in Chapter V, not all of their data were suitable or available for further analysis. The procedure used in the first study on tunnels yielded data unsuitable for this analysis. The individual data of the normal subjects in study III (H/D ratio experiment concerned with ratings of perceived enclosure) were unfortunately no longer available, but the data for normal subjects on depth estimation as a function of the same H/D and B/D ratios of architectural spaces were available. Although not strictly comparable then, I have used them to illustrate the point I wish to make. In study IV (collative variables of complexity in abstract stimuli) only phobic patients participated. The data from these subjects cannot be compared with the data from the normal subjects, but they are included also because they further illustrate my point. Only the data from study II (tunnels and tunnel-like situations) and study V (perceived complexity in street situations) include phobic responses and the responses of normal controls. To limit ourselves only to a consideration of these might be sounder (statistical) strategy, but would considerably weaken the argument, which is based on its demonstrability in different patients of different categories of complaint, over different years, and under different task conditions. The data from study II are considered last, because a deviating procedure was used (method of constant stimulus differences), in which the stimuli in a series were compared with a standard or anchor lying within the series and near the centre of the series. This procedure, as Helson predicts, gives more similarity in "strategy" within a series between persons (that is, generally results in an overestimation of low ratios and underestimation of high ratios of stimulation).

Only after analysing all of the data in all the experiments in the way which I will shortly present, did I consult the intake-cards of the patients to determine the nature of the individual complaints. The nature of the complaint classification was formulated in intake-reports made independently by the psychiatrist in charge of patient admittance, and transferred to intake-cards which were filed, by the secretary for therapy affairs, in the dossiers of our departmental clinic.

I first converted all the raw scores of all the subjects in a given investigation into standardized scores, that is, their individual scores were expressed as deviations from the means for the whole group (normals and phobics; or phobics only in cases where no normals participated), for each stimulus (ratio or level of stimulation) in the series, and relative to the distributions of the scores for the particular ratio or level of stimulation concerned, for the relevant groups of subjects. These z-scores are therefore an expression of the distance of the raw score from the mean, measured with the standard deviation as the unit, for each stimulus. In other words, these z-scores give the relative sizes of deviations about the mean (the absolute sizes of deviations depend on artefacts of measurement). By this conversion, the scores can be compared in a satisfactory way. This also means that z-scores of positive value define overestimations (or have the meaning of "above the mean") for a particular stimulus (ratio); and z-scores of negative value define underestimations (or have the meaning of "below the mean") for a particular stimulus (ratio). One should also bear in mind that in these experiments, the raw score does not represent one observation of an individual in response to a given stimulus; but depending on the study, may be based on the mean value of three, or as much as eight, observations per individual, obtained in a randomized and counterbalanced procedure in the presentation of the varying stimulus levels or ratios.

I formed the subgroups in the different investigations after this conversion of their raw scores and before knowing their complaint classification (except for the group as a whole), by grouping together those subjects who appeared to manifest the same "strategy", that is, by subjects manifesting overestimation or underestimation as defined, or combinations of overestimation and underestimation, over a series of stimuli (or ratios of stimulation). Analyses of variance, using the raw scores as the bases for analysis, were later carried out on the data of the different subgroups. We will now consider these strategies of control, for each study separately.

In the study of *architectural spaces* (Study III, Chapter V), as one may recall, the 32 phobic patients and 22 normals rated the openness-enclosure of these spaces; and 33 normals also estimated the depth, as a function of H/D ratios present in the spaces. Each stimulus ratio was viewed for 10 seconds, and judged three times in a randomized order, on a five-point bipolar scale (in the study "perceived enclosure"), and in the depth estimation task, by using a comparison stimulus representing 30 units, which did not appear in the series. The subject was asked to say 60 if the size of a space seemed to be twice as large as that of the standard with which it was compared, to say 15, if it seemed half as large, etc. In Table 6.2a and b, in Appendix B, the means and standard deviations for the groups are given (normals: depth estimation; phobics: perceived enclosure of the spaces) as a function of H/D and B/D ratios; as well as mean z-scores for the subgroups, showing different "strategies".

Figures 6.1.2a and b illustrate these response strategies of the normal subgroups (depth estimation) and the phobic subgroups (perceived enclosure). ([N1–N4 and P1–P7 refer to the subgroups of normal and phobic persons. N5 and P8 belong to subgroups N4 and P5 respectively, but are lifted out to illustrate how extreme some individual responses are.]

Among the *normal* subjects (psychology students) we see that eighteen students (subgroup N1) underestimate the depth of the spaces, regardless of the H/D ratio levels (that is, their standardized scores fall below the means, for all four levels). Six students (subgroup N2) overestimate the depth of the spaces when H/D ratios are low and underestimate it when H/D ratios are high. Four students (subgroup N3) underestimate depth when H/D ratios are low and overestimate it when H/D ratios are high. Five students (subgroup N4) overestimate the depth, regardless of H/D ratio levels. One of these students (subgroup N5) shows a highly erratic pattern of overestimation of all H/D ratio levels. In fact, three of the five overestimators of all levels (subgroup N4) show highly deviating responses.

Among the *phobic* subjects, in the experiment with varying B/D ratios, when the B/D ratio is high (= 1.00) four patients (subgroup P1) underestimate the enclosure of spaces, regardless of H/D ratio levels. Three patients (subgroup P2) overestimate enclosure when H/D ratios are low and underestimate enclosure when H/D are high. Six patients (subgroup P3) underestimate enclosure when H/D ratios are low and overestimate it when H/D ratios are high. Three patients (subgroup P4) overestimate

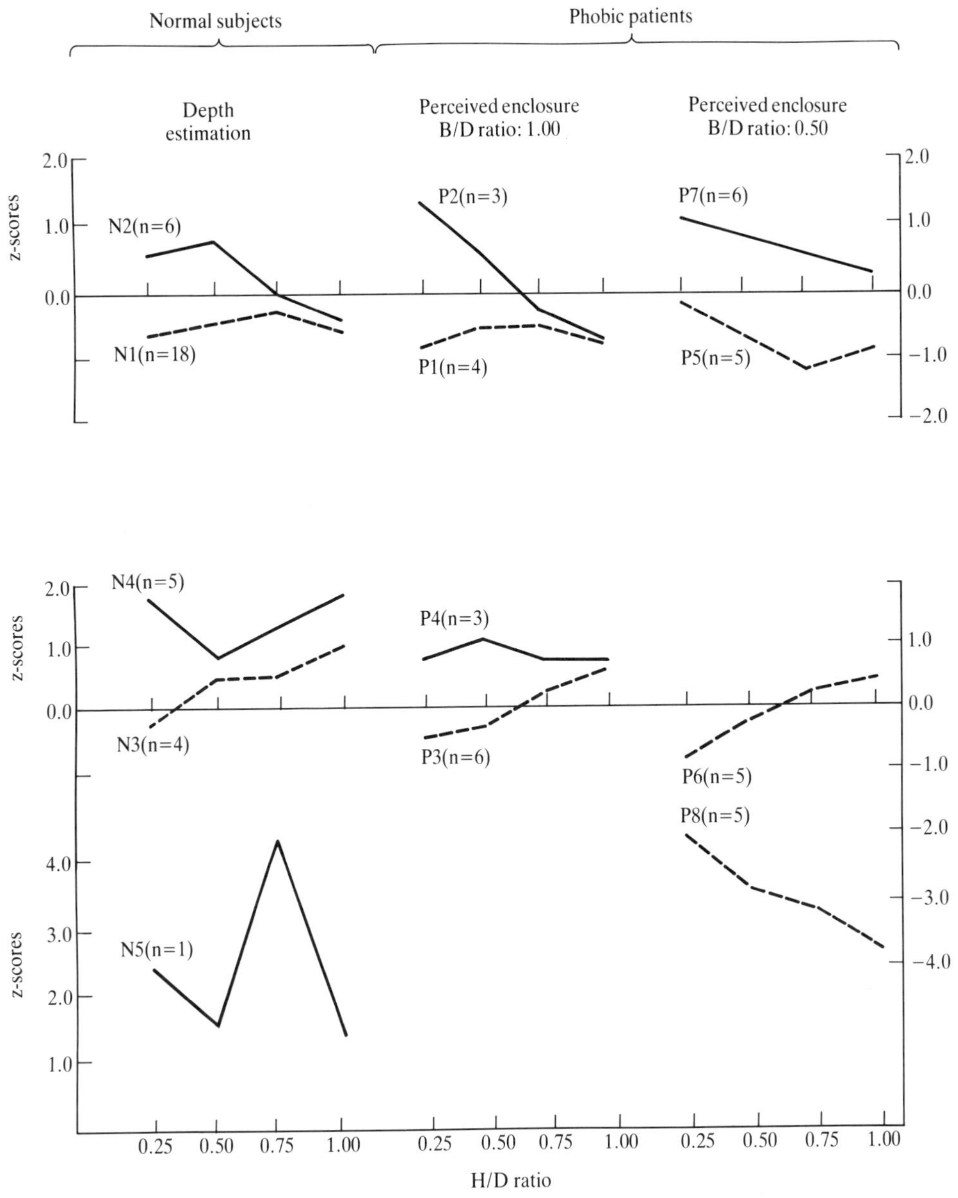

Figure 6.1.2 (a) Strategies of perceptual control (normal subjects); (b) strategies of perceptual control (phobic patients) (Study III)

enclosure, regardless of H/D ratio levels. When the B/D ratio is halved (= .50), five patients (subgroup P5) underestimate enclosure, regardless of H/D ratio levels, and one patient especially [subgroup P8] underestimates enclosure of the spaces to an extreme degree. Five patients (subgroup P6) underestimate enclosure when H/D ratios are low and overestimate it when H/D ratios are high. Six patients (subgroup P7) overestimate enclosure, regardless of H/D ratio levels. In fact, four of these patients responded to all changes in levels of H/D ratio with the maximum possible response (a score of 5 points), and the other two with a near-maximum response (a score of 4). These extreme responses are not reflected in the tables as extremely high deviations, because the group means are based on the scores of only the phobic subjects, the data for the normals in the same experiment being no longer available at the time of this analysis.

For the purpose of analysis of variance, to obtain as large groups as possible, subgroups of these patients were formed, on the basis of apparent strategy, now using the raw scores as the basis (in case of eventual contamination of the data in the conversion into z-scores). This analysis of variance (with subjects nested under strategy) show that the *four subgroups of patients* differ significantly in strategy (F: 42.42, df 3/28, p = .001); also, significant differences between strategies (F: 13.84, df: 3/84, p = .001) are found. And significant interaction effects exist between groups, levels and kind of strategy (F: 10.05 df: 9/84, p = .001). Analysis of variance (with subjects nested under strategy) were also carried out for the normal subgroups (depth estimation). Again, this analysis showed that the *four subgroups of normals* differ significantly in strategy (F: 30.16, df: 3/29, p = .001); that significant differences exist between strategies (F: 3.10, df: 3/87, p = .031); and that significant interaction effects exist too (F: 3.51 df: 9/87, p = .001).

In the study on *collative variables in abstract stimuli* (Study IV, Chapter V), the 24 phobic patients judged two sets of slides representing six classes of complexity, each set depicting a simple and a complex level. As one may recall, the mainly geometric figures represented six dimensions of complexity (number of elements, heterogeneity of elements, irregularity of shape or contour, irregularity of arrangement of elements, incongruity, and incongruous juxtaposition). Perceived complexity was determined by the mean ratings of the individual on *three* seven-point complexity scales. Table 6.1 in Appendix B shows the means and standard deviations for these stimuli, according to the class and level of complexity, and mean z-scores for the different subgroups (again, formed according to similarity in strategy, as earlier defined). Figure 6.1.3 depicts the relations of overestimation and underestimation of the different levels of complexity for the subgroups.

Sixteen, mainly agoraphobic, patients (subgroup P1) underestimate both simple and complex levels of stimulation across *all* classes of complexity. Five other patients (subgroup P2) overestimate both simple and complex levels in the lower categories of complexity and underestimate the higher categories. Two patients, with mixed complaints of agoraphobia and claustrophobia, show similar overestimation of both simple and complex levels in the lower categories, and underestimation of levels of complexity in the higher categories, but do so more extremely (subgroup P3). One patient, a claustrophobic (subgroup P4) greatly overestimates all but one of the stimuli, whether these are simple or complex, regardless of the category of complexity.

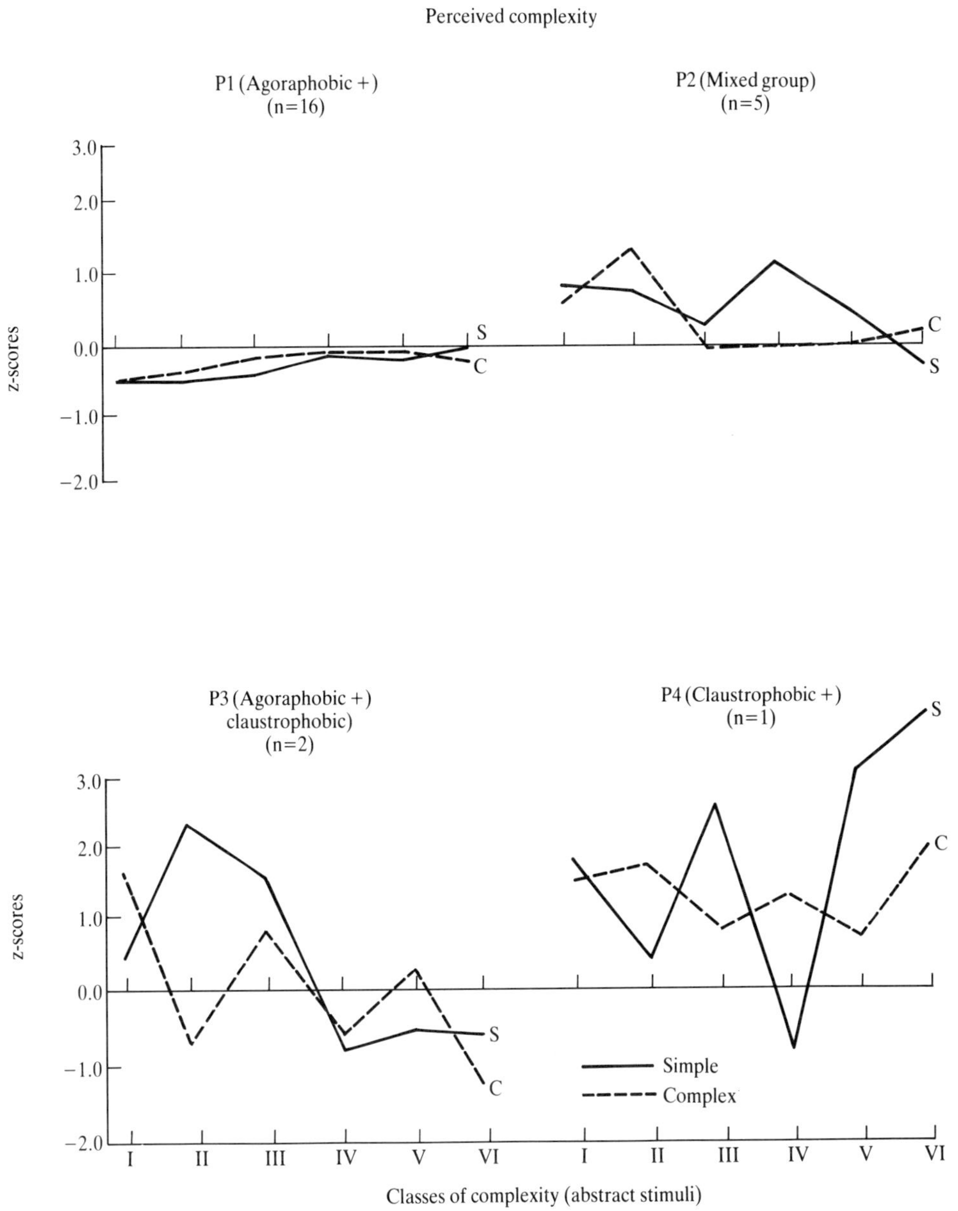

Figure 6.1.3 Strategies of perceptual control (Agoraphobics) (Collative variables, Study IV)

Analysis of variance (with subjects nested under strategy), also based on the raw scores of the different individuals in the subgroups, shows that the *three phobic subgroups* differ significantly in kind of strategy (F: 20.43, df: 2/21, $p = .001$); that significant differences exist between these strategies, as a function of "simple" and "complex" levels of stimulation (F: 144.20, df: 1/21, $p = .001$); and significant interaction effects between levels and strategies (F: 4.33, df: 2/21, $p = .027$) too.

Significant differences also exist between classes of complexity (F: 8.65, df: 5/105, p = .001); between classes of complexity, levels simple-complex, and kind of strategy (F: 10.82, df: 5/105, p = .001); and significant interaction effects (F: 2.30, df: 10/105, p = .018).

A note to the reader: In the different studies the main effects of subgroups in the analyses of variance are all highly significant. This is of course not surprising, given the fact that they have been grouped together according to apparent differences in response strategies. But, bearing in mind that the mean scores for individuals in each subgroup are based on at least three, and in some studies eight observations per person, this suggests a certain stability in the strategy of the individual.

In the investigation on *complexity of street scenes* (Study V, Chapter V), 50 normal persons and 12 phobic patients rated these pictorial stimuli (15 street scenes) on perceived complexity. The stimuli were presented in randomized order and in a Latin square sequence to control for order and sequence effects. The individual persons viewed each scene for one minute and then rated each on *three* seven-point complexity scales. The individual's perceived complexity score for each complexity level is the average of the ratings on three different stimuli per category, on the three seven-point scales. Table 6.1d in Appendix B shows the means and standard deviations for the stimuli on perceived complexity in streets, for normal and phobic groups, and mean z-scores for the different subgroups, classified according to similarity in perceptual strategy, as earlier defined. Figure 6.1.4 depicts the relationships of overestimation and underestimation in perceived complexity for the normal and phobic subgroups.

Twenty-two *normal* subjects (subgroup N1) overestimate the perceived complexity of relatively simple street scenes and underestimate the complexity of the highly complex street scenes. Two of them (subgroup N4) greatly overestimate the lower levels of complexity and underestimate greatly the higher levels. Seventeen other normals (subgroup N2) underestimate the complexity of all the street scenes, in all categories of complexity. Nine normals (subgroup N3) underestimate the levels of complexity in the lower categories and overestimate the levels in the higher categories.

Among the *phobic* patients, three (subgroup P1) underestimate the levels of complexity in the lower categories and overestimate those in the higher categories of complexity Four patients (subgroup P2) greatly underestimate all levels of complexity in all categories. Three patients (subgroup P3) underestimate the level of complexity in the lowest category, and greatly overestimate all other levels in the other categories of complexity. And two other patients (subgroup P4) overestimate all levels of complexity in streets, but particularly those of the two highest categories of complexity.

For purposes of analysis of variance, subgroup N4 was placed in subgroup N1, since these persons show the same strategy, only in more extreme form. For the same reasons, and because of too small groups otherwise, subgroups P1 and P4 were combined. Because normals showed no pattern of overestimation of all levels of complexity, and phobics showed no pattern of overestimation of low levels of complexity and underestimation of high levels, the normal and phobic groups could not be compared as to strategy by analysis of variance, but they were compared by means of Chi-square analysis. Analyses of variance (with persons nested under strategies) show that the *three normal subgroups* differ significantly in kind of strategy (F: 27.94, df: 2/47, p = .001); that significant differences exist between the five different

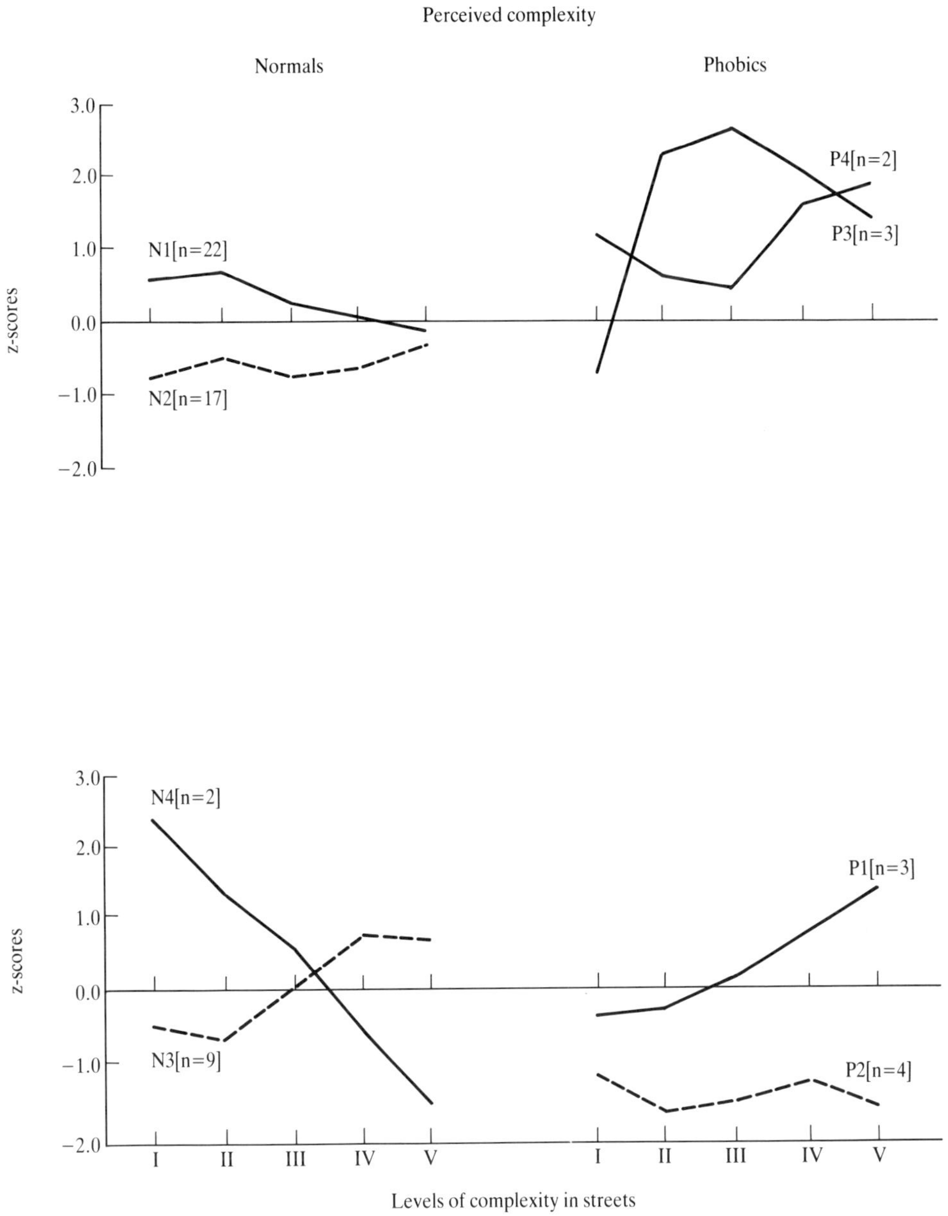

Figure 6.1.4 Strategies of perceptual control (Street experiment, Study V)

levels of complexity (F: 115.02, df: 4/188, p = .001); and significant interaction effects exist between groups, levels, and kind of strategy (F: 3.51, df: 8/188, p = .001). The *three phobic subgroups* differ significantly too in kind of strategy (F: 13.56, df: 2/9, p = .002); significant differences exist between levels of complexity (F: 31.86, df: 4/36, p = .001); but no significant interaction is found between groups, levels and strategy. Chi-square analysis shows further that the normal and phobic groups differ

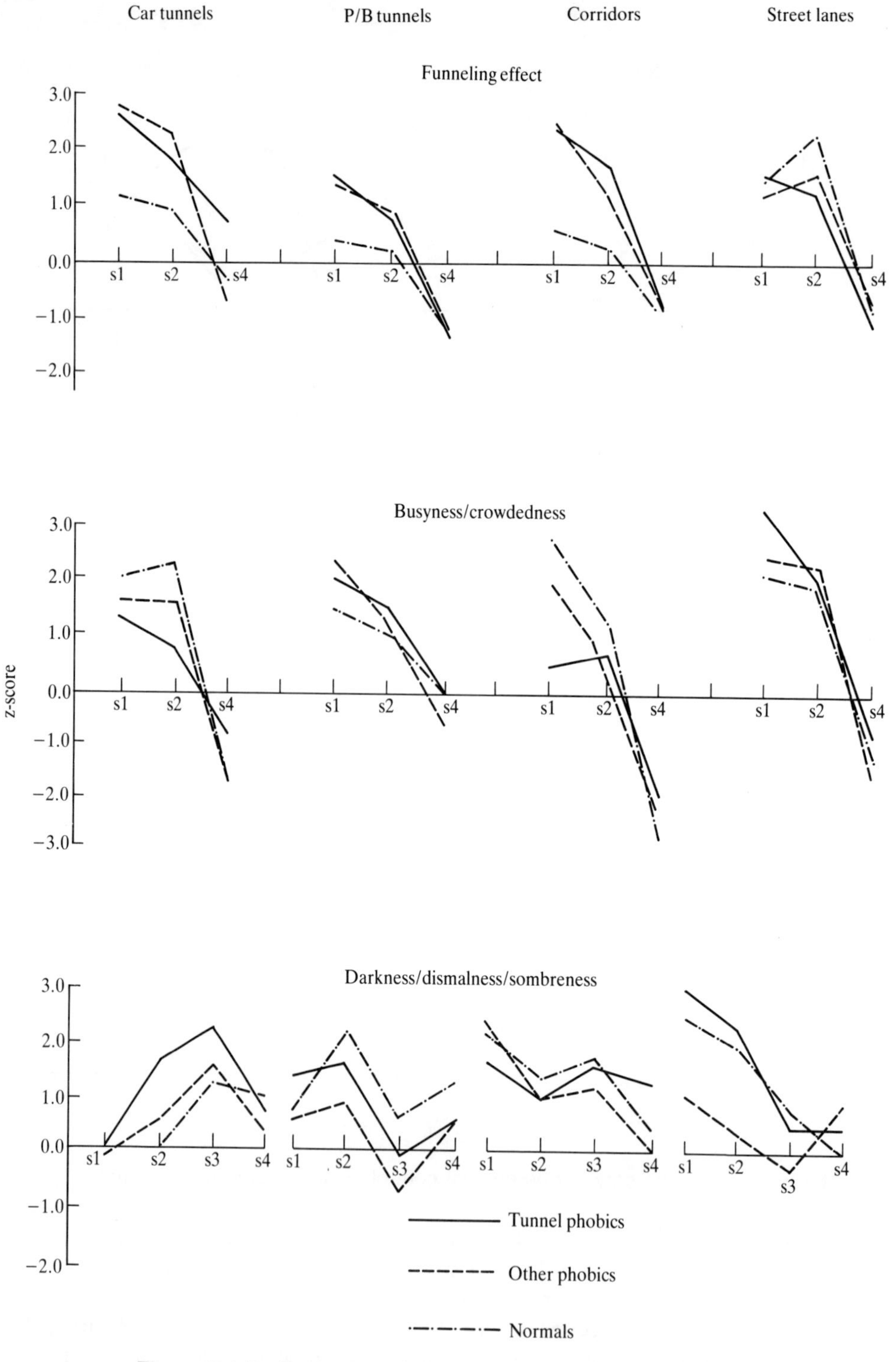

Figure 6.1.5 Strategies of perceptual control (groups) Study II

significantly in strategy (χ^2: P/N: 20.677, df: 3, p <.001). This difference is due to the fact that phobics, but no normals in this study, use a strategy of overestimation of both low and high levels of complexity, and normals, but no phobics, use a strategy of overestimation of low levels of complexity and underestimation of high levels.

In the investigation of *tunnels and tunnel-like situations* (Study II, Chapter V), five tunnelphobics (all with claustrophobia as main complaint), five other phobics (two social phobics, two with a fear of death, disease and/or blood, one animal phobic for snakes and reptiles), and five normal persons judged different characteristics of the above-mentioned situations in a paired comparison design (method of constant stimulus differences). The judged experiential characteristics were, as one may recall, "funneling effect", linked to H/D and B/D ratios of these spaces, "busyness or crowdedness", linked to number of people or vehicles present in the spaces, and "darkness, dismalness or sombreness", linked to illumination ratios. Each level of each variable was judged by each individual eight times in randomized order and counterbalanced for sequence effects. The person was asked merely to say which of the two stimuli presented contained *more* of the characteristic in question. The scores for each individual, for each experiential level, were expressed in percentage correct for that level. These percentages were then converted into z-scores. Table 6.1e in Appendix B shows the mean z-scores for the phobic and normal subgroups for the different classes of situations, and for the three experiential variables investigated. (One should keep in mind that when the subject has a 50% correct response rate, this yields a z-score of 0.00, and a 75% correct response rate yields a z-score value of .68. All negative z-scores indicate <50% error; z-scores of + 3.30 indicate maximum correct, z-scores of – 3.30 indicate maximum error on this task.)

We are already familiar with the graphic relations between the experiential values obtained in this study, and objective ratios or magnitudes of stimulation present in the different situations. These are repeated as a means of comparison with the data of the individual phobic patients and normal subjects with strongly deviating values. Figures 6.1.5 and 6.1.6 depict these relations for all three experiential characteristics in the four classes of situations. (Each point on the graphs for phobics represents the mean of 80 observations; for normals the mean of 40 observations).

From the graphs we can see more clearly that on the experiential variable "busyness or crowdedness" in car tunnels and corridors normals and phobics, as a group, err highly in their judgments on the highest level present. Individual deviations from the general trends, which do not follow the stimulation at all well, are shown in Figure 6.1.6. We see that three of the five normals (but especially n1), in different situations, and for different variables, err greatly in their judgments of the levels of the variables present in the scenes, especially on the lowest and highest levels. To obtain an error score larger than 50% (negative z-value) on the lowest level of a given variable, one must overestimate the level of the variable present, since the standard with which it is compared is fixed at level 3 (excepting for the variable "darkness"). In other words, one in fact says more than 50% of the time that level 1 has *more* of the given characteristic than level 3. It follows that to obtain an error score larger than 50% on the highest level of a given variable, one must underestimate this level, in comparison to level 3. Overestimation of low, and underestimation of high levels occur when the standard stimulus lies within the series being judged and near the centre of the series (Helson, p. 220). Among the phobic patients, we see that two tunnelphobic patients

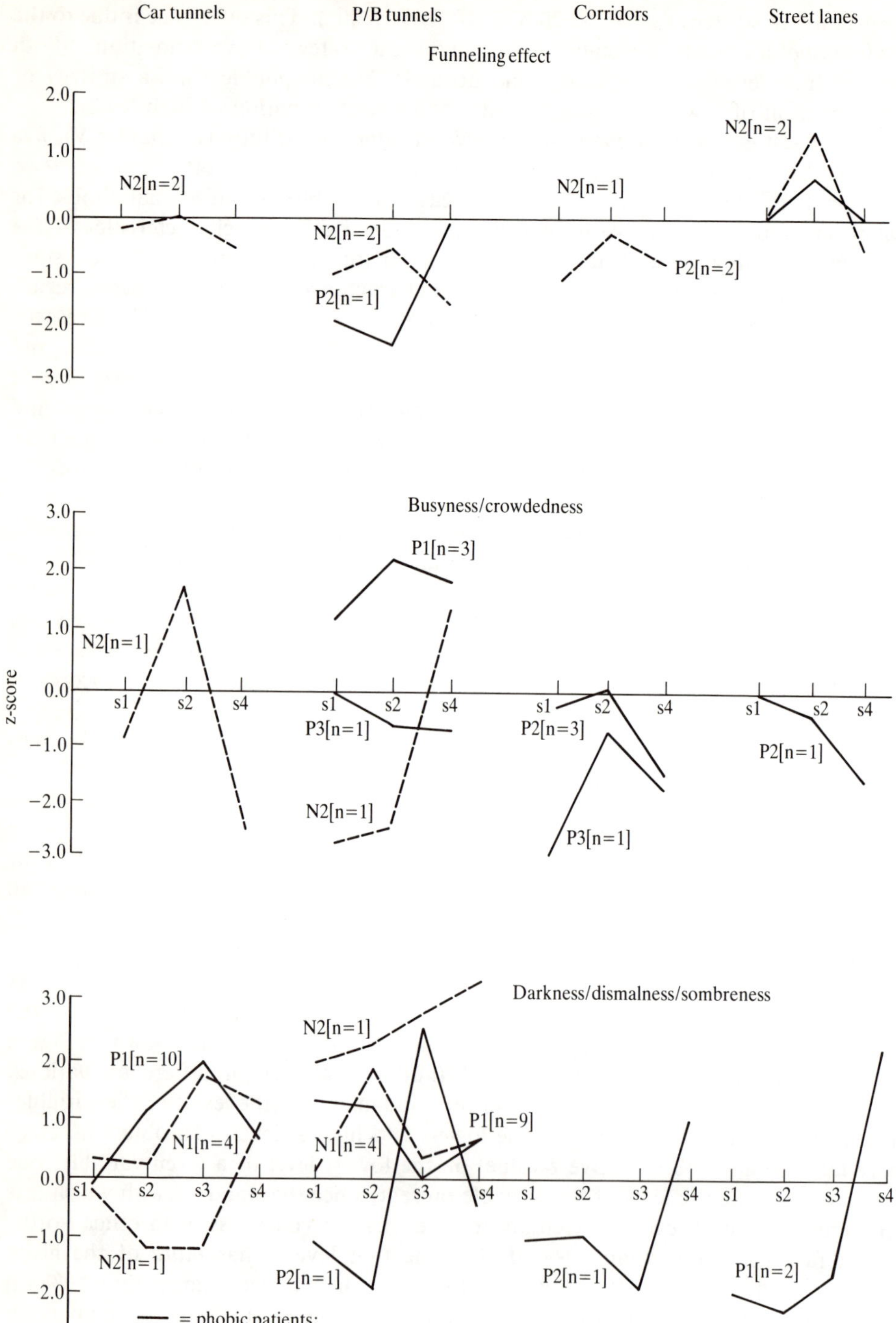

— = phobic patients;

--- = normal subjects; see text for clarification of these individual strategies

Figure 6.1.6 Strategies of perceptual control (individual subjects) Study II and two social phobic patients show large error (that is, extreme overestimation or underestimation of the variables) of some of the variables in different classes of situations, particularly on the variables "busyness or crowdedness", and "darkness, dismalness or sombreness". Some show sometimes near maximum or maximum error in their judgments, although not always on the same variables.

When we consider these deviations from linearity and the different strategies they seem to reveal, over all the investigations, certain relations between under- and/or overestimation of ratios, magnitudes, or characteristics of stimulation and the nature of the main complaint of individual phobic subjects come to the fore. Table 6.2. shows the number of persons in each category, their main complaints, and the strategy of adaptation to the stimulation. Although the numbers of persons in the different categories are relatively few, there does seem to be more than a coincidental relation between main complaint and strategy. It is also possible that the fit is not a better one because so many of these patients suffered from mixed complaints.

The distribution of the phobic patients and normal subjects over the strategy categories is not due to chance but highly significant (X2: P/N: 21.072, df: 3,

Table 6.2 Strategies of adaptation to stimulation (overestimation and underestimation) found in phobic and normal persons in the different experiments, showing number and percentages of persons per category

Response strategy to stimulation	N	O-low & U-high stim. n	%	O-low & O-high stim. n	%	U-low & U-high stim. n	%	U-low & O-high stimulation n	%	%
Phobic patients	78	12	15.4	20	25.0	29	37.2	17	21.8	100
Normal subjects	88	35	39.8	5	5.6	35	39.8	13	14.8	100
Strategies of phobic patients differentiated according to the nature of the complaint:										N
Main complaint + subsidiary complaint										
Agoraphobia + death + disease + travel + claustro/social phobia		5	41.7	8	40.0	22	75.9	6	35.3	41
Claustrophobia + acro- + social + agora-phobia + depression		5	41.7	10	50.0	4	13.8	4	23.5	23
Social phobia + agora- + claustrophobia + death/disease phobia		0	0.0	2	10.0	3	10.3	6	35.3	11
Other phobias: storm + wind + animal phobia + death/blood phobia + neurotic depression + aggression anxiety		2	16.6	0	0.0	0	0.0	1	5.9	3
No. & % phobics per category		12	100	20	100	29	100	17	100	78

O = overestimation of stimulation; U = underestimation. Classification of the different subjects over the categories is based on their response patterns to different levels of stimulation in the series (z-values)

$p = .0001$). The distribution of the phobic patients over categories is also highly significant (X2: 25.74, df: 9, $p = .005$). Significant differences also exist between phobics with different *main complaints* (Ag./C1: X2 = 8.59, df: 3, $p = .035$; Ag./SP: X2 = 8.581, df: 3, $p = .035$; C1./SP: X2 = 10.136, df: 3, $p = .015$) in response strategy. Compared to claustrophobics and social phobics, agoraphobics adapt significantly more often to stimulation by underestimating all levels of stimulation. Compared to agoraphobics and social phobics, claustrophobics adapt significantly more often to stimulation by overestimating both low and high levels of stimulation. And compared to agoraphobics and claustrophobics, social phobics adapt significantly more often to stimulation by underestimating low levels and overestimating high levels of stimulation. In contrast, compared to phobics, normals seem to adapt significantly more often to varying levels of stimulation by overestimating the lower levels and underestimating the higher levels; and significantly less often by overestimating both low and high levels of stimulation. From the tables and graphs we saw too that the normal subjects respond less extremely than phobics to different levels or ratios of stimulation.

If one may say then that slight overestimation of low levels, ratios or characteristics of stimulation and slight underestimation of high levels, ratios, or characteristics (that is, less than 30% over- and underestimation) is much the best way to cope with varying and often extreme ratios of stimulation in daily life (see Helson, 1964; Gregory, 1974; Ross, 1974), then it would seem that other variants of this theme, especially when these include extreme over- and/or underestimation of stimulation, will sometimes lead to gross misperception of stimulation, or yield distortions in the perceived environment. To my mind, one can understand well enough that if behaviour is to be optimal, one must increase the discriminability of low energy levels (by a process of contrast or a highlighting of differences) and defuse the impact of high energy levels (by a process of assimilation or reducing differences). In this way one will undoubtedly keep a greater range of stimulation within manageable bounds, thereby achieving a proper control over differing or varying stimulation. Of course, in doing so, some loss of information inevitably will be incurred. But the loss may well be worth the advantage gained, that is, control over many more situations. Other strategies, though not without advantage in adverse situations or under extreme conditions (think, for instance, of environments at the polar circles; floods; hurricanes; electric storms), may have disadvantages even more severe. For instance, when one repeatedly and greatly overestimates both low and high ratios of stimulation, this implies that the effects of all energies impinging on the person will be maximized. For the internal reference condition (or adaptation level) is not being readjusted as the stimulation changes, and perception, being a continuous process, inevitably will show substantial error between (the matching of) actual input and the internal reference level. Objects and structures in the environment may then begin to appear unstable, fluctuate, "loom" or close in rapidly on one (and thereby seem to threaten), as a result of the increasing error in the output.

The opposite phenomenon may take place when one repeatedly and greatly underestimates both low and high ratios of stimulation. In this case, all incoming stimulation is thereby reduced, and the discriminability of environmental relations will be substantially poorer since fewer differences are discerned. Again, the internal reference condition, matched with the incoming stimulation, may yield large error, since it does not adjust as the stimulation changes. The stability of objects and structures may become at risk too, because of the large discrepancy that might exist over time. Objects and structures may then appear to be unstable, as if being sucked into a black hole. Under such conditions, feelings of disorientation, derealization and depersonalization may, perhaps, arise. Extreme underestimation of low, and overestimation of high ratios of stimulation will combine the disadvantages of the other two strategies, with little advantage in doing so, for only a small range of intermediate stimulation might remain under control. The world may appear to such a person as full of contrast and conflict, and fluctuating; now coming up close, now receding or disappearing. One might well feel as if there is no place to rest one's head or body, being either underwhelmed to a point of extreme boredom, or overwhelmed by opposing effects. In all three cases, perceptual control is either defective, in danger of being lost, or lost. Performance must then deteriorate as the actions of the person become more disorganized and his or her orientation disturbed.

Environmental Structure, Adaptation, and Perceptual Experience: Is Scaling-misapplication, or Conflict Control the Heart of the Matter?

What has just been postulated to be the case in the experience of the world if one greatly overestimates or underestimates ratios or magnitudes of stimulation sounds plausible enough, but it is not at all clear *why* this should be so. Nor, in spite of almost a century of interest in illusions and distortions of a perceptual nature is there any certain answer to the why of this (Von Helmholtz, 1890; Stratton, 1896–7; Kohler, 1951; more recently, Gregory, 1973–81; Epstein et al., 1977; Harris, 1963a–1980, to name a few researchers).

There is a growing understanding of *what* changes, about the *outcome* of adaptation, but not so much that we know how to predict whether and when these changes will occur. To say nothing about the lack of consensus on the influence of many variables in the interactions between visual and haptic systems on this behaviour (see also Harris, 1980).

Yet it does not seem to be mere coincidence that the "cues" in the environment that assist us (or hinder us) in achieving and maintaining stability and constancy of our environment are exactly those which we found in our investigations to be good predictors of anxiety and avoidance behaviours. Some of the variables investigated by us, and others, have long been the focus of interest in the study of illusions, and been shown to be greatly effective in achieving constancy and stability of objects and other spatio-temporal relations.

For instance, height-distance ratio expresses the relation of object size and distance, and is positively correlated to retinal angle size. Height-distance ratio is thus but a different index of retinal angle subtended by an object, one of the most vital of constancy scaling cues. But also cues to linear perspective and density texture are givens in these relations. Illumination ratios, aerial perspective or relative brightness of surfaces are other potent constancy scaling cues. So is overlap, shadow or occlusion of objects in space. If too densely spaced, this can lead to compactness, which will work against achieving constancy. Unoccluded space too (that is, wide, open spaces free of objects or shadow) is prohibitive of constancy, since few cues exist to enable us to judge distances, sizes, shapes, slants and slopes in the terrain. Heterogeneity of arrangements will undoubtedly hinder the achievement of constancy, because this may provide distraction or induce conflict.

Gregory (1973–1981) and Ross (1974) suggest that when environmental structure is systematically distorted, this may be due either to some calibration upset in perceptual mechanisms which remains uncorrected, thus generating error; or due to the fact that perceptual models or "hypotheses" remain unmodified because the information available is inappropriate to the prevailing reality, thus generating distortion illusions (see Chapter II). The representation of three-dimensional settings in a two-dimensional way (as in all our experiments) will yield distortions of this kind, for the abovementioned reasons. They show how this could occur. Normally, real objects become optically *smaller* in the distance. However, the brain enlarges distant objects so as to compensate for the decrease in retinal image size: the result is that the apparent decrease in size is much less than might be expected from the smaller image. Similarly, the brain reduces (minimizes) near objects so as to compensate for the increase in retinal image size, so that the apparent increase is much less than might be expected from the larger image. This compensatory mechanism is known as "size-constancy". When there is a discrepancy between the true distance and the apparent distance, the apparent size is correspondingly distorted. These compensatory mechanisms are postulated in all perceptual systems. According to Gregory, the constancy principle is apparently the work of primitive, lower-order perceptual mechanisms which enable animals and human beings to adapt effectively to varying stimulative effects in the environment. Found in all our perceptual systems, they are presumed to be open to influence from higher-order cognitive systems, though not under intellectual control. Generally, we are not aware of these operations in our perceptions, probably because the mechanisms are "tuned" at very early ages. Slight overestimations and underestimations in this compensatory activity should not be understood as errors, however, since they help to scale the environment in an appropriate way for life. But if these compensations exceed a certain limited range, say about 30% of the impinging stimulation levels, then presumably illusions and distortions arise which can be curious or intriguing, but also frightening or dangerous. Ross discusses several kinds of illusions and distortions common to natural life situations. For instance, if an object appears to be beyond its physical distance (as in a fog), its apparent speed will be increased. If, as is often the case in clear water at close distance, an object appears both nearer than its physical distance and enlarged, there will be different speed distortions depending on the line of travel. An object travelling along the line of sight, over an apparently short distance, will appear to move too slowly. An object moving diagonally, or moving from the region where it appears too near to the region where it appears too far, would of course vary from slow to fast. What we become aware of then, and only when their result no longer "fit", are the sometimes curious, sometimes alarming phenomenal experience, the appearance of things.

In the foregoing the assumption is that distortions and illusions of perception are due to visual scaling mechanisms. But how flexible is the human visual system really? There is growing evidence which casts doubt on the pliability of the visual system, which would appear to be limited to the early formative years, when neuronal pathways are being laid down. Harris (1980) argues that the confusing variations found in investigations of perceptual activity are not due to calibration upset in the visual system but may be due to "change in the relation between physical position of a body part (relative to other parts) and perceived or registered position, regardless of whether afferent input or efferent outflow provides the necessary information" (p. 137). This change he defines as "proprioceptive change" or change in "felt position" given by the position sense. This sense, seeing that it includes not only "fatigue" or "muscle potentiation" effects but also sense of change in limb, head or eye position, is equivalent to what Gibson calls the haptic system and its components. The effects of this system on the visual one may be of particular importance in phobia, as I shall argue later on. Whether distortion is *within* the position sense, as Harris assumes, or comes about in the interaction between, for example, visual and haptic systems, as Gibson, and Powers postulate, is still a matter of conjecture.

Some Interim Positions

Powers' analysis of control in (perceptual) conflict (1973; see also Chapter II) brings into better focus the reason for and the mechanics of the large discrepancies found in the judgments (perceptions) of individual phobics regarding environmental stimulation. Many of them, far from being sensitive to error (that is, following the stimulative effects with "tight" control), show little or defective control over large areas of the stimulative fields. If it is so that when two perceptual systems are in conflict because both attempt to control the same quantity from widely separated reference conditions or levels, as Powers states, then a large dead zone around the virtual reference level (the compromise position) exists, within which there is little or no control, then their behaviours become understandable. Supposedly, the reference levels to which he refers are equivalent to what Helson denotes as the adaptation levels. The new aspect of Powers' contribution is in the rivalry that can arise between different reference conditions, so that reference levels and reference signals operating on the same perceptual signal from the controlled quantity are opposed. Disturbances acting on this controlled quantity (whether external to the person, or internal) no longer can be effectively removed, since the output systems are responding at maximum. Hence the extreme overestimation and underestimation which reveal the large error driving the output systems. Hence, too, the complaint of many of these patients that the world around seems to have "gone out of control", or is in danger of doing so. But what is being controlled? And which systems are in conflict in trying to control the same input but from widely differing reference conditions? As yet, we can only guess, having only an inkling of this, from the qualifications attributed to some objective ratios of stimulation by the patients.

These qualifications, possibly what Gibson might justifiably call the affordances of these structures, are the feeling of being pressed down by the ceiling or thrust through the shaft of certain spaces (the "funneling effect"), common to tunnels, certain architectural spaces, such as corridors, especially narrow, dark ones, a feeling often generated by low H/D ratios combined with small B/D ratios; the busyness or crowdedness of these spaces (occlusion or dense overlap, and milling crowds), which generate feelings of unsafety or of being crowded out; illumination ratios (low and high ratios), which arouse feelings of dismalness, sombreness or darkness, and make these spaces difficult to oversee too; heterogeneity of arrangement of objects and structure;

wide, open spaces, which seem to trigger feelings of loneliness, bleakness or solitariness. All these affordances or variables which describe the "felt" components of these situations have something in common: the self-referent aspect, and the direct experience of spatial relations in reference to oneself. This gives us a hint about the perceptual systems that are probably in conflict. In Gibson's terms (see chapter II), this would be in visual and haptic systems (optical structures, ecological events which yield information about the objective world and of oneself-in-it at one and the same time). The level(s) in the hierarchy of perceptual control at which such conflict may exist is still unclear. It does not seem to be at higher-order levels, given other behaviours of these patients. Possibly such conflict may be at the level of control of configurations; but not necessarily with regard to other objects in the environment, given the lack of systematic difference between phobics and normals in their discriminative behaviours, though perhaps in configuration control with respect to one's own body. If Harris is right about the position sense being the disruptive partner in the interaction of visual with proprioceptive or haptic systems, this may well be so. But as yet the evidence is insufficient to risk a firm hypothesis.

What other interim positions might we reach on the basis of this analysis? Two points concerning diagnosis and clinical intervention can be made. The first concerns the observed tendency of phobics and other neurotics to "complain" at length. Often, in psychological laboratories, this takes the form of making exclusive use of extreme scoring categories on rating scales. We now seem to have an alternative explanation for this behaviour. Their behaviour may be betraying not so much a need to complain or to manipulate the therapist (though this cannot be entirely ruled out); rather, this behaviour may represent specific response patterns (strategies) in dealing with stimulation, which may be the result of malfunction of constancy scaling mechanisms, earlier tuned to the then appropriate stimulation but no longer appropriate to current levels of stimulation. Or they might be the inevitable effect of large dead zones existing around the virtual reference level when two reference levels in conflicted systems give opposing directions; or both.

This brings us to the second point concerning clinical intervention. In this light one can better understand the effectivity of *in vivo* training in the treatment of phobic patients. Walking around in the environment, touching objects and surfaces not only gives one a chance to become more familiar with different aspects of the environment which had been avoided. But by making the person vitally aware of parameters of change in different perceptual systems at one and the same time, the visual-kinaesthetic feedback as the person changes position in space, and the "feel" of things as he or she touches surfaces or objects, will help to bring internal reference levels nearer together, thus eradicating the large error between systems. On the other hand, one often finds that psychotherapy relieves a phobia that is not actively treated. In this view, a partial explanation may be that talking about one's problems and paying attention to the ways in which one deals with different situations may influence and eventually change the cognitive orientations which, at higher levels, influence lower-order perceptions. However, unintended results might also ensue. Whatever the case, perception theorists (e.g., Gregory; Gibson; Powers) agree that since perceptual mechanisms or process are not under intellectual control, are generally unconscious and resistant to change, their "re-tuning" or reorganization cannot be anything but a slow process. The success of therapeutic intervention may then depend, at least in part, on the ability of the therapist to influence perceptual and/or cognitive strategies underlying perceptual control, by providing support over a relatively long period of time to the patient, in helping him or her to pay more attention to parameters of change in the environment and in oneself. This said, it is time to return to questions of more immediate concern. Can we find evidence which may help us to understand the *why* of perceptual control, and give us a firmer idea of *which* perceptual systems are immediately involved in control failure? The next chapter opens new perspectives.

VII

When Control Fails: Perceptual Disorientation, Derealization, and Depersonalization

Distortions of Perception (and Thought) in Normal and Phobic Persons

Nowadays, in a world haunted by the excesses of the different drug cultures in which we live, the disorders of perception and thought which form the subject of this chapter have become commonplace, even among the populace. But this was not always so. Hardly two decades ago the notion that normal persons experience perceptual distortions spontaneously, and just as much as disturbed persons do, was strongly resisted in clinical circles as well as by the man-in-the-street. For instance, in 1960 one psychiatric investigator (Roberts, 1960) found that 39% of a group of college students actually had depersonalization experiences; but he doubted the generalizability of his findings to a normal population. As he wrote: "It is fairly clear that brief, repetitive, depersonalization cannot occur in the general population as frequently as it did in this sample. If it did so, its existence would have been recognized and its incidence acknowledged in the literature" (p. 484). Yet only a few years later, two other psychiatrists (Cappon & Banks, 1961, 1965, 1969) carried out a series of studies into the phenomena of perceptual distortion in clinical and normal persons, and found that these were as common in natural life situations as in psychiatric syndromes. They remarked on the fact that, given non-threatening conditions of inquiry, normal persons even reported more disturbances of this nature than the patients. Of 97 subjects drawn from different sources, they found that 86% of the nonpatients (students) reported orientational percept distortions, compared to 44% of the mental hospital patients, and 73% of the ambulatory patients. Other researchers (e.g., Dixon, 1963; Silverman, 1975; Noyes & Kletti, 1977) found too that in one-third to one-half of the normal population depersonalization and derealization occur spontaneously, during periods of fatigue, illness, sadness, anxiety, and in life-threatening situations; but also under conditions of euphoria, as in peak-experiences.

The cardinal symptom of these disorders seems to be a subjective awareness or feeling of change in oneself or one's body (depersonalization), or in the surroundings (derealization), or in one's orientation in space and time (perceptual disorientation). These feelings of change may be fairly mild and relatively pleasant: "Literally floating on a pink cloud", feelings of weightlessness, with extended body boundaries; or more alarming: a feeling of "being in a room with receding and expanding walls", a feeling of "spinning, sinking or expanding into space"; or even more extreme: an awareness of having separated from one's body (out-of-body experiences). Quite often these perceptions of change in oneself and/or in the surroundings are accompanied by feelings of high anxiety and a sense of impending doom.

As one may recall, in Chapter III, depersonalization phenomena are considered by Barendregt (1982) to be the linchpin upon which phobia revolves; but also of other forms of repersonalization, such as "falling in love"; moments best described in terms of "courage de luxe"; and peak-experiences in normal life. Barendregt & Frijda (1981) suggest furthermore that these phenomena are probably best understood in terms of a failure or a falling-short of cognitive schemata to match reality as it is experienced.

What is a cognitive schema? Neisser's (1976, p. 252) definition of the concept *schema* for the central cognitive structures in perception, a concept derived from Bartlett, accords with what Barendregt and Frijda refer to, and may help to clarify what is meant here:

> "A schema is that portion of th[illegible] perceptual cycle which is internal to the perceiver, modifiable by experience, and somehow specific to what is being perceived. The schema accepts information as it becomes available at sensory surfaces and is changed by that information; it directs movements and exploratory activities that make some information available, by which it is further modified."

In his commemoration of Barendregt's ideas on anxiety and depersonalization, Frijda (1982) elaborates on their ideas on this subject:

> "There is no alignment and no foothold, neither on the part of thought, nor on that of expectation or action, both of which are based on 'categorisation', the applicability of schemata. Our perceptions are made out of recognition, and this recognition forms the basis and ordering of our action(.) This falls away, or does so in part, in the experience of depersonalization ..(.).. what remains is: strangeness, elusiveness, incapacity, chaos" (p. 5).

And again:

> "Depersonalization and anxiety coincide (merge) when, in the absence of reflection, the experience of anxiety merges with the experience of the world, the perception of the world: in the experience of strangeness, emptiness, confusion impervious to reason, overpoweringness, and unpredictability (p. 7) ... This failure of classifying schemata or categories is usually not complete. It is mostly directed to a certain domain: the perception of the external world, or that of orientation in space and time, or of one's body" (p. 10).

The ideas put forward by Barendregt and by Frijda seem to accord well with the assumptions made in this thesis on the nature of phobia, and especially of the part played in it by inadequate perceptual control. Cappon et al. also subscribe to the same school of thought, viewing as they do perception in terms of "a set of variables intervening between sensory stimulation and awareness" (the representational standpoint). Their primary aim in the studies mentioned was to try to provide a sound basis for the assumptions arising from this, that disturbances in orientational perception precede more severe disturbances such as derealization and depersonalization, seeing as, and I quote: "as reality (or at least in its basic physical aspects) can only be mediated through perception and more particularly appreciated through orientational perception" (Cappon et al., 1961, p. 381).

Although, as argued in chapter II, there is room to doubt whether the representational point of view adequately describes the nature of the perceptual process, whatever the case, we can certainly agree on the point that, in the early formative years perceptual systems are unstable because their neuronal substrata are still being developed; and learning still being deficient, perceptual disturbances of an orientational kind may well be quite general in childhood. Besides, if one is to adapt with success to varying levels of stimulation, the mechanisms of perception must necessarily be relatively flexible. But, if as was argued in chapter IV, specific perceptual distortions underlie phobic complaints (e.g., the expansion and contraction of reversible optical structures and visual events), and if no repressive mechanism *per se* is operating in phobia, despite the findings of Cappon et al. that normals report more orientational percept disturbances than patients, we would still expect more phobics than normals to experience these more frequently (or more intensely), even though the incidence is the same in clinical and normal populations.

A Choice of Method for Investigating Distortions of Perception

The studies carried out by Cappon & Banks (1961–1969) made use of different methods to register disturbances of perceptual orientation, derealization and depersonalization, since it was also their aim to replicate in the laboratory conditions such as have been described in the literature. These methods were: caloric labyrinthine stimulation, sensory deprivation, gas inhalation (CO_2 and N_2O), sleep deprivation, and an anxiety situation, taking a final oral exam. Data were collected from all the conditions by having the subjects record their responses on a questionnaire form. (A control study was also carried out to determine whether the questionnaire itself tended to influence the subjects to over-report. It did not.) In general, they found that reports of orientational percept distortions occurred with high frequency in the replicated situations.

Since our study had not the pretension of trying to replicate Cappon's work, or the results in the literature, but merely the more modest one of determining whether, in Dutch samples, differences might exist between phobic and normal persons, inasfar as *spontaneous occurrence in daily life* is concerned, we decided to dispense with the different conditions. The questionnaire used by Cappon et al. seemed suitable to our needs for several reasons: it was formulated in simple language and fairly briefly, contained only 19 questions in all, and had the advantage that the questions asked applied to changes in environmental relations, especially spatial ones, changes in one's body or self, and in people and objects in the surroundings, of a kind that is postulated in this book (see Chapter IV) to be of particular importance in phobia. These changes in perception describe apparent disturbances in space and time (appearing infinite or nonexistent, expanding or contracting); size or weight changes in one's body or body parts (expansion and/or contraction, weightlessness or heaviness); or of one's movement in space (for example, sinking down into the earth or in space, floating in a strange or unreal way, out of the body, disappearing in space); of other people and objects changing in similar ways; and changes in position relative to others in space. One of the questions referred to feelings of unreality or strangeness related to thought disturbances ("as if I am someone else"), but the main concern was those changes in one's perceptual experiences that are labelled in the clinical literature experiences of disorientation, derealization, and depersonalization. Because their main aim was to establish a relation between disturbances in orientational perception prior to more severe disturbances, whether in childhood or adolescence, their questionnaire also inquired into the occurrence of these disturbances before and after one's thirteenth year. The disturbances in orientational perception were also worded to fit those of derealization and depersonalization, in similar categories of experience. Although our concerns were different, we were also interested in possible relations between early years and later, as regards these experiences. So this part was incorporated too. See Appendix C Table 7.1 for an overview of all the items in our questionnaire.

Hypotheses

Our hypotheses were four:

H1: Phobic persons differ significantly from normals ($\alpha = .05$, one-tailed) in the frequency of their experiences of disorientation

H2: Phobic persons differ significantly from normals too ($\alpha = .05$, one-tailed) in the frequency of experiences of derealization and of depersonalization, which are more frequent in phobics.

H3: The differences in frequency of experience concern specifically changes in the experience of spatial relations, of one's own body or self in space, and of other bodies which describe expansion and contraction phenomena, and strange and unreal movement. (The test for this null hypothesis is derived from the first two null hypotheses.)

H4: Furthermore, phobic persons differ significantly from normals ($\alpha = .05$, one-tailed) in the awareness of frequent lack of control over themselves, or danger of losing control.

H0: No systematic differences exist between phobic and normal persons in the frequency of perceptual distortion, nor in kind (whether these be orientational, in the perception of the external world, in self or own body in space, or in control over oneself in space).

Procedure

The investigation was carried out in two phases. We first tried out the feasibility of using the questionnaire with phobic patients by administering it in a group session to first-year psychology students during the test-week. We hoped that the results would also give us some idea of the number of experiences of this kind that occur spontaneously in a normal Dutch sample. In the second phase the questionnaire was revised and administered individually to phobic patients newly being treated, during their diagnostic phase; and also to an older group of normal persons who had earlier participated in the experiment concerned with dimensions of complexity in streets.

Subjects

a. A group of 140 normal, first-year psychology students, consisting of 76 women and 64 men, who participated in the test-week in 1981. Their ages ranged from 18–38 years (mean age: 22.4 yrs).

b. A group of 48 normal persons, consisting of 26 women and 22 men, ranging in age from 21–65 years (mean age: 37.1 yrs). Thirty of these persons (12 men and 18 women, aged 23–62 years, mean age: 34.2 yrs), varying in occupation: housewives, skilled and semi-skilled technical and manual workers, and a few academically trained persons, had also participated in the street experiment. The other 18 persons (8 men and 10 women, aged 30–65 years, mean age: 36.9 yrs) were members of the scientific or administrative staff, two graduate students and one external accountant.
c. A group of 63 phobic patients, consisting of 44 women and 19 men, varying in age from 21–65 years (mean age: 39.8 yrs). These patients had been accepted for treatment in the years 1980–1983. Unfortunately, few were monosymptomatic: 36 patients suffered from agoraphobia as main complaint, with various subsidiary complaints; 11 were social-phobics with mixed complaints; 5 suffered from fear of animals; and 11 patients from complaints as: fear of disease, storms, claustrophobia.

Material

In deciding to use Cappon's questionnaire for somewhat different goals (for instance, the question whether orientational distortion precedes or is concurrent with derealization and depersonalization was of less concern to us), in translating it we changed it in certain particulars to better fit our needs. Cappon had allowed the subject a response to the questions of only "Yes" or "No". For our purposes, where the frequency of response was crucial to our hypotheses, this was much too limited. So we changed the scale to a five-point one, giving the subject the choice of five responses: Never; seldom; now and again; often; very often. Where Cappon inquired into "feelings" of change in the "I" form, we preferred the term "awareness" (*gewaarwording*), as less vague and more relevant, and questions formulated in the less direct "you" form. Where Cappon spoke of the "as if" experiences, we preferred the more neutral "seem to" (*lijkt*), because we expected some awareness of the clinical connotation of the former term, at least in the normal and academically trained subjects. This fact might predispose them to deny having such "pathological" experiences. We changed too the wording of some of the items: Instead of describing changes in space as "seeming infinite or nonexistent", we spoke of space "seeming infinite or collapsed (*ineengeschrompeld*), a perceptual experience more in line with what phobics sometimes describe to be the case, and agreeing better with our hypotheses. Also, to "strange or unreal movement in space", we added the formulation "(objects or people) coming up close", again more in line with phobic experience. Further, to avoid confusion arising in the subject as to what was being asked of him or her, in the first phase (with psychology students) two items, in which seemingly incompatible behaviours were described as happening at one and the same time were split up (items 1 and 6). Although we acknowledged the fact that these fluctuations go together, we did this to facilitate clarity in the respondent, who might have one but not the other experience. In fact, in the second phase, (with other normals and phobic patients) all items describing opposite behaviours were split up into separate items. Also, items were added which described changes in attributes of objects (items 27 to 32) and in control over self (item 33) and others (item 34), because of their relevance.

Instructions

The questionnaire was administered with the following written instruction:

"The following questions are intended to find out if, in *normal* situations, **spontaneous** changes take place in your perception and experience of the outside world, in your own body, and in that of others. Questions do **not** refer to changes in your perception and experience which might take place under the influence of drugs, such as heroin, marijuana, alcohol, and so on. They refer only to those experiences in your everyday life which happen of themselves (for instance, when you feel tired or unhappy), and over which you seem to have little control.

In some people such experiences occur often and can last long; in others only a few of these changes take place and last for very short periods of time. But it is quite possible that you have never experienced any of the changes described here. Whether or not this is so, please answer all questions, otherwise your answers cannot be processed. Next to each question you will find five statements with which you can indicate *how* often these experiences occur. Please indicate which by encircling the answer of your choice."

After completing the questionnaire, the person was then asked to indicate on an attached form which of the experiences had occurred before, and which *after* his or her 13th year of age; and, where possible, to write down in which situation the experience had occurred.

The administering of the questionnaire took, in the main, no more than 20 to 30 minutes, although some patients took up to 45 minutes to complete it. Care was taken by the tester, in replying to any questions put by the person filling in the questionnaire, to avoid referring to psychiatric descriptions, such as derealization or depersonalization.

Data Analysis

The null hypotheses are tested by means of Chi-square analysis for *k* independent samples (level of significance: α.05, one-tailed). For each group (phobics; normal, employed adults; psychology students), the scores are trichotomized in three categories: In category 0, all negative responses; in category 1, the answers "seldom" (1), and "now and again" (2); in category 2, the answers "often" (3), and "very often" (4). The items in each class of experience (perceptual disorientation, derealization, depersonalization) are analysed per pair (those split up beforehand), or per item. The region of rejection of the null hypothesis is, for $df = 1$, $\alpha = .05$ (one-tailed), $\chi^2 \geqslant 3.84$; and for $df = 2$, $\alpha = .01$, $\chi^2 \geqslant 5.99$. For small samples < 30, Fisher's exact probability test is used. The analyses concern the positive responses only (categories 2 and 3). (On the Perceptual disorientation scales, for psychology students (Normals II) the items on space, time, body/body part, and objects/people seeming smaller or larger were not split up; so only one score is available per pair items. Also, the items relating to attributes of objects or people (sound, colour, "feel") and to control over self, and other persons or objects (DR & DP) were added to the questionnaire later; so no scores on these items are available for the students.) Because we were also curious whether sex or age, or kind of phobic complaint, might play a rôle in these experiences, differences are also computed for these and tested by Chi-square analysis. Three age categories, 30 years or less; more than 30 years up to, maximally, 40 years; and more than 40 years old are distinguished, and computed over groups. The patient group is divided into "Agoraphobic" and "Other phobic" groups. In the Agoraphobia group were thirty-six patients whose main complaint was agoraphobia. Eighteen were dominantly agoraphobic, eleven suffered from mixed complaints of agoraphobia and social phobia, two from agoraphobia and claustrophobia, two from agoraphobia and fear of death and disease, and two from fear of travelling and agoraphobia. In the other phobic group were twenty-seven patients, seven of whom suffered from social phobia as main complaint, two from social phobia and agoraphobia, two mainly from claustrophobia, five from fear of animals, three from fear of death, cancer, and disease, two from mixed neurasthenic complaints with specific phobias (fear of travel), two from fear of heights, one from fear of water, and another from a fear of storms and thunder. Product-moment correlations are also computed for the data on reports before and after age thirteen, for all groups; and their differences tested by Chi-square analysis.

Overall Results: Response Totals. Proportions and Distributions of Positive Responses

In Tables 7.1a and b., the proportions and distributions of the positive responses of the different groups are shown, as these apply to the three classes of perceptual experience: disorientation, derealization, and depersonalization. Only a very small percentage of all the subjects say that they have either never had any of these kinds of experience (3.6%), or have experienced one kind but not the other (10.4%). Of the latter, 8.4% belong to the student group. Table 7.1a shows the proportions of persons who report at least one, two or more, and four or more experiences in the three classes. These percentages of the spontaneous occurrence of perceptual distortions are somewhat higher than one generally finds in the literature, except for the student sample, which accords well with other findings.

Table 7.1a. Proportions of persons who report at least one, two or more, and four or more experiences in the three classes: Perceptual disorientation (PD), Derealization (DR) and Depersonalization (DP)

Class of experience	No of experiences	Phobics (n = 63)	Normals I (n = 48)	Normals II (n = 140)
	at least one	88.8	93.8	88.6
PD	2 or more	81.0	87.5	64.3
	4 or more	52.4	58.5	22.9
	at least one	90.5	97.9	77.9
DR	2 or more	87.3	93.7	55.8
	4 or more	66.7	81.2	22.1
	at least one	88.9	89.6	74.3
DP	2 or more	69.9	75.0	47.9
	4 or more	34.9	22.9	15.0

P = phobic patients; NI = normal, employed adults; NII = psychology students

Table 7.1b. Proportions of persons in the different groups who report experiences of perceptual disorientation, derealization and depersonalization, per item

Source:	Phobics (n = 63)	Normals I (n = 48)	Normals II (n = 140)	Mean
Perceptual disorientation				
PD13. Space seems to become smaller	47.0	20.8		34.2
14. Space seems to become larger	34.9	22.9	27.9]	28.9
19. Time seems to pass faster	77.8	85.4		81.6
20. Time seems to pass slower	73.0	85.4	82.4]	79.2
15. Body/part seems smaller	36.5	14.0		25.5
16. Body/part seems larger	33.3	29.2	13.6]	31.2
21. Body/part seems lighter	46.0	31.2		38.6
22. Body/part seems heavier	47.6	47.9	42.9]	47.8
23. Body/part seems to move (e.g., whirl) in space	33.3	27.1	17.1	25.8
25. Body/part seems to change position/place in space	17.5	29.2	6.4	17.7
17. Objects/people seem smaller	25.4	18.7		22.1
18. Objects/people seem larger	23.8	10.4	17.9]	17.1
24. Objects/people seem to move	17.8	8.3	8.6	11.6
26. Objects/people seem to change position or place in space	17.5	14.6	5.7	12.6
Derealization				
DR 1. Space seems to be infinite	68.2	70.8	50.0	63.0
2. Space seems to be collapsed	46.0	27.1	22.1	31.7
5. Time seems infinite/nonexistent	52.4	70.8	61.4	61.5
4. Objects/people seem to disappear or melt into space	20.6	16.7	10.0	15.8
9. Objects/people seem to float in strange, unreal way, come up close	28.6	12.5	10.0	17.0
12. In an unreal world in which obj./people seem strange or unreal	47.6	43.7	47.1	46.1
27. Colour/brightness of objects seems stronger than usual	38.1	66.7	–	52.4
28. Colour/brightness of objects seems weaker than usual	46.0	54.2	–	50.1
29. Sounds seem duller, farther, etc.	61.9	60.4	–	61.1
30. Sounds seem harsher, nearer, etc.	65.1	58.3	–	61.7
31. Objects seem warmer, more vivid	34.9	41.7	–	38.3
32. Objects seem chilly, lifeless	33.3	29.2	–	31.2
34. No control over people/objects	57.1	79.2	–	68.1
Depersonalization				
DP 3. Body/part disappears/melts into space	28.6	27.1	17.1	24.7
6. Body/part becomes weightless	41.3	39.6	44.3	41.7
7. Body/part sinks into space	30.1	20.8	15.7	22.2
8. Body/part floats in a strange, unreal way	28.6	27.8	20.7	25.7
10. You are outside body (OBE)	28.6	39.6	28.7	32.3
11. You feel as if someone else	44.4	27.1	43.6	38.4
33. You are losing control self	80.9	81.2	–	81.1

Few differences would seem to exist between phobic patients and normal persons drawn from different walks of life in the number and kind of distortions experienced. First-year psychology students do tend on the whole to report fewer experiences in all three classes considered but, as will later become clear, this is not due to age differences, or to other significant differences between the normal groups.

In Table 7.1b, the proportions of persons with positive responses in all the groups are shown, now split up according to their responses to the different items. From this overview it is clear that the experiences most rarely occurring in all the groups are those relating to nonself (to other people or objects). The most frequently reported distortions are those relating to the passage of time, to losing control over oneself, and others, followed by distortions of space, of attributes of objects, people, animals (such as, sounds, colour, brightness, feel), being in an unreal world, and feeling as if one is someone else, and distortions of body weight, size or movement. Except for the apparent loss of control over self, and distortions relating to the attributes of others, which were not included in the Cappon study (1961), these Dutch responses agree very well (with respect to what is and what is not frequently reported) with those in the Canadian study.

Group Differences in Response Frequency

We turn now to those analyses of more specific concern to our hypotheses, that phobics differ significantly from normal persons in that these experiences are *more frequent* in the former group.

The first hypothesis stated that phobic patients differ significantly ($\alpha = .05$, one-tailed) from normal persons in the frequency of experiences of perceptual disorientation. Table 7.2a shows the behaviours in this class of experience, their response frequencies, and outcomes of the analyses.

As we see, the null hypothesis can be rejected only for those experiences which relate to space seeming to become smaller and/or larger around one, for one's body or body part seeming to become smaller and/or larger, and for one's body or body part seeming to become lighter and/or heavier (although one knows that these changes do not actually take place). Significant differences are found between phobic patients and their normal controls, specifically, phobics experience these conditions much more frequently than normals (Space smaller/larger: $\chi^2 = 12.946$, df: 2, $p = .005$; Body or part smaller/larger: $\chi^2 = 7.778$, df: 2, $p = .02$; Body or body part lighter/heavier: $\chi^2 = 7.402$, df: 2, $p = .03$). (N.B. In all these analyses the category 0 (never) is not included, to clarify where differences in positive responses lie between the groups. Analyses including category 0 yielded similar outcomes.)

For the above-mentioned perceptual behaviours (disorientation), support is found for the hypothesis.

The groups do not significantly differ in those experiences described by time seeming to go much faster or much slower than is usually the case, one's body or body part seeming to move (e.g., whirl) in space, or change its position or place in space, for objects or other people seeming to become smaller and/or larger, or seeming to move (e.g., whirl) in space, or change their positions or places in space. So, for these behaviours, the hypothesis finds no support (see Table 7.2a).

Table 7.2a. Frequency tables showing group differences (group percentages) and the results of the Chi-square analyses on Perceptual disorientation

Source: Perceptual disorientation	category	P (n = 63)	NI (n = 48)	NII (n = 140)	Chi-square	df	p
Space seems to become smaller or larger, while you know it has not changed (Items 13 + 14)	0	58.7	78.1	72.1			
	1	30.2	21.9	26.4			
	2	11.1	0.0	1.4			
	N	126	96	140	12.946	2	.005**
Your body or some part of it seems to become smaller or larger, etc., (items 15 + 16)	0	65.1	78.1	86.4			
	1	23.8	19.8	12.9			
	2	11.1	2.1	0.7			
	N	126	96	140	7.778	2	.02*
Your body or some part of it seems to become lighter or heavier, etc., (Items 21 + 22)	0	53.2	60.4	57.1			
	1	35.7	36.5	39.3			
	2	11.1	3.1	3.6			
	N	126	96	140	7.402	2	.03*
Time seems to pass much faster or slower, etc., (Items 19 + 20)	0	24.6	14.6	17.1			
	1	52.4	57.3	53.6			
	2	23.0	28.1	29.3			
	N	126	96	140	0.549	2	.75
Your body or some part of it seems to be moving in space/or change its position in space, etc., (Items 23 + 25)	0	74.6	71.9	88.2			
	1	22.2	27.1	10.4			
	2	3.2	1.0	1.4			
	N	126	96	140	1.60	2	.40
Objects or people around you seem to become smaller or larger, etc., (Items 17 + 18)	0	75.4	85.5	82.1			
	1	21.4	13.5	15.8			
	2	3.2	1.0	2.1			
	N	126	96	140	0.312	2	.85
Objects or people around you seem to be moving in space/or change position or place, etc., (Items 24 + 26)	0	82.5	88.5	92.8			
	1	17.5	11.5	6.1			
	2	0.0	0.0	1.1			
	N	126	96	140	5.252	2	.075

Table 7.2b. Frequency tables showing group differences (group percentages) and the results of the Chi-square analyses on Derealization

Source: Derealization	category	P (n = 63)	NI (n = 48)	NII (n = 140)	Chi-square	df	p
Space seems to be infinite or collapsed (Items 1 + 2)	0	42.9	51.0	63.0			
	1	38.9	44.8	30.7			
	2	18.2	4.2	5.4			
	N	126	96	280	12.288	2	.005**
Space seems to be collapsed (Item 2 only)	0	54.0	72.9	77.9			
	1	30.1	27.1	22.1			
	2	15.9	0.0	0.0			
	N	63	48	140	17.581	2	.0002***
You are in an unreal world in which objects and people around seem strange and unreal (Item 12)	0	52.4	56.2	52.9			
	1	38.1	41.7	45.0			
	2	9.5	2.1	2.1			
	N	63	48	140	6.771	2	.034*
Time seems to be infinite or nonexistent (Item 5)	0	47.6	29.2	37.9			
	1	41.3	58.3	51.4			
	2	11.1	12.5	10.7			
	N	63	48	140	0.233	2	.837
Objects or people around you seem to disappear or melt into space (Item 4)	0	79.4	83.3	90.0			
	1	19.0	14.6	10.0			
	2	1.6	2.1	0.0			
	N	63	48	140	1.627	2	.443
Objects or people around you seem to float in a strange or unreal way, and come up close (Item 9)	0	71.4	87.5	90.0			
	1	22.2	12.5	10.0			
	2	6.4	0.0	0.0			
	N	63	48	140	4.967	2	.083
Colour or brightness of objects in surroundings seems to become stronger/weaker than usual (Items 27 + 28)	0	57.9	39.6	–			
	1	35.7	53.1	–			
	2	6.4	7.3	–			
	N	126	96	–	0.035	1	.85

(*continued*)

Table 7.2b. *(Continued)*

Source: Derealization	category	P (n = 63)	NI (n = 48)	NII (n = 140)	Chi-square	df	p
Sounds of people, animals, objects seem duller, muffled, farther away/harsher, more penetrating, nearer than usual (Items 29 + 30)	0	36.5	40.6	–			
	1	47.6	52.1	–			
	2	15.9	7.3	–			
	N	126	96	–	0.622	1	.40
Objects seem to feel warmer, look more vivid/feel chilly, look more lifeless than usual (Items 31 + 32)	0	65.9	64.6	–			
	1	30.2	32.3	–			
	2	3.9	3.1	–			
	N	126	96	–	0.000	1	1.00
You have little control over people or objects in your surroundings (Item 34)	0	42.9	20.8	–			
	1	44.4	64.6	–			
	2	12.7	14.6	–			
	N	63	48	–	0.014	1	.907

The second hypothesis stated that phobic patients differ significantly too from normal persons in the frequency of their experiences of derealization and depersonalization, these being more frequently experienced by phobics.

Table 7.2b shows the results of the analyses for derealization experiences, and Table 7.2c, the results for depersonalization experiences. The null hypotheses can be rejected for those experiences of derealization in which space seems to be infinite and/or in which it seems to be collapsed (*ineengeschrompeld*), the differences between phobics and normals being highly significant (Space infinite/collapsed: $\chi^2 = 12.288$, df: 2, $p = .005$; Space collapsed: $\chi^2 = 17.581$, df: 2, $p = .0002$). A glance at the tables shows that the normal control groups do not differ. Significant differences exist too between phobics and normals in the experience that one is in an unreal world in which people or objects seem strange and unreal ($\chi^2 = 6.771$, df: 2, $p = .034$). Phobics experience this more frequently, and again no differences exist between the normal control groups.

Only for these derealization experiences do we find that phobic patients experience these significantly more frequently than normals. No significant differences are found between the three groups in the following experiences: the awareness of time seeming infinite or non-existent; in the awareness of disturbances in the movement of people or objects in space (e.g., seeming to disappear, floating in a strange or unreal way, and coming up close); or in the awareness of having little control over people or objects. Nor do they differ in the experience of changes in attributes of objects (e.g., in colour or brightness, sounds becoming harsher or more muted, or in the feel of objects).

Table 7.2c. Frequency tables showing group differences (group percentages) and the results of the Chi-square analyses on Depersonalization

Source: Depersonalization	category	P (n = 63)	NI (n = 48)	NII (n = 140)	Chi-square	df	p
Your body, or some part of it disappears or melts into space (Item 3)	0 1 2	71.4 20.6 8.0	72.9 25.0 2.0	82.9 17.1 0.0			
	N	63	48	140	8.347	2	.015*
Your body, or some part of it becomes weightless (Item 6)	0 1 2	58.7 30.2 11.1	60.4 37.5 2.1	55.7 40.0 4.3			
	N	63	48	140	6.033	2	.049*
You are outside you body, or apart from it (Item 10)	0 1 2	71.4 20.6 8.0	60.4 39.6 0.0	71.4 26.5 2.1			
	N	63	48	140	8.407	2	.015*
You feel as if you were someone else (Item 11)	0 1 2	55.6 33.3 11.1	72.9 22.9 4.2	56.4 42.2 1.4			
	N	63	48	140	9.739	2	.007**
You are losing control over yourself or in danger of doing so (Item 33)	0 1 2	19.0 52.4 28.6	18.7 79.2 2.1	– – –			
	N	63	48	–	12.318	1	.0005***
Your body, or some part of it sinks into the earth or space (Item 7)	0 1 2	69.8 25.4 4.8	79.2 18.7 2.1	84.3 14.3 1.4			
	N	63	48	140	0.478	2	.787
Your body, or some part of it floats in a strange or unreal way (Item 8)	0 1 2	71.4 20.6 8.0	72.9 25.0 2.1	79.3 17.9 2.8			
	N	63	48	140	2.526	2	.232

N.B. Category 0 = never (not included in Chi-square analysis); category 1 = seldom or now and again; category 2 = often or very often;
P = phobics; NI = normal, employed adults; NII = psychology students

The hypothesis finds support then only for the experiences of the seeming expansion and/or contraction of space, and of being in a strange and unreal world in which people or objects seem strange and unreal; but not for other experiences of derealization.

In Table 7.2c we see that in the class of depersonalization experiences, the null hypothesis can be rejected for the following experiences: the awareness of one's body, or some part of it, disappearing or melting into space; of one's body, or some part of it, becoming weightless; of being outside one's body, or apart from it; of the feeling as if one were someone else; and of losing control over oneself or in danger of doing so. For all these experiences phobics differ significantly from normals in the greater frequency with which they experience these forms of depersonalization (Body/part disappearing: $\chi^2 = 8.347$, df: 2, $p = .015$; Body/part weightless: $\chi^2 = 6.033$, df: 2, $p = .049$; Outside one's body (OBE): $\chi^2 = 8.407$, df: 2, $p = .015$; Feel as if someone else: $\chi^2 = 9.739$, df: 2, $p = .007$; Losing control over self: $\chi^2 = 12.318$, df: 1, $p = .0005$). The normal control groups do not differ significantly. Thus, the hypothesis finds support for all the above-mentioned experiences of depersonalization. The null hypothesis may not be rejected, and thus no support is found for those experiences of depersonalization in which one is aware that one's body, or some part of it, sinks into the earth or into space, or in which it floats in a strange or unreal way. Nor do the normal control groups differ in the frequency of these experiences.

The third hypothesis, that the differences in frequency of experience between phobics and normals concern specifically those changes in the experience of spatial relations, of one's body in space or self in space, which describe expansion and contraction phenomena, in being in a strange and unreal world (objects and people strange and unreal), finds support in these data.

Finally, the fourth hypothesis, that phobics differ significantly from normal persons in the awareness of losing control over themselves, or of being in danger of doing so, finds emphatic support in these reports, since we can reject the null hypothesis at a level of significance of $p = .0005$ ($\chi^2 = 12.318$, df: 1).

Other Differences

We also carried out Chi-square analyses on the data which were sorted on the bases of sex, age and kind of phobic complaint (agoraphobic versus other phobic complaints). No differences at all were found between these groups. This lack of difference was a little disappointing, given Barendregt's postulate that "nothing is so personal in phobia as the depersonalization". But, on considering the fact that we had limited ourselves to those depersonalizations of a perceptual nature only, and the varied composition of the two groups, which might have cancelled out more personal effects, this result is in hindsight not so surprising. Nor can it be considered to be a fair test of Barendregt's postulate.

The variables Sex and Age did not, in the main, affect responses in the different classes of experience. Two significant sex differences were found: men experiencing more frequently than women that objects or people seem to move in space or change position, while knowing this to be not so (χ^2: 4.746, df: 1, $p = .035$); and women experiencing more frequently than men the awareness of losing control over oneself (χ^2: 4.630, df: 1, $p = .03$). Age differences were found on two variables: persons younger than 30 years or of exactly that age have more frequently than other age groups the experience of objects or people seeming to become smaller or larger; and persons older than 40 years of age seem to have less frequently than younger persons the experience that sounds fluctuate (respectively: χ^2: 7.182, df: 2, $p = .035$; and χ^2: 6.086, df: 2, $p = .05$). Bearing in mind the fact that these were the only differences found in all the comparisons, one may reasonably conclude that age and sex do not play any important rôle in these behaviours.

Product-moment correlations were computed for the data on the reports of the different groups between the experiences remembered before their thirteenth year and after their thirteenth year. For perceptual disorientation experiences, a high correlation is found in all groups between the number of reports before, and after age thirteen (Phobics, $r = .80$; Normals I, $r = .88$; Normals II, $r = .93$). For derealization experiences, the correlation between the number of reports before, and after age thirteen is low for phobics ($r = .34$), but high and positively correlated for normals (NI, $r = .75$; NII, $r = .77$). For depersonalization experiences, there is no (or no linear) relation between the number of reports before and after age thirteen for phobics ($r = .04$), but a fairly high, positive correlation for normals (NI, $r = .51$, NII, $r = .77$).

Chi-square analysis on the Before age thirteen and After age thirteen reports of distortions in these classes of experience show significant differences between phobics and normal, employed adults (NI) with respect to changes in the attributes of things or people (colour or brightness fluctuation: $\chi^2 = 4.27$, df: 1, $p = .035$; sound fluctuation: $\chi^2 = 6.284$, df: 1, $p = .015$; Warmth/cold changes: $\chi^2 = 6.218$, df: 1, $p = .015$), significantly fewer phobics reporting remembering such changes before age thirteen. Also, significantly fewer phobics than normal, employed adults report being aware of little control over other people or objects before age thirteen ($\chi^2 = 5.565$, df: 1, $p = .015$). Significantly fewer phobics than both normal control groups report too the awareness before age thirteen of their body or body part becoming weightless ($\chi^2 = 6.733$, df: 2, $p = .035$). A near significant difference is also found between phobics and normals in the same direction (that is, fewer phobics reporting remembering before age thirteen awareness) of: Being in an unreal world in which objects or people seem strange and unreal ($\chi^2 = 4.84$, df: 2, $p = .075$); body or body part becoming smaller or larger ($\chi^2 = 5.386$, df: 2, $p = .075$); body or body part becoming lighter or heavier ($\chi^2 = 5.651$, df: 2, $p = .075$); and objects or people seeming to move (whirl) in space or change position or place ($\chi^2 = 5.00$, df: 2 , $p = .075$).

For both phobic patients and normal persons, the kinds of situations in or normal conditions under which these experiences of distortion in self or world *spontaneously* arise are in moments of stress, and when consciousness is temporarily lowered: before falling asleep, after long periods of lack of sleep, when bored, tired, unhappy, sick, during fits of anxiety, while dreaming, after a car accident, panic, and so on. This accords well with what one would expect from the findings in the literature.

Discussion

The first noteworthy result is the finding that a large number of phobics and normals experience the distortions of perception commonly labelled disorientation, derealization, and depersonalization. But these experiences occur only incidentally ("seldom" or "now and again"), and generally under conditions of stress, or when consciousness is temporarily lowered. The majority of the reported distortions are those relating to the passage of time, to losing control over oneself, and others, followed by distortions of space, of attributes of objects and people (colour, brightness, sounds, "feel" of objects). In this lack of difference in incidental occurrences of these distortions between phobics and normals there may, however, be a little snag. We do not know if phobics differ from normals in the *intensity* with which these are experienced, for we did not ask. Assuming from Barendregt's publications to be established that phobics differ from normals in the intensity of their transient depersonalization experiences (included in his classification are derealization experiences), we did not wish to complicate the issue of our concern (or lengthen procedure) by inquiring about this parameter of experience.

What we do know now is that up to about thirty per cent of these phobic patients are subject to frequent or very frequent perceptual distortions in daily life, which occur spontaneously. This might come as a surprise to some clinicians, who assume that phobia can be distinguished from psychosis by the relative lack of distortions of perception (and thought). Nor is it all that long ago (as we saw in the introduction to this chapter) that psychiatrists struggled against the idea that perceptual distortions, far from being limited to psychosis syndromes, form part and parcel too of normal, everyday experiences. Of course, one might argue that this high frequency may be due to a rather liberal selection of patients for treatment in our department. But, according to the intaker-psychiatrist (see Chabot, 1975) who was still the intaker at the time when these patients were in treatment, only 3% of the patients screened by him were borderline (psychotic) patients too. And it was, and is, the policy to keep this percentage as low as possible, in view of the fact that students-in-training carry out therapy.

One of the specific hypotheses of this study (hypothesis three) finds strong support in these data: that phobics differ significantly from normals in changes in the experience of spatial relations, of one's own body or self in space, and of other bodies which describe expansion and contraction phenomena, and strange and unreal movement. The results show that the changes are related to self, rather than to other objects, and to space: Space seeming to become smaller or larger; seeming to be infinite or collapsing in on itself; and to one's body in space (becoming larger or smaller, lighter or heavier, disappearing or melting into space, separating of self from body, becoming weightless). Phobics differ too from normals in the frequency of experiencing some alienation from self ("as if one were someone else"); which is not really surprising in its generality, being an emotional or thought disturbance that can be expected to go with such perceptual distortions as described. A significant difference is also found in the frequency of the experience of being in a strange world, in which objects and people seem strange and unreal. And, most significant of all, the frequency with which phobics, in contrast to normals, feel that they are losing control of themselves, or in danger of doing so (hypothesis four).

These results suggest that it is not the strangeness of objects or of other people that is the main concern of phobics. What is, is the strangeness of space, and of one's own body or body part, the strangeness of one's movement, size, weight or weightlessness in space. Here we would seem to have significant evidence of the intrinsic interactions between the visual and haptic perceptual systems. But in their case not working smoothly or in tandem, and thus with pernicious effect. Curiously enough, these same patients report remembering fewer incidences of these distortions of body weight, or body disturbances, or of lack of control over others, or in attributes of objects, than normal persons before age thirteen. But after age thirteen, they report bodily distortions (one's body disappearing or melting into space, one's self separating from the body, and its becoming weightless) much more frequently than do normals.

All this gives support not only to the conceptions of Barendregt and of Frijda, that characteristic of these experiences is the experience of having no foothold and no alignment with thought, experience, or action; that is, the failure or falling-short of one's (cognitive) schemata of reality, as it is experienced. This is certainly true. But something else seems to be suggested also in these data, and more in line with the theoretical analyses of perception in phobia (in Part One). Namely, that the perception of spatial and temporal relations may differ. Time, being the stuff of asymmetrical relations, of conceptions of succession and duration obtained by reasoning and thought, does not frighten, not in this elusive way. Space does. For space is experienced directly, as inseparate from one's own being. It is the direct experience of symmetrical Being, and the fusion of ourselves with it (to paraphrase Matte-Blanco). Perceptually, visual and haptic experiences seem to coincide. With a little imagination one can recognize that space is the primordial experience, and I shall return to this idea after discussing the experiences of different phobics, as told to us during personal interviews in chapter IX. But before doing so, we will briefly consider whether phobics differ from normals in other time functions than the ones considered in this study.

VIII

A Little Intermezzo on the Experience of Time

Varieties of Time Experience

Before the previous study on the phenomena of perceptual distortion got under way, it occurred to me that in the Cappon study the experience of Time had been treated rather like a stepchild. In our questionnaire, which had been modelled on theirs, only two references were made to distortions of time, and these two referred only to one of the different modes of time experience known from the literature, namely, simultaneity and succession. The items inquired about time seeming to be infinite or nonexistent; and to time seeming to pass much faster or much slower than one knew was objectively so. In fact, besides simultaneity and succession, other modes of the experience of time are distinguished in the literature, some of perhaps more relevance to neurosis than the abovementioned. Philosophers and scientists have been concerned with the perception of present, short-term time (which includes (a) the perception of short intervals, and (b) rhythm or *timing*); the perception of duration, the past, long-term memory; temporal perspective – philosophical, social, cultural constructions of the world and their effects on the interpretation of time experience – "becoming", the future; and simultaneity and succession (e.g., James, 1890; Bergson, 1910; Dunne, 1934; Michotte, 1963; Fraser, 1966, Michon, 1967; Ornstein, 1969; and Melges, 1982, to name a few of the more prominent works). Of these, the last work on *Time and the Inner Future*, a temporal approach to psychiatric disorders, has some relevance to our investigation. In this work, Melges states that different attitudes to time exist in the psychoses, in depression, and in the neuroses.

These different distortions of psychological time disrupt, in different ways, the person's sense of control over the future and lead to psychopathological vicious circles (spirals). Correction of time distortions and the harmonization of future images, plans of action, and emotions restore the sense of control over the personal future.

In the psychoses there is a marked loss of control over the future, future images, plans of actions, and emotions being confused and disorganized. In depression the future seems blocked. The depressed person believes that his plans of action are no longer effective for reaching future images and goals. In neurosis the future seems uncertain and foreboding. The neurotic person feels that something catastrophic might happen. This dread of the future, and his future images are coloured by catastrophic expectations stemming from the past (Melges, 1982, pp. x–xxi). Barendregt, too, stressed in his work this sense of impending doom in some phobics.

These ideas suggested to us that phobics might not differ from normal persons in the experience of simultaneity and succession, but might well differ in their perception of duration, and especially in their temporal perspectives.

The Chosen Procedure for Examining Time Attitudes in Phobics

What was now needed was a vehicle for examining other time experiences than simultaneity and succession, to use as a supplement to the Cappon questionnaire. We found this in some work of Calabresi & Cohen (1968).

In their work on the relations between personality and time attitudes, they administered sets of personality and time attitude items to 100 psychiatric hospital patients, 100 psychiatric patients in a mental hygiene clinic, and to 308 college students (116 males and 192 females). The sets were factor analysed in the total sample and the data factor scored. They found substantial relationships between personality attitude (restless dysphoria, extraversive adjustment, tense dependency and excitement seeking) and time attitude factor scores within samples; and moderate relationships of both kinds with diagnostic and demographic variables. The Time Attitude factors found were: Time Anxiety, Time Submissiveness, Time Possessiveness, and Time Flexibility.

Time Anxiety was found to be "a very large and meaningful factor. Anxiety about the flow of time and need to control time are its striking characteristics...(.) They are reflected in the uncomfortable feelings that go with thoughts of the future and in the frustrated longing for the past. The future is threatening because it cannot be controlled; the past cannot be truly comforting because it is not mastered through the chronological sequence of memories. (.)"

Sixteen items loaded on this factor Some examples of the items with high factor loadings are: "It makes me a little uncomfortable to think about my future"; "When I am by myself, my thoughts often drift back to the past"; "I find waiting in line, even for a short time, very annoying", "I get almost panicky when I don't have enough time".

Time Submissiveness was a factor in which "is reflected an extremely dutiful and conforming attitude toward time. Orderliness does not allow the confusion of rushing and the dread of being late. One should make efficient use of time,..(.)Thus, no freedom or initiative is allowed."

Eight items loaded on this factor. Examples of some of the items are: "I am almost never late for work or appointments"; "I would rather come early and wait than be late for an appointment"; "I like to have a definite schedule and stick to it."

Time Possessiveness was "a weak factor that portrays a possessiveness and greedy attitude toward time. Those who score high are disturbed by the rapid flow of time. ... (.) thinking of the past is useless and upsetting. ( )."

Six items loaded on this factor. Examples of the items are: "It bothers me to think how fast time goes"; "Time spent sleeping is wasted time"; "I try to save minutes during the day by rushing."

Time Flexibility was found to be "a factor that embodies an accepting and flexible attitude toward time. (.)..wondering about the past and planning or fantasizing about the future have an equally positive quality. The same is true for the experience of leisure and time pressure. Thus the present can be enjoyed in contrasting situations. (.)."

Nine items loaded on this factor. Examples of items with high factor loadings: "I can spend hours working at a pasttime, like a puzzle or a workshop project, and lose track of time"; "It is fun to plan for the future, even though the plans may not work out." (See Calabresi and Cohen, 1968, pp. 435–436, for more information on the items, their factors and loadings.)

Calabresi and Cohen argued that their results provide empirical support to the long-held conjecture that attitudes toward time reflect basic features of the individual personality. The factor items on these time attitudes (especially those of the factor Time Anxiety) seemed particularly relevant, since individual phobics often complain about these experiences (e.g., "I find waiting in line, even for a short time, very annoying"; "I get almost panicky when I don't have enough time"; "When I am by myself, my thoughts often drift back to the past"; etc.). The factor Time Flexibility contained items which seemed to be able to differentiate between phobic and normal experiences too; for in other studies phobics and other neurotics were often found to differ from normals in their rigid attitudes, in their inability to flexibly alter course when this is called for.

Since we were less interested in replicating Calabresi & Cohen's findings, and in fact only interested in the part of their study concerned with time attitudes, specifically with the use of the scales for discriminating differences in time attitudes between phobics and normals, we dispensed with basic procedure, that is, any attempt to determine the reliability and validity of their factors in a Dutch population. For use in our study, we sufficed with translating all items verbatim into Dutch. We made no effort to capitalize on these by giving weights to different items. Calabresi & Cohen found that "Factor A scores (Time Anxiety) are of good alpha reliability (.79) for the total sample and for all four groups. Patients score significantly higher than students in this factor ($p < .01$). Factor B (Time Submissiveness) is moderately reliable (.56) in the total group ...(.) Factor C (Time Possessiveness) has low reliability in the total group (.47) ...(.) Reliability for Factor D is fair (.51) for the total group, with considerable unevenness among groups (patient samples .32, .34; student samples .46, .49)" (1968, pp. 435–436).

Response scale. For their purposes Calabresi & Cohen needed a response scale of a fairly high differentiation. They made use of a six-point "agree-disagree" response continuum: Strongly agree; agree; not sure but probably agree; not sure but probably disagree; disagree; and strongly disagree. For our purposes, however, this response continuum seemed rather elaborate, since what we wished to know was if other experiences relating to time than the ones incorporated into the Cappon questionnaire needed to be taken into account in perceptual dysfunction in phobia. So we opted for a simple bi-polar response: "Yes" or "No".

We *hypothesized* that phobic patients would differ from normal persons on the Time Anxiety scales, being significantly more anxious than normals. We expected phobics to differ too from normals on the Time Flexibility scales, being significantly less flexible than normals. Although Calabresi and Cohen had found only a significant interaction on Factor B (Time Submissiveness) of Diagnosis and Site (hospital *versus* clinic: borderline outpatients being less submissive than outpatient psychotics but their standing being reversed among the hospitalized patients), we expected phobic patients to have a more submissive attitude to time than normals. We expected normals to be more possessive of time (fearful of time passing unfruitfully) than phobics, that is, to score significantly higher on these scales. Our null hypothesis stated that no significant differences exist between phobics and normals in these time experiences ($\alpha = .01$, two-tailed).

Subjects. Since the patient sample, and the normal control samples are identical to those in the preceding study on disorientation, derealization, and depersonalization, their descriptions are omitted here.

Procedure. The procedure was also the same as in the preceding study. Only the instruction to the subjects was different. They were simply asked to indicate, by underlining the response of choice or by deleting the response that was not relevant, whether or not the statements in the Time Attitude questionnaire were relevant to their experience. In this questionnaire too they were required to respond to all statements. Only two students returned an incomplete form, and their data are not included in the study.

Data Analysis

Analyses of variance were performed using the different scale scores (Time Anxiety, Time Submissiveness, Time Possessiveness and Time Flexibility) as dependent variables to yield comparisons between the three groups, phobics, normal, employed adults (NI) and psychology students (NII). The variables sex and age were introduced as covariates in these analyses, to check for eventual differences due to these.

Results

Tables 8a and b show the means and standard deviations for Time Attitude scale scores for the three groups, and the results of the analyses of variance, the F-ratio test comparisons for the Time Attitude scale-scores of the different groups. In Table 8b we see that the only significant differences at a 1% level are found on the variable Time Flexibility. There is a significant main effect on the scale Time Flexibility (F: 3.718,

Table 8a. Means and standard deviations for Time Attitude scale-scores of phobic patients (P), normal, employed adults (N I) and psychology students (N II)

Source	Phobics (n = 63)		Normals I (n = 48)		Normals II (n = 140)	
	M	SD	M	SD	M	SD
Time Anxiety	7.63	2.99	8.92	3.37	7.86	2.80
Time Submissiveness	3.97	1.41	4.06	1.45	3.86	1.30
Time Possessiveness	2.98	1.35	3.23	1.08	2.90	1.13
Time Flexibility	4.19	2.05	5.69	2.02	4.81	1.80

Table 8b. F-ratio test comparisons for Time Attitude scale-scores for the phobic and normal groups (Analyses of Variance)

Source	Main effects	df	Groups	df	Sex	df	G × S interactions	df	Age	Explained	*p*
Time Anxiety	2.209	3	3.076*	2	.720	1	2.720	5	1.951	2.213	.043
Time Submissiveness	.285	3	.426	2	.000	1	1.952	5	.001	.876	.513
Time Possessiveness	1.327	3	1.424	2	1.124	1	3.404*	5	.007	2.039	.061
Time Flexibility	3.718**	3	5.574**	2	.055	1	2.275	5	.812	2.754	.013

$^{*}p < .05$; $^{**}p < .01$

df: 3, p = .01) and a significant group effect (F: 5.574, df: 2, p = .004). No interaction is found between Groups and Sex, or with the covariate Age. The true variance is explained by these two effects only (F: 3.141, df: 5, p = .009). Phobics differ then from normal, employed adults (NI), but not from psychology students (NII), in being less time flexible. Thus the null hypothesis can be rejected, and the alternative hypothesis supported.

A systematic group effect (at 5% level) is also found on the variable Time Anxiety (F: 3.076, df: 2, p = .048), but neither the main effect nor the interactions between Group and Sex reach significance. This difference is due to a difference between phobics and normal, employed adults, the latter being more time anxious than the former. The hypothesis that phobics are more time anxious than normals finds no support in these data.

No differences are found between groups on the variable Time Submissiveness or on the variable Time Possessiveness. A significant interaction effect (at a 3% level) is found on Time Possessiveness between Groups and Sex (F: 3.404, df: 2, p = .035), but no other significant effects are found. Apparently, normal, employed men are more time possessive than other men or women (Pw: M: 3.16, s.d: 1.19. NIw: M: 3.08, s.d: 1.05; NIIw: M: 2.72, s.d: 1.09; Pm: M: 2.60, s.d: 1.60; NIm: 3.41, s.d: 1.09; NIIm: M: 3.11, s.d: 1.15) in this sample.

Comments

In their attitudes to time, phobic patients differ from normal, employed adults (but not from psychology students) on two counts. They are significantly less flexible in their attitudes towards the past and in planning for the future, and in the ability to relax and lose track of time. A finding that is not at all surprising, given earlier clinical findings (e.g., Barendregt, and Melges). On the other hand, normal, employed adults seem to be more time anxious than phobics (and than psychology students) about the passage of time, the need to control the flow of time, in adhering to schedules and routine activities, etc. This, too, is hardly surprising if one considers that these persons are actively participating in jobs, often with tight time schedules to be met and heavy demands on their ability to organize their time efficiently. For the same reason, one might expect psychology students indeed to be much more relaxed about the passage of time and time schedules, not yet being part of the 'rat race' in earnest. Patients, on the other hand, because of their being through illness temporarily "shunted aside", may be less concerned about the efficient organization of their time, even apart from the fact that they are more absorbed by the workings of unconscious or partly conscious effluences of their psyche.

With these additions to the findings on time in the previous study, we can now say with a little more confidence that, on the whole, time functions or time dimensions are not of great concern in the phobic experience.

IX

Children of Space and Time

Dangerous Alliances and Disturbances in the Field

If the findings of the preceding studies have more than face validity, the implication may be that in a profounder sense than I had supposed (chapters II to IV, Part One), pathologic functioning may be tied in with different orientations to space and time. For at more than one level of reality we are the children of Space and Time.

At the mythological level, and in the beginning, as Hesiod tells us, there was Chaos, vast and dark space.

"From Chaos were born Erebus and Night who, uniting, gave birth in their turn to Ether and Hemera, the day. Then appeared Gaea, the deep-breasted earth; and finally Eros, 'the love which softens hearts', whose fructifying influence would thenceforth preside over the formation of beings. Gaea first bore Uranus, the sky crowned with stars, 'whom she made her equal in grandeur, so that he entirely covered her.' Then she created the high mountains and Pontus, 'the sterile sea', with its harmonious waves. Gaea then united with her son Uranus and produced the first race, the Titans" (Guirand, 1935, 1963).

After a series of bloody offspring, whom Uranus regarded with such horror that, as soon as they were born, he shut them up in the depths of the earth, he was disenthroned and emasculated by Gaea and her last-born Cronus, in an act of terrible vengeance for his rejection of her offspring. Cronus (or Time), after liberating his brothers, with the exception of the Cyclopes and the Hecatoncheires, became chief of the new dynasty. Under his reign the work of creation continued; and Doom, Death, Sleep and Dreams, Misery, and all the Fates came into being.

Similar tales and mythologies of space and time can be found not only in Greek mythology but in almost all cultures (Cavendish, 1980). In these tales are reflected the foam and the sediment of human experiences. These are regularly summoned to explain the vicissitudes of the unconscious and conscious components of our being (see Freud; Matte-Blanco; Barendregt; quoted earlier).

Originally, the term "chaos" (from the Greek root meaning "to gape") simply designated "open space". Only later, because of a false derivative from the word meaning "to pour", was "chaos" considered to mean "the confused and unorganised mass of the elements scattered through space". To my mind, in the way Barendregt uses the term (1982, p.168) to describe the disorganization in the experience of "it", he is more true to the original meaning than to the later, false derivation:

> [*Het is niet de complete chaos zoals die in sommige acute psychoses benaderd kan worden. Ook onze patiënten weten gedurende 'het' geen orde te scheppen, maar er is een groot verschil: hun aandacht is niet verstrooid over losstaande gewaarwordingen. Integendeel, die is gefixeerd op het ontbreken van samenhangen*]. "It is not total chaos (in phobia), like in some acute psychoses During (attacks of) 'it' our patients also cannot achieve any semblance of order, but there is a great difference: their attention is not dispersed over an unorganized mass of sensations. On the contrary; it is fixed on the lack of relations (between their sensations.)"

Space then surrounds and supports us, as a Mother. She is felt, if not perceived, is inhaled and exhaled. She is the pulsating womb from which all forms arise. Time, as a Father, infuses fire in us, takes our hand, and teaches us the rhythm of life. A poetic formulation, perhaps; but one that seems to do some justice to what Matte-Blanco designates "symmetrical Being" and "asymmetrical Being", concepts which, as we have seen, are closely allied to Freud's "system Unconscious" and "systems Preconscious and Consciousness". Enjoined, as Space-Time, they become the primordial twins; as great a riddle as ever, despite the endeavours of physicists and philosophers (who now even consider space-time to be eleven-dimensional!; Davies, 1984).

The psychological formulations of relations between space and time in terms of "Chaos" and "Cronus", "symmetrical being" and "asymmetrical being", "the unconscious" and "consciousness" may, perhaps, even be mundane. But in this chapter, in which the *appearances* of these relations are the focus of concern, one uses what tools are to hand to impress upon psychologists, who are hardened in a materialistic-statistical view of reality, the real mystery of these profound relations, and the faces that Space-Time may assume. Hence, now and again, little excursions into poetic formulation. From a physical perspective, all that we perceive of Space are her surfaces, tilting, moving, shifting. Some look to us permanent, solid, closed; others appear transient, transparent, open. Some, like the grin of the Cheshire Cat, appear and disappear, seemingly and continually in flux, yet persisting in time. All that we perceive lends credence to her vitality to shape, and to destroy us as, together with all her other creatures, we cling fast to her boundaries while she spins and evolves.

In such remarkable environment, having the power to awe, enthrall and affright, we dare to live; dare to walk on, through, in and around her impermanences, giving hardly a thought to the great feats of imagination that this entails. But what to do when we no longer dare, paralyzed by the thought of taking even one more step? In this, the last chapter but one, we shall perceive the appearances of things to those who dare not take that fearful step, or, taking it, expect catastrophe.

Let us bear in mind too that, like every nuclear family in which children form alliances with one or other parent, so also in the Cosmic one. Such alliances may further one's growth, or stunt it; may engender *souplesse*, or bring about disturbances in the field. Seen in this light, the normal of today is the child who lies easy in the arms of Space, but is hard-pressed by Time. And the phobic is the child who, perhaps, walks indifferently on the hand of Time but is uneasily enveloped, or engulfed, in the primordial embrace.

But where are the children who fear neither parent? They are not the thrill-seekers: the mountain climber, the parachutist, the deep-sea diver, the speed-freak. Like phobics, they experience as much fear but learn to cope with this fear differently (Epstein & Fenz, 1965; Averill, 1971; Baddeley, 1972; Ross, 1974; and also Piët, 1986). Clinicians call them "counter-phobic".

The reader may by now be wondering whether we are concerned here merely with metaphor or with reality. As I hope to illustrate in the pages to follow, we are dealing with a reality much more immanent than our metaphoric formulations can describe. Symbolic, yet actual; but in every case describing perceptual functions of reality.

Gibson says that, in fact, we perceive neither space nor time, though we can visualize the one, and trace the passing footprints of the other. Nevertheless, our omnipresent reality, as will become clear when our patients speak of their experiences.

Space, like Time, does not always wear a terrible face. She has many faces and many functions, as we know from experience. In this she is as many facetted as in all her permutations and combinations. In the following vignette, taken from the literature (see Kaplan, 1964, pp. 311–322 for a full account), a highly articulate account portrays some of these faces. In it are told the experiences of a professor of English literature at the University of Wisconsin in the 1920s, who suffered from an acute anxiety neurosis and phobia, all his life.

One hot June morning, during a long walk with a friend along the shores of a lake near where he lived, he began to feel queer, queerer than he had ever felt in his life. So, after a while, they stopped at a roadhouse for refreshments. Facing a wall, on which hung a huge red-yellow map, in its centre a train, dashing headlong down a track, he suddenly saw it spring out: "Head-on. Right at me. Hideously hostile ..huge ..God ..Death. To destroy me for my guilt, as myself the destroyer of my wife. The objective fact was still there ..But here again was the old split in the personality, creating this split in the objective world: the picture, to the *eye* an old map on a tavern wall; to the *feel* a horrible alien monster...I became panicky over my panic.... I am convinced this is my last hour ... perhaps my last minute ... I say to Brown, "I'm feeling awfully bad" in a low, controlled voice. We get up ... pay at the counter I buy a cigar ... light it in the doorway ... just as a train is passing over beyond the meadows. And my eye, above the match, turns by an unconscious fascination once more to the map. The Locomotive-God, with thrust more malignant still, seems as if leaping out at me across the tavern-room from behind the bar. I suffer the intensest seizure of terror yet. The feel of onrush is so fiercely authentic that my very reason spontaneously omits the rational explanation (i.e., absurd hallucination)... I keep looking to *make sure*. I say nothing to Charlie, try to "walk it off" ... Then on the tracks ... from behind the woods across the lake comes a freight-train, blowing its whistle ... Instantaneously diffused premonitions become acute panic. The cabin of the locomotive *feels* right over my head, as if about to engulf me ... The train *feels* as if it were about to rush over me. In reality it chugs on. I race back and forth on the embankment. I say to myself (and aloud): "It is half a mile across the lake – it can't touch you, it can't; it can't run you down "...

Brought home that evening by his friend with the help of passers-by in an automobile, he sleeps long that night. "In the morning, though feeling strangely weak in body, I start out on a little walk down the street. Within a hundred feet of the house

I am compelled to rush back, in horror of being so far away .. from home and security. I have never walked or ridden, alone or with others, as a normal man since that day (p. 320)".

This poignant narrative tells us not only what "it", the subjective but alarming distortion of space feels like, and the excruciating anxiety and even terror which it can induce, but it illustrates well the functions that space has for the human being. Space allows relations between objects and structures to be seen, so that action is possible; space is a medium that can be traversed, allowing one to get from one place to another; space forms the background, the scene or arena of action; space can become the focal point of attention, the agent whose terrible face induces fright and impels flight; space can function, in an enclosed area, as a protector of one's identity and form and, at the same time, be "possessed" by one (the safety of the home; personal space).

Time, of course, has analogous faces and functions, for it allows the human being to be successively what space allows simultaneously. Experientially though, it may be of another order of magnitude, since as far as we know, where space functions in similar fashion for animals, of time they seem to have little awareness.

An Inquiry into the Spatial Functions that Underlie Subjective Experiences (the "It") of Phobic Patients

Even if the phobic person is space-engulfed, not all spatial functions may be disturbed. When I began to realize the importance of certain optical transformations in the phobic complaint, I already knew that some spatial functions were quite intact. At that time the results of the experiments described in Chapter V were already in, but those in Chapters VII and VIII had yet to begin. Although the patients' perceptions of dimensions of space seemed to be relatively intact, some phobics appeared to add or subtract a constant from spatial ratios or relations (i.e., overestimate or underestimate these); but the perception of their ratios or relations remained unchanged. If this were not so, we could not have obtained such slight differences between phobics and normals on the discrimination or judgmental tasks. Yet, their *experiences of these structures* were significantly different from normals, whether we measured aesthetic experience (hedonic tone), arousal, anxiety or avoidance. I speculated that the added or subtracted constants brought about some disequilibrium, some instability in the visual field which changed the appearances of these structures. I supposed that these strategies yielded error too large to be compensated by the system, thus inducing instability and/or nonconstancy of environmental structure. Work of Ross (1974), and of Powers (1973) had suggested these possibilities of explaining the observed overestimation and underestimation of spatial relations, in the light of the sharp differences in experiences between phobics and normals. However, there was still little hard evidence to support this line of reasoning (see Chapter VI), nor any likely to be found without getting into the deep waters of neurophysiology. Then it occurred to me that there might be experiential evidence of the kind predicted in my hypothesis, which might provide more solid ground to stand on, without actually going into neurophysiological processes. The studies described in Chapters VII and VIII, and the interviews with patients in this chapter were conceived out of this need.

Expectations

In Chapter VI, on reflecting on the meaning of the systematic deviations from linearity (overestimation and underestimation) of response to the discrimination and judgmental tasks, I found some evidence for a relation between these responses and the nature of the phobic complaint. I suggested that the systematic underestimation by agoraphobics of environmental relations (and to the degree that this was done) should result in the vanishing or disappearing of structure, away from the agoraphobic observer, like Alice disappearing down the rabbit hole. The systematic overestimation by claustrophobics of environmental relations should yield a looming effect, as if the structures threatened to crush or engulf one. The evidence for other strategies of a disabling kind, for instance, underestimation of weak or low energies of stimulation and overestimation of strong or high energies, should result in particularly unstable, split, or conflicting perceptual experiences, and be possibly linked to social phobia. But, given the small number of patients investigated, this expectation had little basis in fact.

That some normal persons also appeared to manipulate spatial relations in similar ways, although to a lesser degree, suggested that a basic perceptual mechanism was involved. If so, then it became considerably easier to understand how distortions arose, in normal and pathological experience. To put these ideas to the test, though, was not easy, and for the following reasons: the majority of our patients suffered more than one complaint, and symptoms could change over time as well. Of course, if these perceptual behaviours go together, as Helson supposed, are complementary rather than opposed; and if they are linked to the form that phobia takes, then this was as it should be. The question then became one of ingenuity, to devise a way to induce experimentally the perceptual strategy at will. Pondering this, I came face to face with some of the unsolved problems in perceptual theory, and my Odyssey began.

A simple way out of the dilemma appeared to be to ask the patient, and probe gently, without seeming overcurious. But two arguments against this were (a) the fact that most of our patients are routinists at the kind of information they offer to the clinician. It takes expert technique to sift, from the mixture of much-hashed complaints, what is to the point, and what not; (b) the indoctrinated belief that people do not, or cannot tell the truth about their behaviour if asked (see, for example, Nisbett & Wilson, 1977). How could they answer questions then about their perceptual behaviour and strategies, which more often than not, remained unobserved by them? In thinking thus, we were too sceptical. For when put to the test, even the average person with no special introspective gift comes up with much more knowledge of his or her perceptual behaviours than one could suppose. Best of all, the process of self-observation in this area is enjoyed by most, is experienced as a voyage into *terra incognita* at least as interesting as a voyage down the Amazon of the psyche.

Subjects

We hoped at first to find prime examples of a particular kind of phobia, claustrophobia, agoraphobia, social phobia, etc., by sifting through the dossiers. This proved difficult; and even more so when we added the criteria of more than average intelligence, preferably verbally articulate, and at the beginning of therapy.

When such a person could be found, our hopes were often thwarted by the following criteria: that participation should be voluntary, and with permission from the therapist and supervisor, who should judge whether or not the series of planned talks might interfere with ongoing therapy. We soon had to abandon most of these too liberal criteria and settle for a catch-as-catch-can strategy, retaining only the last of these.

The final catch consisted of three patients diagnosed as claustrophobic (in the intake for therapy), with other complaints such as fear of travelling, fear of disease, the dark, or of blindness; three patients diagnosed as mainly agoraphobic, with other complaints as fear of being alone (at home or in the street), fear of travelling, and various somatic and emotional problems; three patients diagnosed as mainly social phobic but with other complaints such as fear of being alone, fear of disease (cancer); and two patients who feared blushing, and complained of body-image and/or weight problems. (The latter two cases are not discussed here, because one, a young woman, told us little about space or her interactions with it, her phobia being centred on her body images; and the other was a man whose comments on his experiences of space and himself in it were lost through a defect in recording). These nine patients, eight women and one man, varied in age from 19 to 53 years old. All were married or living in concubinage. All were of average or above average intelligence, and some were verbally gifted. None had participated in our earlier studies.

Material

Forty-eight questions were formulated to be put to the patient over a series of three interviews. These concerned different aspects of perceptual experience and of perceptual control: the experience of space as a whole, and of spatial relations; of one's self and body in space, and that of other bodies (people, animals, objects) and structures (buildings, etc.); of attributes of objects (e.g., colour, sound, other sensations); of time changes and time perspectives; perceived control of one's relations to others and of self-control; the kind of efforts habitually made to regain or keep control of self or situations when a threat to this arises; finally, the changes that chronic anxiety or the phobia had brought about in one's daily life, and perceived consequences of these.

Each question or area of perceptual function was illustrated by examples of the kinds of behaviour we had in mind, taken from the literature (e.g., from Cappon et al., 1961; Calabresi & Cohen, 1968; Klausner, 1965, on strategies of control). Since most of these have been amply described in the foregoing Chapters VII and VIII, they will be omitted here.

Procedure

I wished to cover as many areas of normal and pathological perceptual functioning as possible, without a special accent on one or other area that might give any clues to my expectations. That, in this roundabout way, more information would be obtained than might be required was all to the good, since little was known about the perception of phobic persons.

The student-interviewer was instructed to ask about all areas covered by the questions but to use the questionnaire as a guideline, rather than as a strict procedure;

to give examples of the kind of perceptual behaviours intended when necessary or asked for, but also to stress that the examples were illustrative and need not represent any experiences of the particular person interviewed. The patient was to be allowed as much leeway as possible in response. The interviewer should avoid at all times leading probes, or laying stress on any particular area of perceptual function. The interviewers, who were kept in the dark about the hypothesis entertained by me, conducted the interviews without interference, and answered questions put to them by the patients as best they could. They were coached only in spotting inadequacies of their interview technique, and in identifying their own prejudices which affected or could affect the responses of the patient. They were allowed complete freedom also as to place or time in which to conduct an interview, the only restrictions being that it should be quiet, not distracting to either patient or interviewer, and private. Some interviews were carried out in the patient's home, some at the laboratory, and some out-of-doors. With the permission of the patient, all interviews were recorded. The patient could, on request, listen to the previous tapes and change anything he or she wished to say differently, or erase anything of a particular, intimate nature. Few made use of this provision.

Instruction to the patient. Having arranged a series of three interviews, each to last not more than 1 1/2 hours, the patient was told that we wished to talk about her (his) way of perceiving and personal experiences, not of conceptions on how perception functions. The body of the instruction follows:

> "It is quite difficult for most people just to talk about their perceptual experiences. We aren't used to thinking about how and what we see, feel, hear, smell, etc. Nor if there is anything remarkable about the way we experience these perceptions. In the conversations to come, I shall ask you a number of questions on how you perceive things, and illustrate my questions with examples. These examples are quite arbitrary, are given merely so that you will have an idea of what is meant by the question. Always keep in mind that they are only examples, which may or may not accord with your own experiences. If they do not, just forget about the example, and tell me what you actually experience. Some of these examples are formulated in extreme changes of perception; this is also to make clear that all your experiences may be mentioned, even when these seem strange to you. Of course, it is quite possible that your own experiences are never as extreme as our examples. We are as much interested in the subtle, less remarkable changes, as in the sudden, remarkable or strange ones. So take all the time you need to think about these before replying".

The areas described above were then mentioned, and the person told that in the coming talks the questions would revolve around one or more of these perceptual behaviours (some of these data are in Kok & Lowich-Russell, 1980; Dreesmann, 1982; and Lohmann, 1984 – master's theses, University of Amsterdam).

In the coming pages not all of the information gleaned from the patients on their perceptual behaviours will be given. For instance, the information on time changes and time perspectives, and on the perceived lack of control over self, and others, accords well with what has been found from the larger studies using rating scales, in the preceding chapters. To avoid duplication, these data will be omitted unless they are particularly relevant. The information on the experiences of space relations, of one's body or self in space, and the interactions with other objects or structures, are presented at some length; because the patient's personal experiences prove to be immensely clarifying.

The Inner World of the Phobic

The Claustrophobic Experience

Patient A, a business woman, is 33 years old, married, has no children. Her main complaints are a phobia for flying, for elevators and for disease (cancer). *Patient B*, a 23-year old woman, is married, has no children, and a profession in metal crafting. Her main complaints are fear of the dark, of becoming blind, and claustrophobia. *Patient C*, a housewife, is 53 years old, married, with one child. Her main complaints are fear of travelling in public conveyances, and claustrophobia.

Experiences of Space Itself, and/or Objects or Structures in Space

(Patient A): "Sometimes the whole world seems to close in on me, for instance, when a storm is approaching. I feel then like a tiny wisp of a girl, a nothing ... Sometimes I get this feeling too in streets where the buildings are high ... or in very high mountains. It's like they will fall down on me, crush me. I feel completely helpless. That great, massive, strong ... enormous, colossal aspect of mountains ... it would be easy to sweep me off the face of the earth. At night too when I'm afraid, of the dark. What I notice then is how quiet everything is. If you screamed, nobody would hear you; again that feeling of being puny, of no significance ... I feel so impotent, so weak.

... Sometimes people overwhelm me too, annoy me. I feel almost threatened by them. The whole environment seems to threaten me, as if it would flatten me. Not kill me or annihilate me exactly, but very threatening nevertheless. I know it sounds like nonsense, but I often wonder if I'm going mad. I realize with my intellect that this is not so, but emotionally I'm sure of it; I know they threaten me ... Crowds overwhelm me, always someone next to you, in front of you, behind you. Sometimes I get this idea that if I had a mitrailleuse, I'd mow them all down ... I wouldn't really, but I do find it horrible that I even think it ...

... In my case, hearing is even more important than seeing. When I'm not feeling well, then I often find that sounds irritate me. Even those sounds which, normally, would not distress me ... the sounds of the tram going by, or the telephone ringing ... they sound much more penetrating, and irritate me unbearably. No, they never sound muted. Even voices sound much louder. Sometimes things and people seem to me so unreal ... the elevator that creaks; the plane that changes gear, the sound of voices ... and at night too when I feel afraid, I hear things which I do not perhaps really hear".

(Patient B): "Yes, when I feel anxiety, then yes, space seems so large, and it closes in on you, a very suffocating feeling ... space takes on quite other forms ... I feel this especially in a small room that is suffocating ... I sometimes got this feeling in a disco- (dancing). It wasn't even busy, only a few people were there ... and yet I became anxious because the whole room affected me in a suffocating way.

... Once in a while things seem to move from their place, without actually doing so. For instance, when I was a child, just before going to sleep, when the lights went out, I'd close my eyes and then open them again ... I had the feeling that the wallpaper would start to move. It was just a striped wallpaper, or with little blocks or small stripes, but they'd move up and down, or diagonally, sometimes it was just as if it was raining, but I no longer have that. (A little later she tells the interviewer): This afternoon, in the museum, I was looking at a poster. It was a strange light ... there were these large, thick, black letters on that paper, and a strange light ... and then it was just as if the letters began to fan out ... I can't explain it, it was a very strange effect ... I asked myself: 'Am I seeing things? Is it the light, or is it me?' ... It became a bit misty, as if a filter had been placed over the lines I was reading, and the letters of the text just began to fan out, in a streak like, fanning out ... but I think it was the light that did it.

... Just before falling asleep, the feeling of falling into a deep hole ... I have that often. I used to dream often as a child that I was being pursued by a witch, and I'd run and run and run, and then I'd fall into a large, black hole; then I'd become dizzy, and suddenly I'd wake up. Or I'd fall from a high tower, and wake up with a shock. Now I often dream of falling off a very shallow pavement, a short step ... what does that mean? (laughs). I am often extremely angry in my sleep, my boyfriend wakes me up because I've been kicking and punching him in sleep".

(Patient C): "I once had the experience of walking in the street, a cobbled street, and suddenly I had the feeling as if the stones were very near to me, and that I was very, very small ... I don't remember my emotional state, but I remember I was in a great hurry. I wanted to go somewhere, to get away quickly, and return home quickly.... Another time I went to a reception which I had been looking forward to, and how it happened I don't really know, but suddenly I felt, in the middle of a pleasant talk with others, where I was the centre of attraction, 'I have arrived'. I felt on top of the world. And suddenly it happened. All the people became tiny, like little dolls. It was as if I'd become very large, something very big with large ears, which could really cope with much harder sounds, but the voices of the people, their jokes, their music, everything sounded much softer, muted, as if they came from very tiny people (the patient describes this as a peak-experience of happiness). Even the light seemed to be much brighter than normally is the case.

... When a migraine's coming on, I find light and sound unbearable; and when I'm getting tired sounds become harsher, and irritate me. Then I'm not able to listen to anything at all. When I'm tired the glaring colours of the television irritate me; but I'm never irritated by sunlight, even in a migraine attack. I can't get enough of the sun. When I'm tired too even my own voice sounds different to me. I hear it and think: 'Is that my voice?' It sounds so harsh.

... At night, when I have an anxiety attack, I have to rush out into the street, I feel so suffocated in my room (this need she says has much to do with her experiences in World War II, when she was forced to stay inside as a young Jewish girl).

... Once I fell asleep, and when I woke up ... it was dark in the room, and I thought: 'Something is in the room'. So I turned on a large lamp, and I saw something dark red in the corner next to the chimney ... my husband is a witness to this. I thought: 'Now something is going to happen to me. I have to get out of the room'. But it was only a mass of hate. HATE. I woke my husband up, showed it to him, and he said: 'What is it?'. Then it just dissolved, and he said: 'Perhaps we are just imagining things'. But it was a mass of hate that wanted to assault me".

Experiences of One's Self and One's Body in Space

(Patient A): "Sometimes I think: isn't the human body strange. Two eyes, why not three or one ... there they go again, all those strange things with strange clothes on. What an absurd form we have ... I sometimes look different to myself, but it's more a psychical thing, than a bodily one. When I am not feeling well, then I look at my mirror-image and think sometimes: 'You don't look pleasant ... you are a peculiar human ... too fat, too'. Looking in the mirror, I feel that I am not I ... I am two persons on the inside ... one who thinks realistically, and the other who thinks quite differently ... there are two opinions in me. Nowadays, I don't seem to know anymore what is 'good' and 'not-good' ... that duality that is often contradictory ... the strange thing is that I appear to other people as a very self-sure person, as a calm person who knows what she is talking about ... yet inside I am very unsure of myself ... and those inner uncertainties don't seem to appear to others. Now and again, when I imagine myself back in my childhood, only in thought, I see things much more clearly than then. As a child I was teased quite a lot, very much, by other children, because of my large nose. I remember especially those slanging-matches. The whole scene comes back, and I can get very angry about it now. Then I always crawled into my little shell, made myself small, and ran away. And they teased me a lot, hit and kicked me even sometimes, those children. I can even see the faces of those children still, very clearly.... My mother is 'a very strong personality', knows always what's best, is always right. You accepted everything she said to be good and right. Now I'm much more critical of her ... and that's rather a shock for me".

(Patient B): "I often have the idea that my body is a part of how I think, my face, my hands, or any of my movements ... In therapy I learned that I have these anxieties exactly because I did not identify feelings of anger (in my body) and express them.... Through Yoga training I have learned to do this, and am no longer alarmed at 'things happening' in my body (e.g., heart palpitations, arms becoming heavier through tension).... When I am quite relaxed, or tired, I slouch and hang my head ... Tense, I pluck my hair and pick my toes. My father told me this".

(Patient C): In her "peak-experience", apart from her body expanding, while those of others became very small, she noted other kinaesthetic experiences. "My hands were so cold, as if they were made of glass. As if needles of ice tingled in them. And in my feet too. Not pricking them in the sense that you feel when your foot 'goes to sleep', but as if they were crystal clear, made of ice-cold glass. Sometimes the point of my nose also became like that ... When I am tired, and out walking, not only does the road seem much longer than usual, but my legs become so heavy that I can't raise them ... as if I'm dragging elephant legs. All the objects in my hand, bag, bicycle, the dog, feel much heavier too, impossible to drag them any further ... but this has to do with my mood at the time.

... To be shut up in your own anxiety is like ... not like an iron-cloak ... but like a tough mass around you, because if you try to shift it from your breast, it slips down to your belly.

... After an attack of panic, I feel different the next day. My rhythmic movements seem faster ... but I feel as if I'm trudging behind myself ... as if all of me is made of lead ... I feel clumsy, ungainly. And my midriff especially is inflexible. It is as if my arms have become terribly long and will sweep everything out of their way, and as if I have large legs which bump into everything ... one of the ways I cope with this anxiety is to pass my finger-tops over all kinds of ledges or ridges ... or I hit myself ... like someone would do who says, 'Hé, am I awake? Pinch me then to check' ...

I want to feel pain to be able to wring myself thru' it, through that anxiety-chute in which I am enclosed, from which I can't emerge".

The Agoraphobic Experience

Patient D, a housewife, is 37 years old, married, has two children. Her main complaints are street phobia, fear of travelling in public conveyances, fear of disease (heart and cancer), acrophobia and hydrophobia. *Patient E*, a housewife, is 51 years old, married, with one child. Her main complaints are street phobia, and a number of somatic and emotional complaints. *Patient F*, is 19 years old, unmarried, has no children, and is without a profession. Her main complaints are fear of going anywhere alone, and hyperventilation.

Experiences of Space Itself, and/or Objects or Structures in Space

(Patient D): "When I suffer from my phobia, then everything appears blurred. People seem to be much farther away from me than at other times, and their voices sound muted ... But just before the attack begins, before I arrive at this point, their voices sound extremely harsh. I want to say: 'Please, don't shout like that', but nobody's shouting.

... It's as if I'm sitting next to myself. I know what's going on, but I experience everything as if it is at a great distance. It's just as if there is a barrier between me and the others, as if I'm not really next to them ... Suddenly the whole world has changed ...

... I'm not only afraid in the street, but also when the sun shines. I find that even more frightening than when it rains. I'm also afraid of the dark. Sometimes, at night, I have to let the dog out; then no one is in the street, and it's dark and I am paralyzed with fright. ... I walk close to the houses to feel a bit protected. A street with a broad sidewalk I find worst of all. I simply hate those kinds of streets. And when I look into the distance, I get the feeling, 'O God, what a distance it is from me'. It seems as if such a street, which is often no longer than one with a narrow sidewalk, is miles and miles longer, and I think, 'I'll never make it, never', and I panic again.... It's just as if the whole street becomes smoky. I don't know how else to explain it ... it's as if the street becomes deeper. I feel like I am walking in a thick mist ... and I swear to myself that if I get home safe, I'll never, ever go out into the street again".

(Patient E): "Outside ... space seems a little weird ... and huge ... When I have to go out in the streets with my dogs, I take them one by one otherwise I can't manage, when I reach the corner, I become frightened to death and go back. I don't dare to go any farther ... It's as if I'll fall over ... I don't even dare to cross the street alone at a zebra crossing ... at such times I can't even think ... only about the fear ...

... The whole neighbourhood is so noisy where I live, and when I am not feeling well ... then sounds seem much louder and jar my nerves. If my husband puts down a cup harder than usual, I get annoyed ... he says that he didn't put it down harder than usual, but to me it sounds very hard ...

... In the street it is just as if the stones dance, going up and down".

(Patient F): "Walking in the street is terrible ... the street seems much longer and larger than it is in fact, when I am feeling bad. I walk, but it feels as if I am standing in one place and raising my feet up and down. Then, yes, the street seems very long, because it goes so slowly ...

... No, I don't feel that space is larger. If you said that space becomes smaller, everything becomes smaller, I'd agree. At least, this is so in my room when I'm in a bad mood. I have the feeling that everything gets in the way, that everything has become smaller. Because you bump into objects that are standing in the way. Yes ... I don't feel really shut up, or closed in, but rather as if I'm sitting in something, sitting inside something.

... When I am tense, it's just as if everybody shouts at me, instead of talking. That is not exaggerating ... sometimes I wish to say, 'Stop shouting, please!', although they are not really shouting, just talking. On the other hand, when it's quiet, I can't bear it. It's so deathly quiet".

Experiences of One's Self and One's Body in Space

(Patient D): "I begin to see badly ... that's always one of the first symptoms. It's just as if I can't see straight. Then I become afraid that I'll faint. I hear what people say, I even answer them too ... but their voices sound far away. So does my own voice, and that frightens me terribly. You never know what will happen then ...

... Often when I'm like this I bump into things too, even at home. It's as if I no longer can estimate the distance of things to myself. It's as if my eyes have suddenly become bad, no, it's more like ... this sounds crazy, but it's how it feels ... as if my eyes were not in front of my head, but at the back on the inside. Like having to look past something, through the head. I also fear heights. When this panic comes over me, I don't even dare to go out on the balcony, because I stumble over the threshold, and everything is turning around fast .

... Sometimes I have the feeling that I'm not walking normally in the street, but waggling, stumbling around like a drunk. My legs refuse to go where I want them to, they shake, I feel as if I'll fall, that they'll slither out from under me. I seem to have no control over my limbs.

... That feeling, it's a bit like having a bee in your bonnet. It buzzes around and around ... the feeling that you are falling sometimes. This happens quite often in the kitchen, that I turn round ... and I feel bad ... that I clamp onto the kitchen sink, I think, 'I need support'. And when you turn around again, you have the feeling, 'hold fast, if you don't want to turn', but it is just as if you keep on turning. I hold fast, but my body keeps on turning ... that's the feeling I have. I went to visit my mother last week, feeling terrible ... and I heard her talking, as if she were far away ... it's just as if you aren't really there ... as if you are on automatic ... My mother is a fine woman, but if you need her, she is never there. She can't cope ... As a child, if something happened that I didn't like, and I went to cope with it myself, I found that my mother had already taken care of it ... Now I have to learn to say what I don't like. I have never had to do that ... But if I say now to my mother that I don't like something, she says: 'You're wrong.'"

(Patient E): "I used to ride a bicycle, but I don't anymore, because if I did now and a tram came along or a car I would ride straight into it, so attracted I feel to it ...

... it's the same with the ditch. I was walking on the little path next to the ditch, with my dogs ... and when I do, I always feel so attracted to it that I started walking slantedly towards it. That's strange, because I was just walking, not even on my bicycle.... When I'm walking with my husband in the street, and he says to me, 'Look, so-and-so just past us, won't you say hello?', I think: 'Good heavens, I didn't even see her'. All my attention goes into concentrating on walking. I have no time for looking around anymore, like I used to do ... If I don't concentrate on walking in a straight line, I know an accident will happen ...

... My hands shake so much, I can't hold a cup and saucer anymore ... the saucer starts rattling around, and it falls ... I've broken a lot of things that way ... I spend hours staring in front of me at nothing. Then my husband says, 'Don't worry so much', and then I realize that I've been staring ahead at nothing ... Sometimes I start scratching myself, and go on scratching until my skin breaks. I even do it in bed, and in my sleep. My whole back is sometimes full of the scratches I give myself in my sleep.

... My mother died two-and-a-half years ago. I still can't get accustomed to it. For months after she was dead, I used to ring her up every day. I kept thinking, 'She's still there', and then I'd ring and get no answer. Before she died, I used to see her a lot, I visited her a lot ... I sometimes ask myself what it's all about ... when I was a child, my mother wasn't at all kind to me ... but when she died, I couldn't get it through my head that she was dead ... not at all."

(Patient F): "I never feel really fit, neither physically nor mentally fit. I'm always tired, tired, tired. My head feels heavy. I have continuously the feeling that there's a brick in my head ... Sometimes I become so light, so light, that I feel like a feather. Sometimes I walk across the street with the idea that I could just blow away, so light am I. Then at a crossing, I become quite crazy, and have to hold on to a lantern pole. Once in a tram I became dizzy and since then it's got worse.

After that I became more and more afraid of trams. I didn't dare to go out anymore, because I thought, 'I'll faint in the street. I am all alone, and I'll just lie there'.... I had another peculiarity. I kept walking to the left, I had to. It was as if I was pulled that way. Not that I was waggling about the street, but very slowly I was pulled to the left. I would start on one side of the street and end up on the other side ... was it to the left ... or to the right?. I don't remember exactly. But after that I started becoming afraid ... and dizzy. It was just as if you were shut up in yourself ... swallowed up ... The people in the street, I saw them, but they seemed so far away, the people and the surroundings ... rather peculiar, strange. When people spoke to me, I didn't connect ... it just didn't come through. I started to hear badly too, but the doctor said there was nothing wrong with my ears, either.... It was just as if my body walked outside, but my mind was asleep. I felt very, very tired ... and with a lot of noise in my ears ... I was deafened in a way. When I got up in the morning, I was very unsteady on my feet ... so I would lie down on the couch all day and do absolutely nothing. I think I didn't leave the house for eight months. Afterwards, I had to take a taxi to my work. I knew most of it was psychical, but I was sure too that there was something wrong with me ... and then I started to hyperventilate; and after one or two panic attacks in the neighbourhood, I would start running so hard that I'd almost trip and fall down ... I saw everything as if through a mist, as if I had a filmy substance in front of my eyes ... things were clear and not clear.

... I used to see stars and lights before I fell into sleep ... I don't have it all the time, but sometimes, before falling asleep, I would fall in space, into a bottomless space, and then wake up with a shock. I found it so awful that after a while I didn't dare to fall asleep. But after a while you fall asleep, and at the moment you fall, you fall and fall into space without a bottom to it.

... When things irritate me, I wait a long time without saying anything, but at a certain moment it all becomes too much, and then I explode! My father and mother never really fought ... it was limited to wretched words, answered by silence ... sometimes my mother, sometimes father ...'

The Social Phobic Experience

Patient G, a teacher, is 25 years old, unmarried, has no children. His main complaints are fear of disease (cancer), and social phobia. *Patient H*, a housewife, is 31 years old, married,with two children. Her only complaint is that she is afraid to sign her name to anything (e.g., cheques in a bank). *Patient I*, a housewife, is 30 years old, married, with three children. Her main complaints are fear of people, and of being alone.

Experiences of Space Itself, and/or Objects or Structures in Space

(Patient G): "When I am feeling disturbed, agitated, then buildings, especially those in industrial surroundings become unbearable ... and I dare not go near them. You should know that industrial landscapes have always fascinated me, I love them, the cranes, the oil tanks, the lines of the industrial landscape. But at such times they take on a fearful quality, a threatening atmosphere, a prelude to Death. The metal of the tanks looks as if it is worn thin by the chemicals inside, breakable, transparent, on the point of disintegration.

... I don't think I see things differently, rather I feel things differently, my moods change. The whole landscape becomes grey, sombre, the colours dimmer, more muted, less discriminable. The grasses look more uniform, light brown and white, not like these really are.

... Music is my hobby, especially Gluck's music; but when these fears come over me, then any sound at all takes on an extremely sad tone, like death marches, only dissonances, only minor keys, very, very low.

... Once I felt really bad, turned in on myself, very isolated, unable to make contact with anyone. My girlfriend and I decided to go for a walk. What do you think happens? All conversation is impossible between us, because I begin then to hum Bruckner's Ninth Symphony and I go on for two hours, up until the walk has ended ... just as if I am a blind man, I've walked through the whole countryside, and seen nothing of it ... you see it ... but you don't take it in ... or are able to talk about it.

... When I feel really bad, it's as if everyone is looking at me, staring at me, invading my privacy. I have the feeling that the houses come closer, stand closer together. The buildings, the balustrades, the cornices of the houses, they all tilt over, as if they'll fall on me ... and I have to get out into the streets.... But even the houses across the way from my apartment seem to come closer, very near to me, and I feel worse than I already feel. It seems as if the people in them stare down my neck, watch everything

I do, take a special delight in butting in on my affairs, have their noses on my lips ... and I panic, and have to go out for a walk, or on my bike. Then I tear through the streets at terrible speed, like a madman, cycling to Alkmaar and back, in one-and-a-half hours.... Distances become enormously minimized, but time strangely enough seems to go slower.... It began two years ago ... I remember it as if it were yesterday, and know exactly what kind of weather it was, where we were cycling, everything ... Now I have this fear ... to see industrial compounds ... if I see them, it leads immediately to digressions, strange notions, and the like".

(Patient H): "It is very difficult when I am angry to see things ... I also perceive differently then ... if I don't feel well, I am not aware of my surroundings, I am turned inward. I can walk or bicycle for long distances without having taken in anything of what I have passed through. I notice nothing else, but my feelings at that moment. Afterwards I more or less know where I've been, but at the time you don't take it in.... If I don't feel good, and I have to go somewhere, the distance does not seem longer, but just the opposite, it's shorter ... because I don't notice it ... suddenly I am where I had to go ... In town, I mostly have some purpose, and I think of that. But if I don't feel well, I can't keep my mind on that purpose, and then you feel as if you are walking around without any aim ... the idea comes up, 'What am I doing here?' ... I walk through the town and the other people do too, but I am alone, and the rest is a big mass, the rest belongs together, but I am alone, I walk next to them, between them, but I am not part of them ...

... I do have that at the times when I don't feel well sounds irritate me more ... the radio can become really annoying ... you are trying to get yourself under control, and it distracts you, prevents that ... sounds become harsher, harder, and besides they become sharper ... then you wake up with a shock ... If I'm not feeling well, then I sometimes feel in a group of persons as if I am on the outside of it ... I perceive things less clearly, a bit vaguely, I don't really register what they say or do, ... things seem farther away ... in a bank or at a reception-desk, the railing of the counter isn't next to me anymore but has moved off at a distance, sometimes even a metre away. So everything else becomes a bit vague, a vague cluster, and I am separate from it".

(Patient I): "When I am tense, then everything seems to loom at you, then you see more things too ... I mean, I used to see little mice out of the corner of my eyes ... I always see something when I am tense, and it suffocates me. When I'm not tense, I don't see much of what's around me, but what I see looks nicer ... but when I don't feel well, then it is as if there is a veil over everything ... When my husband asks me to go to the market with him, in my mind I go there and back ... and then it seems too far to go, because I've already been there and back, down the stairs, out into the air, through the garden ... it all seems too far away ..Sometimes I can stand before the window for hours and stare outside, although I don't see what is happening outside. I see the houses, I see the people, but I don't see who is walking around. If there was even a fight going on outside my door, and you'd ask me who took part in the fight, or even if there was a fight, I wouldn't know.... If I go down to the greengrocer's and one of the boys there makes some comment or other, I blush terribly, and then I avoid the greengrocer's after that. What do I do? I flee, turn my head away but I still feel his gaze, and so I try to get away altogether.

... When I day-dream, I don't fantasize about myself, I am as I really am ..not shy at all. I feel fine in these day-dreams. Other people in my day-dreams?. Yes, but they don't have faces ... I don't know what I'd do if they had faces..If my husband has gone to bed, and I feel anxious or suffocated, sitting in the sitting-room, then I rush off to bed too because I'm terrified of sitting there alone while I'm afraid".

Experiences of One's Self and One's Body in Space

(Patient G): "When people look at me, or when I am feeling sick, then my body changes too. It is like a harlequin feeling, as if my limbs, my legs, feet, arms and hands are made of wood, and my movements feel like those appear in the harlequin, a wooden doll, without the suppleness that one normally has, very wooden, very mechanical. In stages too, like this: turn to the left, a bit to the right, a step forward, arm down, and yet quite co-ordinated .. but it's difficult to grasp hold of a (sauce-) pan.

... I feel very unhappy, inferior with people I don't know ..afraid that I'll make some catastrophic mistake; feelings of shame too, about what I don't know, but I feel them. I am afraid that the other will find me strange, pushy, but uninteresting ... I am more turned in on myself when I am feeling low and I creep into my shell, become terribly indifferent to the outside world, avoid contact with it. When I feel low, I don't find a number of people sympathetic. Perhaps I start noticing their unsympathetic side, become intolerant. I have that often".

(Patient H): "I am afraid to put my signature to anything, and every time I have to do this, then I become not myself to myself. Then I look at myself as if I am a thing. I find it unreal that I am doing what I'm doing, that I am who I am with that behaviour. Then I say to myself: 'That isn't you' . I don't feel myself anymore, doing that that's not me that is a piece of me apart from me ... a sort of 'flu that will pass. Once, a few times I have had a feeling of having enormous hands, very large hands and very large feet, very soft material, not wooden, not hard, but all of it very light, very heavy ... but like boxing gloves, soft but heavy too. But gloves with fingers. When you're going to sleep, when you can't see anything, only feel ..Then you get an anxiety reaction, a very intense feeling ..you have the idea: 'They are so big' ..I have the feeling that signing my name to me is more or less the same as 'I am showing whom I am, this is me' it is something very personal".

(Patient I): "Before I was an insignificant person, of no account I wouldn't even look at my figure in the mirror. In my mind I was horrible to look at, but others were beautiful, but I wasn't I noticed that that hand became smaller and smaller. I had that feeling, that your fingers became shorter and shorter ..I would look at them for a long time, and then I would think: 'I probably never looked at them before when I was a child'. I thought I was different to what I am; but other people seemed different too. Now when I look at them carefully....

As a child I was always afraid before I went to sleep. When I shut my eyes I saw spirals, and everything swam before my eyes, and then I sank into a deep well ..I was terribly afraid of this. In my dreams I see all the people I dream of but I am not there myself. I never see myself, but I take part in the dream. I never see myself walking or doing anything in my dreams ... if anyone would come up to me to give me a kiss, then that face would only come closer and closer to me, but I never see me. I think I've always been afraid, I think I have to have something to be afraid of, to exist".

Concluding Remarks

These experiences of individual patients, occurring often when they are feeling "down", seem to bear out the findings of the larger study in which the answers were determined by ratings on different scales (Chapter VII). The most remarkable of these experiences, shared by all the patients interviewed, is the awareness of the expansion and/or contraction of space around them, of their bodies (or body parts) expanding or contracting in space, and of the awareness of the instability of spatial surfaces supporting them. These strange distortions of spatial surfaces, of inflow and outflow patterns of movement and of self-in space seem to go together, though not in a smooth, consistent way. In some experiences (for example, in the claustrophobic experience) visual and haptic perceptions seem to coalesce. The patient feels unable to separate what is haptically perceived (the "feel") from what is visually happening, and loses control of herself (or her body) in space. Spatial structures loom, come up close, threaten to engulf one, consume one's personal space, or seem to crush the integrity of one's body. From this seeming intrusiveness the claustrophobic, becoming anxious (and angry), takes recourse by retreat into "the little shell", the little bubble of space that is projected to protect.

In others (for example, in the agoraphobic experience) haptic and visual perceptions seem to yield experiences of separation or disintegration, as structures zoom away from one, seem to disappear into an unbridgeable distance, leaving the person abandoned, washed-up, like a beached whale, alone and defenceless before the expanding and retreating void. Becoming increasingly anxious, the agoraphobic tries to escape from the harsh experience by retreat into disconnectedness, into "being-not-there".

In still other experiences (for example, in the social phobic experience), haptic and visual perceptions seem to merge and then separate in a rhythmic, pulsating fashion, as the two flow-patterns of space, expansion and contraction, combine to yield the appearance of a world in which one is enclosed, but threatens one by this uncontrollable instability. Against these terrifying experiences the social phobic tries to defend himself (or herself) by a further turning inwards, away from the horror of space, to sole preoccupation with his (her) haptic experiences and the concomitant, negative emotions.

The suddenness with which these "switches" take place in change of experience of the outer world and of oneself in it, and the rising panic that the seeming loss of control engenders, are characteristic of all the experiences, as reported by these patients. They all describe the suddenness of the experiences in terms of the *feel* of things or of themselves, as the change occurs: "Suddenly it springs out, right at me, head-on, it feels as if about to engulf me" (the professor of English literature); "It's like they will fall down on me, crush me ... I feel almost threatened" (a claustrophobic woman); "Suddenly it happened. All the people became tiny ..and it was as if I'd become very large" (another patient with claustrophobic and travelphobic complaints); "Suddenly the whole world has changed ... it's as if I experience everything at a great distance ... as if there's a barrier between me and the others" (an agoraphobic patient); "My head feels heavy ... like there's a brick in it ... but sometimes I become so light that I feel like a feather ... I could just blow away" (another agoraphobic patient); "I don't think I see things differently, rather I feel things differently ... (at times) the whole landscape becomes grey, sombre, colours dimmer, more muted, sounds very very low

... at other times it's as if everyone is looking at me, staring at me ... even the houses come closer ... they all tilt over, as if they'll fall on me" (a social phobic patient); "If I don't feel well, I am not aware of my surroundings, I am turned inward ... am aware of nothing else, except my feelings at that moment, long distances seem much shorter ... suddenly I am where I had to go ... but the town and other people ... are a big mass, belonging together ... but I am alone, not part of them" (another social phobic patient).

These experiences, especially those of looming structures, bring to mind the series of experiments described by Gibson et al. (1962, 1965) in which a small, dark silhouette was projected at the centre of a large, translucent screen, with a point of observation close to the screen. After the shadow filled the screen, observers (both human and animal) experienced the virtual object as not increasing in size but as suddenly coming out of the screen, as visually colliding with them. So impelling was this impression that all observers dodged or ducked to avoid the oncoming object. The rate of magnification was proportional to the imminence of the collision, and the accelerated portion of the sequence was called "looming" by the investigators, specifying as it did impending collision (see Chapter II).

This suggests that, in both the experiences of the patients and in the experiments, constancy scaling mechanisms are operative, determining their impelling effects. The sustained attention to a certain part of the visual field, thereby blotting out other relations which might be necessary to correct these scaling effects (and behavioural action), and/or the triggering of earlier patterns of adjustment in the haptic system, may be part of the explanation for the frequency of these illusions in phobic patients. As earlier suggested (Chapter VI), there seems to be a tendency in phobic patients (and in some normals) to adjust to stimulation in ways that are not congruent with stable perception. Perhaps, under the sustained attention to bodily (or personal) matters characteristic of these patients, and/or abased levels of awareness of external happenings or events, these constancy scaling mechanisms automatically revert to ("switch back to") earlier adjustment levels, determined in infancy or childhood. Hence the suddenness of the perceptual change. It is certainly intriguing that these patients, while reliving or remembering their experiences in the retelling, spontaneously mention or hark back to early childhood experiences, hinting (sometimes broadly) at intrusive, inadequate or overprotective responses from the mother. Another curious and, for the patients, rather inexplicable tendency in two (agoraphobic) patients, to deviate inadvertently from a straight line while walking on the street, starting on one side and ending up on the other, brought to my mind the image of a little child being dragged along by the parent on the street, trudging reluctantly away from items of interest to her but not to the parent.

Did some such thing often happen in the child's past? A more probable explanation may lie in the fact that, when visual cues fall away, and one relies solely on bodily cues (tactile, kinaesthetic, or vestibular) one tends to veer or circle. Apparently, bodily cues are inadequate to detect small changes of direction; a slight bias is sufficient to produce veering over a short distance (Ross, 1974, p. 115).

All speak too of felt distortion in body size, weight, movement when feeling low, and some hint at simultaneously perceived (felt) distortion in the parent's body, for instance, in an embrace. While reading through their reports, time and again one receives a strong impression of young children experiencing contacts with the parent in which inadvertently too little, too much, or too conflicting room was allowed the child. These relations between mother and child possibly describe what Gibson indicates as the (negative) affordances of environmental structures or relations, picked up directly by the observer (*in casu*, the child). The immediacy of these affordances triggers behavioural action (for instance, strong emotion, escape or avoidance). But affordances are perceptual effects that *precede* action. What the person or object *stands for* is first felt or perceived by the person paying attention to the event, object or relation. Also, affordances control or constrain behaviour but do not cause it.

Several of the patients recall too, just before sleep or in dreams, experiences of falling into a bottomless space, horrific and paralyzing. These experiences, common enough hypnagogic illusions to which we are all subject, arising as these do from the involuntary relaxation of one's muscles on the edge of sleep, were unrecognized as such by the child (and uncorrected by the parent in talks with the child), thus remaining a source of horror, sufficient in some to trigger anxiety responses, even in adulthood.

What all the patients seem to have in common, apart from the experiences of spatial distortion and distortion of self-in-space, is the feeling of being caught up in a dynamic (and involuntary) interaction with this Other, held in the ban of an omnipotent, omnipresent, greater Whole. But as a prisoner, caught on a treadmill, or on a roller-coaster. All try valiantly to escape, although excited by this at the same time. It is as if there is a longing to become an integral part, an eager participator in the drama, on centre stage. Instead, one is overpowered or rejected, crushed or relegated to the shadows. Hence the anger, anxiety, distress, and increased focusing on one's sorry state, as one turns away from the phenomenon, into one's little shell or fragile bubble of space.

Such descriptions suggest very strongly that we are dealing with a subjective experience of a very intimate, fundamental nature: the intrinsic bonding of mother and child, a bond that can easily become a millstone around one's neck (incidentally, as much so for the mother as for the child). The importance of the interactions between the haptic system and its components (touch, position sense, bodily movements, etc.) with the visual, and other perceptual systems is underlined. Although several patients mention how abrasive and disturbing sounds of everyday objects, or of persons become when they are not feeling well or happy, we know from the larger study (Chapter VII) that phobics do not differ herein from normals, at least in the frequency of alterations in the experience of sounds. But they may differ in the intensity of such experiences. Nor may we rule out potent effects from internal organs, affecting these states. Vestibular function too, being part of the basic orienting functions, undoubtedly plays some part in these disturbances. But, on the basis of what our empirical inquiry brings to light, we may now postulate with a little more certainty that at least two major perceptual systems, the visual and the haptic, must be taken into account, if we are to gain a proper understanding of the nature of perceptual dysfunction in phobia.

Throughout, I have also spoken of the claustrophobic, agoraphobic, and social phobic experience, rather than of experiences of specific phobics. This is done to bring out more clearly that the interactive effects of person with space yield certain basic experiences, which may take on other forms, depending on the nature of the relation, or the focus of attention. Many patients suffer from more than one type of complaint, which suggests that within the same individual and at different times, one or other pattern of spatial (self) distortion might be experienced. If the distortions as described in the foregoing are linked to the different experiences of phobia, it becomes easier to understand why some symptom substitution may arise; even without recourse to other psychodynamic explanations. For these could appear spontaneously, as the focus of attention changes in the patient, or as a result of different stimulation and triggering of adaptation effects in the course of treatment. But the essential point is not that certain types of phobics generate, or adjust to, stimulation in ways peculiar to their specific problem, however interesting this is in itself. Rather, that the forms such adjustments take (or the complaint that may result from these) are probably a direct consequence of the fact that, in humans and animals, certain patterns of response (or strategies) are built into our perceptual systems to ensure adequate and effective responses to the remarkable environment in which we live, for survival ends.

To live happily in the awe-inspiring transformations, permutations, and fluctuations of Space, the primordial Mother or, in Gibson's formulation, the ecological events of our planet, one must not only control to some extent the appearances of these relations, by maximizing some and minimizing others. One must develop a sense of (the feel of) being an integral part of her. In adjusting her relations and being adjusted by them, perceiving all her faces and being perceived in them, one ensures her beneficence.

Codetta

After writing this chapter, a friend and colleague who had suffered from agoraphobia as an adolescent wrote to me about his experiences then, which had in part been relived while reading my work. An excerpt from his letter may form an apt conclusion, an independent and yet congruent commentary on what has gone before, like the coda of a sonata.

"It's very strange: when it gets dark, the phobic threat diminishes, in my case. How does that happen? I remember that I formulated it for myself then, like this: 'Because I and everything else are enveloped in that darkness'.

When it snows, when the world lies under a white carpet of snow, a heavy pack of snow, the phobic tension lessens too, and finally disappears. Why? Because without exception the snow covers every single thing, it brings everything into contact, in one big grasp that encloses everything. In some way or another this enormous, threatening visual space (let's say, the fields in front of me, the village silhouette in the distance) becomes connected by the pack of snow, and loses its threatening, empty infinitude.

Music too works like a magic wand. When my ear, my eardrums are stimulated by intelligent, warm, well-formed sound, creating order in my universe, the balloon of expected phobic tension is pierced and bursts. And I relax....

When I think about it, it seems to me that phobic states – at least, agoraphobic reactions – come about through the separation or falling apart of one's haptic and visual perceptions. I no longer experience the synesthetic quality of my primordial perceptions. How I long for this again ! But it is gone forever. As a baby, as a child it was always there, I know it was so".

X

General Discussion

Optical Structures, Visual and Haptic Events that Evoke Derealization and Depersonalization, the "It" of Phobia

Let us briefly retrace our steps to see more clearly where we now are, and by which route we arrived. In Chapter I, we started out amid a portent of hints, allusions, uncertainties and guesses about the (perceptual) nature of phobia. I suggested, after reviewing what phobic patients have told us down the ages, and what psychodynamic theorists have concluded from their experiences, that perhaps the theories have given too little weight to one link in the chain that might be essential to a proper understanding of the complaint: the environmental. We had taken into account the intrusions of the unconscious, the emotional and physiological distress, developmental aspects, and learning and social contributions. But we had discounted something that all seemed to experience, an uncontrollable instability and nonconstancy of their external world, and of themselves in it. We had discounted this because, with our greater insight and knowledge of interactive effects between person and world, we had attributed these experiences merely to a wrong coding of the stimulation received from the external world. As Aretaeus (ca. A.D. 30–90) said, and Barendregt (1974) expressed in similar terms (see his definition, Chapter I, p. 2) without knowing about Aretaeus (as he told me, when I pointed out the similarity between their formulations): "Persons who are mad see as others do but do not form a correct judgment on what they have seen."

In Chapter II, I decided to take a closer look at what is known about perception. For if we learn to perceive, like we learn to think, or like we learn to identify and properly code our sensations, then the psychodynamic theorists might have a point. But if perception, unlike sensation, is a more direct process, then this argument might not be as relevant as it seemed. In contrasting the two main standpoints in the field, the representational approach to perception with the ecological approach, I found out that the field of opinion was still undecided. The former approach, long the established position, which states that perception is indirect and achieved by complex representations of reality in the brain, seemed now to be losing a little ground to its leading rival. Far from being established as definitive, the ecologists (Gibson) argue that the process of perception is direct, and that the age-old conceptions, though hoary with age, are wrong.

I took heart from this. And, though enjoying the confusion of the Establishment through the cogently argued standpoint of the ecologists, I hedged my bets a little by taking one important concept from the representationists – constancy scaling (Gregory), – and another from the ecologists – reversible optical structures (Gibson)

– to form the two cornerstones of the building I was about to erect on the nature of perception in phobia.

Armed with a little more knowledge of perceptual affairs, I returned to the psychodynamic theorists and clinicians, in Chapter III. With eyes cleansed, it became easier to see where, in their theoretical constructs, they might be relying too much on perceptual ideas that had still to be definitively established. Still, a deeper understanding of the uneasy relations between the unconscious and consciousness, or symmetrical and asymmetrical being, and the complicated intertwining of their processes was gained in exploring the theoretical ideas of some well-known clinicians (Freud; Matte-Blanco; Barendregt). This weight of knowledge received a partial integration in Chapter IV, as I tried, by drawing together the skeins of knowledge on perceptual theory and psychodynamic theory, to combine their ideas in a sensible way, to form the bricks of the house. Though still not much more than a scaffolding, this attempt yielded an hypothesis about the probable nature of perception in phobia, which took into account many aspects of the problem, including the environmental one. This hypothesis states that reversible optical structures and the visual (and haptic) events they give rise to, e.g., occlusion phenomena, expansion and contraction, inflow and outflow patterns with locomotion, etc., will be effective in evoking "it", because of their "affordances" and consequences for control of self-in-space, from infanthood on.

In the next pages, we will draw up the balance, to see what has been achieved by what might have seemed an unnecessarily circuitous route. In Part Two, bit by bit, supposed links between spatial relations, perceptual process, and phobic experience took on form. In Chapter V, and by learning from our reproach of the psychodynamic theorists, we started off by asking (in a systematic way) the phobic patients about the environmental relations (variables) which caused them such apparent distress. Taking them seriously, we proceeded step by step to try to substantiate what was found from the first explorations. But, to do justice to both sides, we let ourselves be guided also by what was going on in this field in the mainstream of perceptual inquiry at that time.

Despite a non-Gibsonian approach to the exploration of spatial relations, certain "invariants" of structure appeared as the relevant ones in maintaining phobic responses to the environment. These are: those height-distance (H/D) and breadth-distance (B/D) ratios that elicit feelings of enclosure, the funneling effect of being pressed down or thrust through the shaft of the spaces, of unprotectedness, of suffocation; ratios of illumination (especially dark and extreme light) that elicit feelings of sombreness, dismalness or darkness, and which make the spaces difficult to oversee; moving, occluding objects or people in space that elicit feelings of busyness or crowdedness; massive, compact structures whose heterogeneity of arrangement in space occlude spaces or make spaces difficult to oversee; irregularity of arrangement of elements in space (asymmetry or random distribution), and irregularity of shape and contour. Last, but certainly not least, wide, open, empty or unoccluded spaces that elicit feelings of loneliness, solitariness, or bleakness.

The linking of these aspects of spatial relations is important, and for two reasons: First, the spatial variables exactly describe environmental components long known to psychology to be effective in aiding or hindering us to achieve constancy of objects and/or the layout of space, and by implication, of ourselves or our bodies in space.

The second reason refers to what might be called, in line with Gibson's formulations, the *affordant* aspects of these structural components, which are underlined by the qualifications attached by the phobic patients. Put in another way, they symbolize or embody some relations between parent (mother) and child; but also the relations of the adult person turned to the infinity of Space, as I have argued in Chapters IV, VII and IX. The haptic and visual experiences speak directly of too little or too much space, of a relation seen from the perspective of the child-in-arms, who is repeatedly either too closely embraced, or too often abandoned, or both, by the parent or adult caretaker. Perhaps, because of this embodiment, these dimensions of space have such potent effects on phobics, who strenuously avoid, or are highly anxious in, those situations in which such relations are multiply present. One might recall here that Gibson was of the opinion that it is the affordances of structures that are probably first perceived by the infant, long before colour, size and form are distinguished as such. It may even be that, when phobic patients focus their attention on the affordant aspects, the frightful faces of Space appear, and the functions of spatial relations as footholds (or constancy cues) are lost, or temporarily unperceived.

That phobics, however, are capable of perceiving these ratios of stimulation from a normal perspective, is borne out by the fact that they did not significantly differ from normal persons in perceptual judgments of these variables. But some individuals seemed to add to or subtract from these ratios a large constant. This, though, still speculative, may help to explain why – in spite of the correct perception of the ratios of stimulation present in the environment – their *experiences of these relations* differ so greatly from those of normal persons.

With this observation, I was forced to entertain the idea that some basic perceptual mechanism(s) must be involved. And, for the present, the representational standpoint seemed to clarify this more than the ecological one (although, see Turvey, 1977, for an alternative to how constancy may be achieved in an ecological perspective; and more recently, Pribram, 1991, for a holonomic viewpoint to perceptual and cognitive processes that integrates both constructional and ecological approaches).

A closer look at the individual responses of both normal and phobic persons seemed to bear this out. This link is tentatively forged in Chapter VI. The argument, as put forward, states this: the (strategy of) overestimation of low ratios of stimulation and underestimation of high ratios has been demonstrated to be the best way to cope with (extreme) variations of stimulation in one's environmet (Helson). And this is what normals, in general, do. But this over- and underestimation should not exceed a certain value, generally 10–30% of the actual stimulation impinging on the organism, otherwise distortions will arise in one's perceptions or experiences of these ratios of stimulation (Ross, 1974; Powers, 1973). Helson (1964) noted that psychological studies, whether perceptual, cognitive, motivational, learning or social of nature, show that people generally adapt to stimulation as described above. But other forms of adaptation are also found among normal populations. And it is these other variations on the "constancy-scaling" theme that appear to be more often adopted by the phobic patients (see Chapter VI). Some normals also adapt in these ways, but their overestimation and underestimation behaviours, with a few exceptions, seem to remain within the 10–30% "error range", whereas some phobics exceed these limits considerably (see the graphs in Chapter VI). Considerable overestimation of low and high ratios of stimulation was more often found in claustrophobic patients; a greater underestimation of low and high ratios of stimulation in agoraphobic patients; and a substantial underestimation of low, and overestimation of high ratios was found in some social phobic patients, and in others. I will return to this question in the next section, when considering how speculative this link is in the chain.

In Chapters VII and VIII, some evidence was presented of the importance of spatial, rather than temporal relations in perceptual malfunction in phobia. These findings are intriguing from various points of view. The fact that normal persons seem to be not only much more time-flexible but also more time-anxious and time-aware than phobics is, in itself, not a remarkable finding. One would expect persons who are actively integrated into the schemes of daily life in a time-oriented society to be more aware, anxious, and flexible about time-functions than persons who, through illness, are temporarily shunted aside. But, taken together with the greater awareness in phobics of spatial flow-patterns and experiences of spatial distortion, with relative indifference to time-functions, this suggests different orientations to space and time between normals and phobics. The difference might be explained by the more frequent intrusions of the unconscious in lowered states of consciousness, in which, if Freud and Matte-Blanco are right, time does not exist. But Matte-Blanco also suggested that, in his analysis of the characteristics of the unconscious (from a logico-theoretic standpoint), space also vanishes! Still, we shall see in a moment how this paradox of space relations being vital, but space vanishing or vanished being central to the experience of phobics, can be reconciled.

The results of the data on perceptual disorientation, derealization, and depersonalization phenomena show that normals and phobics report infrequent and spontaneous distortions of these kinds under conditions of lowered consciousness (Chapter VII). Herein they do not differ. But phobics differ significantly from normals *in the frequency of some* of these experiences of distortion. We also know from Barendregt's work that phobics differ from normal persons in the *intensity of their transient depersonalization experiences*. Our data show that the greater frequency of derealization and depersonalization experiences in phobics, compared to normals, refers only to the following experiences: seemingly uncontrollable expansion and contraction of space itself, particularly of space seeming to collapse on itself (a finding which is highly significant); the expansion and contraction of one's body in space; its weightlessness; its seeming disappearance in space; the separation of self from body (OBE); feelings of alienation from self; of strangeness and unrealness of self, and of the environment; and, a highly significant difference too in the experience of not being in control of oneself or in danger of losing control of oneself in space. A difference seems to exist between phobics and normals in recall of some of these experiences before their thirteenth year. Fewer phobics than normals recall lack of control over others, and bodily distortions.

No significant differences were found between phobics and normals in the experience of control over other persons or objects in space, or in the experiences of fluctuating changes in the attributes of objects (sensations). Nor any differences in the experiences of time passing, or in the expansion or nonexistence of time.

Such differences as these cannot be laid solely at the door of malfunction in physiological processes (e.g., dizziness, heart palpitation, the sickness of Menière), although vestibular function and kinaesthetic function, and other haptic perceptual functions are involved. This is clear from the fact that, in several of the investigations (e.g., the interviews), the patients often speak of the *feel* of these perceptions, rather than the awareness of them. And, as if to bear Gibson out, their interactions with spatial relations (flow-patterns) are *felt* rather than *perceived*. Yet, to interpret these as expressions of emotional feelings would be a mistake; from the perspective of the babe-in-arms, it is the *feel* of these interactions with space that is registered, probably more than visual contours. In other words, we have evidence here of the haptic perceptual systems influencing the visual one.

One implication of these findings is that, in phobia, not time but space is of prime concern: spatial flow-patterns and the corresponding pulsation of space through one's whole body, as it expands and contracts, and one's body, or parts of one's body, expand and contract with it. But not all spatial relations are disturbed; not, for instance, the perception of relations of objects, or of their movements in space. This finding brings out the subjective, but also the *intimate nature* of the relations with space mentioned in the foregoing. As if to underline this message given by numbers of phobics in the studies described in Chapters V, VII and VIII, the personal experiences of the patients interviewed, in Chapter IX, who had taken no part in the previous studies, tell us in poignant detail what these mean. And they tell us much more than that. They show how the structural components, described in Chapter V, appear to them, and why these are so menacing. They describe the horror and the alienation involved in these interactions. They hint broadly at the relations between the here-and-now experiences and their experiences as children. In fact, in their experiences, past, present and future flow into one. Time, in this sense, ceases to exist.

Furthermore, and clearer than ever we ourselves could imagine, they describe three variations on the theme of being space-engulfed: the flow-patterns of space, and the accompanying pulsation of one's body (becoming smaller and larger, weightless and heavy, etc.), which are so terrifying.

In the claustrophobic experience, spatial relations loom, come up close, even in expansion, consume one's personal space, and threaten to crush the integrity of one's body. The sole defence is anger at this intrusiveness, and retreat into the tiny, and continually diminishing bubble of space around one ("the little shell"), projected to escape this horrible fate. In the agoraphobic experience, spatial structures zoom away from the person, disappearing into an unbridgeable distance, leaving the person washed-up, beached on a shore of nothingness, abandoned and defenceless before the expanding and retreating void. The sole defence against this horror is retreat into the tiny, extremely fragile bubble of space left around one, into disconnectedness, into "being-not-there". In the social phobic experience, the two flow-patterns of space, expansion and contraction, combine, as the world recedes or comes up close in a threatening way. Inside this dynamic happening, but equally unable to control it, the social phobic projects a little bubble, slightly more opaque than the bubble of the agoraphobic and the claustrophobic, and encapsulates himself in this cocoon. In the illusion of separateness from the world, he perceives even less of its contours and these more vaguely than the agoraphobic and the claustrophobic persons do. The world, and all therein, is an amorphous mass "out there", pitted against his small, cocooned self "in here". The sole defence in the face of these terrible antics of space, is a still further turning inwards, away from these disturbances, to a preoccupation with his haptic perceptions and the concomitant emotions to which these give rise. Dreading the amorphous mass in which he is encapsulated just as much as the other phobics, who see it a little more clearly, the social phobic sees only "as through a glass darkly", never face-to-face.

Seen in this light, Freud may, perhaps, be right about the childhood trauma, but wrong about its sexual specificity. The intrusion of the parent is a spatial, yet an emotional one; at least, that is what these phobics describe, as did the phobics in the larger studies who were not interviewed, except by means of rating-scales. It is the distorted relations between parent and child that are portrayed. Freud may have been wrong too about the repression operating in phobia, for nothing is repressed. On the contrary; the child-adult carries in her fragile body (and in her perceptual processes) the ghastly imprint of (space-) relations gone wrong. More exactly, of relations that have never been right. Space carries every attribute in her of these (parent-child) relations – the wellformed and the malformed. To live at ease in her, one must perceive her relations correctly. If one does not, her terrible faces appear, and one is doomed to look at them daily, and nightly.

These phobics, in this view, are the defenceless children of Space, trapped in a bondage not of their own making (though they perpetuate it). Their malformed accommodations to this omnipotent and omnipresent Other, who was once identical with their own mother, are so fragile, so vulnerable that a mere glance, or a breeze, a harsh word or negating gesture, a storm approaching, or the nightfall, an ambiguous smile, or the sun shining too brightly, all are capable of puncturing and deflating these. In a twinkling of an eye one is plunged back into that bottomless place, dreamed of as children; or experienced in hypnagogic illusions before falling into sleep. Misperception of involuntary muscular relaxation, yielding the common, hypnagogic experience of a deep fall into bottomless space as sleep approaches, has gone uncorrected; and thus become an epitome of horror. Small wonder, the suddenness of the "irruptions of symmetrical being into asymmetrical consciousness" (Matte-Blanco). Perhaps though, a better description might be "a fall into symmetrical being", Space in her frightful aspect. And, with this fall, space also vanishes, for she and the phobic become one pulsating Being.

Hence too the susceptibility to failure, or the falling-short of all too brittle schemata to keep the world at bay (that is, to cope with reality as it is experienced). No foothold, no alignment anywhere, as Frijda and Barendregt observe; none indeed. But this lack is perhaps less due to failure of cognitive or emotional schemata of reality, though these too will have suffered some malformation. Rather, in a very literal sense, the lack signals a failure of *perceptual process*, experienced as direct and immediate, with devastating consequences.

The phobic perception is correct, since this *is* the cosmic situation of these unhappy children, only half-emerged from the nuclear family. But it is incorrect too, because partial; because, without other experiences of the more benign faces of Space, she cannot easily be lived in.

These unfortunates have been telling us of their experiences for centuries. How is it that we have listened, yet have not heard? It is not through lack of compassion with their sorry state of non-being. Are we, clinicians and theorists alike, then too caught up in our pet theories, like the social phobic in his solipsistic bubble? For, in truth, we have discounted the contribution of Space, as the real link, and the symbol *par excellence* of the intimacy of relations between mother and child.

Perceptual Control in Phobia: a Matter of Misapplication of Constancy-scaling, Early "Tuning" in Perceptual (Visual and Haptic) Systems, or Conflict Control?

Of course, this is a pretty tale and, in the way I have told it, the gentle reader might well be willing to overlook the holes in the evidence. But the fact remains: this instability and nonconstancy of space itself, and of oneself (or one's body) in space has not been objectively ascertained. We have only the patients' word for it. From a scientific point of view, the theoretical basis is there (as I have shown in Part One), but the empirical evidence is not solid. None of the investigations described can provide this evidence, for they were not set up to do so. Yet, a good deal of the substance of this argument stands or falls on the demonstration that these experiences of spatial flow-patterns, and of one's body expanding and contracting, inhaling and exhaling (and not only by hyperventilating) are not mere figments of the patient's imagination, not hallucinations, nor illusions of the mind. Or not entirely. Yet how are we to understand that space and oneself can be whirling and turning, yet the object environment remain relatively stable? Which is what they report. Frankly, as yet I do not know. The literature, though, provides us with at least three scenarios that might explain this. In Chapters II and VI these were already put forward, but a brief recapitulation might be in order here.

The first goes somewhat like this. At very early ages, perhaps in the first weeks or months of life, neural mechanisms (constancy-scaling mechanisms) are adapted to the then prevailing stimulation. All perceptual systems have such mechanisms, or so the representationists tell us, which have their own specific territories to command: size, form, weight, colour, sound, movement, speed, and so on (Gregory; Ross). Other researchers (e.g., Coren & Girgus; in Epstein, 1977) have shown that these constancy mechanisms operate with selectivity: A part of the visual field can become distorted, leaving other parts relatively or wholly undisturbed. These mechanisms can be influenced "from the bottom up or from the top down", but are not under intellectual control. But the little snake in the grass in this scenario, as far as accounting goes for what happens in phobic perceptual experience, is that there are empirical reasons to doubt the flexibility (pliability) of these visual (and auditive) mechanisms. Once adjusted, they stay adjusted. How then to explain that sometimes the world and oneself in it is stable throughout (to the phobic), and sometimes not?

The second scenario gets around this minor difficulty by doing away with these unnecessary constancy mechanisms (Gibson). The retinas pick up not images, but "invariants" of structure, that is, relations between stimulative effects. The visual system is not the only one obtaining this information; all perceptual systems are attentional systems and all receive much the same information about the environment. So they can correct each other at any time. Each perceptual system picks up not only objective information about the environment but also of the self-in-environment (the subjective information). Systems are "tuned" to stimulation and hence can become better tuned, by movement in the environment, among other things, and by learning processes.

Turvey (see Chapter II, and Turvey, 1977) suggests that the constancy function is probably the same in perception and action, and that there might be only one class of appropriate structures or appropriate procedures for achieving constancy. His bet is that these are "co-ordinative structures which devolve on separate neuroanatomical systems, that is, reflexes and functional combinations of reflexes, through which the interjection of environmental properties (invariants of a higher order) is brought about". Gibson would certainly agree, for he has always contended that the visual and haptic (proprioceptive) systems go hand-in-glove. In this scenario, Harris' objection that it is the proprioceptive systems, and specifically, the position sense, that can account for all the perceptual distortions found on perceptual, and other tasks, does this scenario no harm at all.

If these systems, because of their pliability, are the culprits it is no more than is to be expected. "To see, one must locomote; to locomote, one must see". To observe persistence *and* change, and to perceive correctly one must observe both, one must literally *not* stand still. Standing still, one may see the perspective of things better but one's perception probably will be more liable to distortion.

Neither of these scenarios needs a postulate of conflict to explain perceptual distortion, though neither discounts it either. Helson, who does not concern himself with the question which is the mischiefmaker under the perceptual systems, does point out clearly that, to understand these overestimations and underestimations of stimuli, one needs to take into account the reference level within the person, the zero error point, or neutral point from which stimulation is judged. In other words, the adaptation level reached by that person as a function of past and present acquaintance with the stimulative effects in question.

This brings us to the third scenario: behaviour as the control of perception (Powers), which postulates that large error in output systems (muscle tensions) comes about when two perceptual systems at the same level in the hierarchy of control systems attempt to control the same quantity (in the external world) from widely separated reference conditions. A large dead zone around the virtual reference level will then exist, within which little or no control will be possible, since both reference conditions or levels are opposed, and the output systems are operating at maximum. Since "disturbances in the field" can no longer be effectively removed, the "controlled quantity" cannot be controlled, and responses might oscillate wildly. Hence the large overestimations and underestimations, and the sense of not being in control, or of a world "gone out of control", or in danger of doing so. Yet perceptual control systems that are not in conflict, whether higher or lower in the hierarchy, can operate (function) perfectly well, so that one's perceptual behaviour (and thus stability in certain areas) will be normal except within the dead zone around the reference levels in conflict.

In this model, although perceptual control is hierarchically ordered, the control systems are relatively independent too, otherwise certain perceptual behaviours could not remain stable and under control, while others are "out of kilter".

Whatever the scenario, in all three versions perceptual change is necessarily a slow process. Change will not come about except through heroic effort (whether through therapeutic intervention or otherwise). One reason, perhaps, why phobia is so persistent!

Through the comparisons it is now clear how close the different approaches to perception are. In Powers' model, we can find place for the ecological approach, since his ideas can only be understood if one takes into account the intrinsic interactions between perceptual systems, trying to control the same (external or internal) quantity from different reference conditions. And constancy-scaling becomes transparent too, if what we observe in experiments (and which made the postulate of scaling mechanisms necessary) is merely the result of feedback processes between input, comparator functions and output. Depending on the closeness with which perceptual signals track the reference signals, perception may be correct or wildly incorrect; even showing the patterns of response observed by Helson and others, and by ourselves in our experiments. Gibson's contention that perception is not based on sensation, but is a direct pickup of invariants of structure (whether lower-order or higher-order) can also be accommodated, if we allow, as Powers does, that *some* of the perceptual control systems are geared to this task (e.g., configuration control, control of transitions, etc.), where others might be geared to sensation control, or control of intensity. And these can proceed independently of one another, though not entirely.

To decide which approach is the best fit of the behaviours observed, fundamental research must be undertaken, aimed at answering these questions: Can we demonstrate instability and nonconstancy in the world of phobics, taking into consideration that the world is not separate from ourselves in it? If so, which perceptual systems are involved? Is a postulate of conflict and control necessary, and sufficient, to understand these behaviours? To answer such questions, one may have to carry out tests for constancy in a laboratory setting, but also in the field, tests for rivalry between perceptual systems, and/or tests for conflict control. The explorations in this study did not address these issues. Designed in a teaching capacity to allow students to fulfil requirements for courses and to learn more about perceptual function in phobia, they cannot provide satisfactory answers to such fundamental problems. Yet, given their modest aims, the yield is quite high, in the power that lies in the hypotheses these have generated, which seem to me fruitful ones to pursue.

I should like to mention here three groups of researchers whose work might be particularly relevant to the problems discussed in this book, and which may enable us to attack some of the fundamental issues involved: First, the work of Lee and Lishman (1975, 1977) and their co-workers, in showing how vision may provide exproprioceptive information which can be used to control balance, may be one way of gaining access to the information in the optic flow, in phobic (and normal) locomotion. Secondly, the new work of Gunnar Johansson and Erik Börjesson (1989) on wide-angle space perception which presents a new type of theory for visual space perception, and shows how wide-angle recording of slants of plane surfaces under self-motion can be achieved, thereby enabling us to explore three-dimensional metric specification of slant information in the optic flow. Thirdly, for a better approach to and understanding of the neurophysiological processes underlying these perceptual behaviours, the work of Pribram (1991) and his co-workers.

Phobia, the (Failed) Quest for Control: Final Comments

Still, the experiential evidence that our phobic patients have presented should not be ignored. In fact, in this may lie the heart of the matter. We now see that though they do not code perceived relations of the objective environment incorrectly (if they did so, their responses to these would have significantly differed from those of normals; which they did not), they may err in their strategies for containing or controlling perception (that is, in wanting to be part of Mother Space and separate from her, at one and the same time).

From this viewpoint we can see that what is crucial in the formulation of Barendregt and Frijda is the clause: (to cope with reality) *as it is experienced.* For we still do not know very much about the "failure or the falling-short of their cognitive schemata"; although we know a great deal more about the experiential clause. If we are to gain a proper understanding of the failure of control in these patients, it is not enough to focus on the haptic system and its components. It would even be misleading to do so, that is, if Powers is right in his analysis of control systems; and/or if the psychodynamic theorists and clinicians are right in saying that it is not the unconscious but the distorting function of consciousness (or asymmetrical being) that is to blame for the misery. For their perceptual instruments, that is, the haptic (in *casu*, of the unconscious) system and the visual (in *casu*, of consciousness), given that they are in conflict about the perceptual ends to be achieved, will interact and "it" will come to full bloom. In other words, it may be the confusion arising from the perception, visually, that the world is stable and ordered while perceiving, haptically, instability and disorder which, in the attempt to reconcile these irreconcilable positions, generates large error and drives the output systems to maximum response in opposed directions.

Recognizing now that we, our bodies, our selves, are not separate from the world but part of her, we may now understand why the profounder aspect of this conflict, the interaction of (primordial) Space with her children, is central to the phobic experience. Space-engulfed as they are, half-emerged from the nuclear family, and still in bondage to the parent, they are most susceptible to her antics. It is highly probable that the vulnerability of the phobic person lies in the fact of having half-emerged, or being half-submerged, if one prefers. The normal person, relatively independent in his dependency, does not suspect how disabling it may be to strive, and not to succeed in achieving an equilibrated stance. For even when the world and oneself in it seem stable, there is always the sense of unsafety, of impending doom, the expectation of catastrophe. Knowing "on the inside, in one's little shell" that something is radically wrong, without being able to pin-point just what is wrong and why, is to live on a precipice with the constant feeling that, at any time, one's precarious balance may be upset, and world and self spin out of control.

This experience, an intensely anxiety-evoking, existential state, deserves not only our sympathy but our respect, for the courage to be that is shown by phobic persons in the face of impending calamity.

XI

Summary

The origin of this study lies in the idea that theorists and clinicians, in assuming that the environment plays only a minor, and at most, symbolic, part in phobia, amounting to little more than being an inappropriate substitute for unresolved psychic conflict, might be overlooking an essential link. The fact that phobic patients, even when enlightened about the "true" source of their troubles, still seemed unable to ignore the environmental contribution, was reason enough to try to find out whether or not it should be given more weight in theoretical formulations.

This study reveals that, though the environment is by no means the only determinant of phobia, in the interaction of person with world, and in the origin and maintenance of phobia, it may be a vital, even an essential link. The empirical inquiry demonstrates the existence of relations between physical characteristics of the environment, their "affordant" or experiential characteristics, and adaptation responses, that trigger and may even control the phobic experience, though they do not cause it. The theoretical inquiry provides us with a better understanding of the roots of these relations.

The main thesis of this study is that phobia, at least in part, derives from some not well-understood perceptual interactions of persons with relatively permanent structures common to all environments in all ages, forms that these perceptual transformations of structures take, and inadequate control of the situations involved. In this context, *perceptual control* is considered in a dual capacity, to refer on one hand to the constraints imposed on perceptual systems by the nature of environmental stimulation and, on the other, to the regulating, guiding, and steering perceptual actions resulting from information thus acquired.

Within this frame of reference, the hypothesis is entertained that in the perception of phobic persons, certain configurations of structure, objects, and/or events that define environmental relations are systematically distorted. This distortion involves substantial over- and underestimation of parameters of environmental conditions, which in turn may give rise to experiences of being overpowered by, and/or alienated from the environment; as well as to experiences of instability in or fluctuations of (parts of) the surround.

The frequency (and/or intensity) of these experiences in phobic patients is such that the higher frequency (and/or intensity) of disorientation, derealization, and depersonalization experiences found in these patients may be understood as following from them. In this view then, part of the problem of phobia lies in inadequate attempts to come to grips with prevailing (perceptual) reality.

The study begins with a brief consideration of some of the problems of definition of phobia, and a comparison of descriptions of phobia down the years up to the present. This comparison yields several working hypotheses: of developmental, emotional, physiological, personality, and perceptual nature. Only the perceptual hypotheses are put to the test in this study. Perceptual aspects relevant to these hypotheses include: (a) differential effects of environmental structure, objects, and events; (b) relative instability of environmental structure and objects, and of the phobic person's own movements in space; and (c) individual differences among sufferers, not only in the degree to which certain structures, objects or events affect them, but also in the range that is effective.

The striking fact, discussed in the clinical literature, of a constant, almost obsessive self-observation in these patients with concomitant disregard for other objects or structures in the environment suggests that their perceptual behaviour cannot be properly understood unless one takes into account developmental and familial conditions in forming such behaviour. Furthermore, since these apparent self- (and object) orientations seem to result from projections of internalized (i.e., subjective) sources of anxiety onto environmental (i.e., objective) sources, the hypothesis further includes that their perceptual activity cannot be properly understood unless one takes into account the complicated intertwining (or confluence) of unconscious and conscious (cognitive) systems in this behaviour.

Part One of this work is therefore concerned with elaborating on the concept of control in some theories of perception, in which specific attention is given to: (a) defining the parameters of environmental stimulation which are deemed essential to a successful and stable organization of the world; (b) the nature of perceptual process; and (c) the rôle of regulatory and adaptive responses of organisms (people, animals) to the natural environment. The representational standpoint (the established position) is compared and contrasted with the ecological approach (its main rival); and the weaknesses and strengths of these theoretical approaches brought out in the ensuing discussion between different (perceptual) theorists.

This controversy is followed by a consideration of the psychodynamic approach to neurosis, and particularly to phobia, in which Freud's ideas on perception and on the rôle that perceptual and ego control plays in the origin and maintenance of the phobic reaction are described and discussed. Through further clarification of his theoretical position by the contributions of other psychodynamic theorists (Matte-Blanco; Barendregt), some emendations of his theory are proposed by them.

Part One is concluded by an attempt to integrate what is substantial in theory and empirical work reviewed in the foregoing chapters, which yields a more full-bodied idea of the different and necessary links in the phobic chain, and of their interactions.

In Part Two some empirical relations are explored between environmental structure, organismic process, and phenomenal experience, as these pertain to the perception of phobic persons and normal controls. First of all, five studies are described which were designed to try to pin-point the characteristics of environmental structure that are effective in phobia. The findings show that some of the important characteristics are defined by the linking of objective components of the environment (e.g., the ratios of height to distance and breadth to distance of architectural spaces; illumination ratios; presence or absence of people and objects; compactness of structure; wide, open spaces) to their "affordant" aspects. An analysis of individual responses to these ratios of stimulation brings out the fact that individual phobics differ in their "strategies" of perceptual control. Some evidence was obtained for the hypothesis that these differences are tied to the nature of their phobic complaints. Differences also exist between phobic patients and normal persons in strategy and/or degree of control. These strategies of control may well determine, in part, the experiences of phobic patients of environmental stimulation, which differ significantly from those of normal persons.

In a further study on perceptual disorientation, derealization, and depersonalization phenomena, the empirical data show that both phobic and normal persons invariably report experiences in all three classes, albeit infrequently. The groups do not differ in overall frequency of experience of these phenomena, except in a few categories. The categories of experience which phobics have significantly more frequently than normals are:

Spontaneous occurrences of distortions in the influx and outflow of space itself, particularly of space seeming to collapse on itself; of the seeming expansion and contraction of one's body in space, its weightlessness, its seeming disappearance in space; of feelings of separation of self from body, of alienation from self, of strangeness and unrealness of self, and of the environment; and of not being in control of oneself or of one's movements in space.

The lack of difference in distortion of time-experiences and, in a little intermezzo on the experience of time, the greater flexibility towards time but also higher time-anxiousness of normal persons, compared to phobic patients, suggest a profound difference between normal and phobic spatio-temporal orientations.

An exploration of the inner world of phobic patients, by means of personal interviews, brings to light that the postulated link, between environmental structure, orientation of self (or body) in space, and perceived lack of control over self, is not hypothetical but securely forged; and the predicted pernicious effects, their bitter facts of life. Furthermore, in the phobic experience, the agoraphobic, claustrophobic, and social phobic variants, though they have something in common, are suggested to yield different experiences of the dynamics of space and of oneself-in-space; which experiences are predicated in their different strategies of perceptual control.

The study is concluded by a discussion of the empirical work in the light of the theoretical premises put forward in Part One.

References

Allport, F.H. 1955 *Theories of Perception and the Concept of Structure*. New York: Wiley & Sons. Inc.,

Averill, J.R. 1973 Personal control over aversive stimuli and its relationship to stress. *Psychol. Bull.*, 80, 286–303.

Baddeley, A.D. 1972 Selective attention and performance in dangerous environments. *Brit. J. Psychol.*, 63, pp. 537–46.

Baird, J.C. 1970 *Psychophysical Analysis of Visual Space*. Oxford: Pergamon Press Ltd.

Bannister, D. 1968. *The Evolution of Personal Constructs*. London/New York: Academic Press, Ltd.

Barendregt, J.T. 1972 Jaarverslag Vakgroep Persoonlijkheidsleer, 1971/72. *Bulletin Persoonlijkheidsleer*, 1. University of Amsterdam.

Barendregt, J.T. 1973 Onderzoek van fobieën. In A.P. Cassee, P.E. Boeke, & J.T. Barendregt (eds), *Klinische Psychologie in Nederland*. Deventer: Van Loghum Slaterus.

Barendregt, J.T. 1974 De relatie van diagnostiek en therapie binnen het Fobieënproject. *De Psycholoog*. Amsterdam: Nederlands Instituut voor Psychologen (NIP).

Barendregt, J.T. 1975 Phobias and Phobics. Paper presented at the International Symposium on Research in Neurosis, Amsterdam.

Barendregt, J.T. 1975 Voor de exacte fobie moet men de fobici afschaffen. *Bulletin Persoonlijkheidsleer*, 4, pp. 47–51. University of Amsterdam.

Barendregt, J.T. 1982 Fobieën en verwante angsten. In J.T. Barendregt, *De zielenmarkt. Over psychotherapie in alle ernst*. Meppel/Amsterdam: Boom.

Barendregt, J.T., & Frijda, N.H. 1982 Cognitive aspects of anxiety. *Tijdschrift voor Geneesmiddelenonderzoek*, Amsterdam, July, 17–24.

Bartlett, F.C. 1932 *Remembering: A Study in Experimental and Social Psychology*. Cambridge: Cambridge University Press.

Bartlett, F.C. 1941 Fatigue following highly skilled work. *Proceedings of the Royal Society of London*, B 131, 247–57.

Békésy, G. von. 1967 *Sensory Inhibition*. Princeton: Princeton University Press.

Bergson, H. 1960 *Time and Free Will. An Essay on the Immediate Data of Consciousness*. New York: Harper & Bros. (orig. publ. 1910).

Berlyne, D.E. 1957 Conflict and information-theory variables as determinants of human perceptual curiosity. *J. Exp. Psychol.*, 53, pp. 399–404.

Berlyne, D.E. 1960 *Conflict, Arousal and Curiosity*. New York: McGraw-Hill.

Berlyne, D.E. 1974 *Studies in the New Experimental Aesthetics: Steps Toward an Objective Psychology of Aesthetic Appreciation*. Washington: Hemisphere Publ. Company.

Berlyne, D.E., Ogilvie, J.C., & Parham, L.C.C. 1968 The dimensionality of visual complexity, interestingness, and pleasingness. *Canad. J. Psychol., I Rev. Canad. Psychol.*, 22(5), 376–387.

Binswanger, L. 1975 Freud's conception of Man in the light of Anthropology. In Binswanger, L. *Being-in-the-World. Selected Papers* (translation: J. Needleman), New York: Basic Books.

Blakemore, C. 1974 Developmental factors in the formation of feature extracting neurons. In F.O. Schmitt & F.G. Worden (eds), *The Neurosciences Third Study Program*. Cambridge, Massachusetts: MIT Press, pp. 105–113.

Bleeker, T., & Velthuizen, J. 1972 *Seeing is Believing*. Een literatuurverkenning en een exploratief onderzoek naar de stimuluskenmerken, die mogelijk een rol spelen in een tunnelfobie. Masters thesis. University of Amsterdam.

Bonarius, H. 1980 *Persoonlijke psychologie. Deel I: Inleiding in de theorie en praktijk van constructenpsychologie. Deel II: Ontwikkelingen in de theorie en praktijk van constructenpsychologie. Deventer*: Van Loghum Slaterus.

Bower, T.G.R. 1974 *Development in Infancy*. San Francisco: W.H. Freeman & Company.

Bower, T.G.R. 1979 *Human Development*. San Francisco: W.H. Freeman & Company.

Bower, T.G.R. 1980 The Object in the World of the Infant. In R.L. Atkinson & R.C. Atkinson (eds), *Mind and Behavior. Scientific American*, pp. 55–63. San Francisco: W.H. Freeman & Company (first publ. 1971).

Bower, T.G.R. 1980 Repetitive Processes in Child Development. In R.L. Atkinson & R.C. Atkinson (eds), *Mind and Behavior, Scientific American*, pp. 64–73 San Francisco: W.H. Freeman & Company (first publ. 1976).

Bower, T.G.R., Broughton, J.M., & Moore, M.K. 1971 Infants' response to approaching objects: An indicator of response to distal variables. *Perception & Psychophysics*, 9, 193–196.

Bower, T.G.R., Broughton, J.M., & Moore, M.K. 1971 Development of the object concept as manifested in changes in the tracking behavior of infants between 7 and 20 weeks of age. *J. Exp. Child Psychology*, 11, 182–193.

Bowra, C.M. 1973/1957 *The Greek Experience*. London: Sphere Books Ltd.

Breuer, J., & Freud, S. 1895 "On the Psychical Mechanisms of Hysterical Phenomena: Preliminary Communication" In: *Studies on Hysteria*. Standard Ed. 2., 3.

Bruce, V., & Green, P. 1985 *Visual Perception. Physiology, Psychology and Ecology*. London: Lawrence Erlbaum Associates Ltd.

Burton, R. 1972/1621 *The Anatomy of Melancholy*. London: J.M. Dent & Sons.

Calabresi, R., & Cohen, J. 1968 Personality and Time Attitudes. *J. Abnormal Psychology*, 73, 3, 431–439.

Cappon, D., & Banks, R. 1961 Orientational perception. A review and preliminary study of distortion in orientational perception. *Arch. Gen. Psychiatr.*, 5, 380–392.

Cappon, D., & Banks, R. 1965 Orientational perception: II. Body perception in depersonalization. *Arch. Gen. Psychiatr.*, 13, 375–379.

Cappon, D., & Banks, R. 1969 Orientational perception: III. Orientational percept distortions in depersonalization. *Amer. J. Psychiatr.*, 125: 8, 1048–1056.

Cappon, D., & Banks, R. 1969 Orientational perception: IV. Time and length perception in depersonalized and derealized patients and controls under positive feedback conditions. *Amer. J. Psychiatr.*, 125, 9, 1214–17.

Cavendish, R (ed). 1980 *Mythology*. London: Book Club Associates.

Chabot, B.E. 1975 105 Intake gesprekken voor gesprekstherapie binnen het Fobieënproject. *Bulletin Persoonlijkheidsleer*, 4, 26–46. University of Amsterdam.

Coren, S., & Girgus, J.S. 1977 Illusions and Constancies. In W. Epstein (ed), *Stability and Constancy in Visual Perception: Mechanisms and Processes*. London: John Wiley & Sons, Inc.

Craik, K.J.W. 1966 (1943) The Nature of Explanation. In K.J.W. Craik, *The Nature of Psychology*, Cambridge: Cambridge University Press.

Cruikshank, R.M. 1938 The development of size-constancy in early infancy. *Ile Congres Int. Psychologie*, Paris: Impremesia Moderns.

Cruikshank, R.M. 1941 The development of visual size-constancy in early infancy. *J. Genetic Psychology*, 58, 327–351.

Davies, P. 1984 *Superforce. The Search for a Grand Unified Theory of Nature*. New York: Simon & Schuster.

De la Mare, W. 1951 From *Dreams* In K. Allott (ed), *Contemporary Verse*. Harmondsworth. Middlesex: Penguin Books.

Dixon, J.C. 1963 Depersonalization phenomena in a sample population of college students. *Brit. J. Psychiatry*, 109, 371–375.
Dodwell, P.C., Muir, D., & Di Franco, D. 1976 Responses of infants to visually presented objects. *Science*, 194, 209–211.
Donaldson, M. 1978 *The Child's Mind.* Glasgow: Fontana Paperbacks.
Dreesmann, W. 1982 *De waarneming en beleving van enkele fobici.* Master's thesis, University of Amsterdam.
Dunne, J.W. 1934 (1927) *An Experiment with Time.* London: Faber and Faber Ltd.,
Ellenberger, H.F. 1970 *The Discovery of the Unconscious. The History and Evolution of Dynamic Psychiatry.* New York: Basic Books Inc.
Epstein, S., & Fenz, W.D. 1965 Steepness of approach and avoidance gradients in humans as a function of experience: Theory and experiment. *J. Exp. Psychol.*, 70, 1–12.
Epstein, W. 1977 *Stability and Constancy in Visual Perception.* New York: John Wiley & Sons, Inc.
Exner, S. 1894 *Entwurf zu einer physiologischen Erklärung der psychischen Erscheinungen.* Leipzig & Vienna: Franz Deutiche.
Fodor, J.A., & Pylyshyn, Z.W. 1981 How direct is visual perception?: Some reflections on Gibson's "Ecological Approach". *Cognition*, 9, 139–196, Elsevier Sequoia, S.A. Lausanne.
Fodor, J.A. 1980 Methodological solipsism as a research strategy in cognitive psychology. *Behavior & Brain Sciences*, 3, 63–109.
Francès, R. 1976 Comparative effects of six collative variables on interest and preference in adults of different educational levels. *J. Personality and Social Psychology*, 33, 1, 62–79.
Fraser, J.T. (ed). 1966 *The Voices of Time.* New York: Braziller.
Frazier, S.H., & Carr, H.C. 1967 Phobic Reactions. In A.M. Freedman & H.I. Kaplan (eds), *Comprehensive Textbook of Psychiatry*, chap. 23, 899–911.
Freedman, A.M., & Kaplan, H.I. (eds) 1967 *Comprehensive Textbook of Psychiatry.* Baltimore: The Williams & Wilkins Company.
Freud, S., & Breuer, J. 1940d (1892) On the Theory of Hysterical Attacks. *Standard Ed.*, 1, 151 (40).
Freud, S. 1894a The Neuro-Psychoses of Defence. *Standard Ed.* 3, 43 (327).
Freud, S. 1954 (1895) Project for a Scientific Psychology. *The Origins of Psycho-Analysis.* New York: Basic Books.
Freud, S. 1976 (1900) *The Interpretation of Dreams.* London: Pelican Books.
Freud, S. (1915) The Unconscious. *Standard Ed*, 14, pp. 158–215.
Freud, S. 1976 (1916–17) *Introductory Lectures on Psychoanalysis.* London: Pelican Books (GS X – German Edition).
Freud, S. (1923) The Ego and the Id. *Standard Ed.*, 19, pp. 1–66.
Freud, S. 1971 (1926/1936) *Inhibitions, Symptoms and Anxiety.* London: The Hogarth Press and the Institute of Psycho-Analysis.
Freud, S. 1977 (1933) *New Introductory Lectures on Psychoanalysis.* London: Pelican Books.
Freud, S. (1940) An Outline of Psychoanalysis. *Standard Ed.*, 23, pp. 139–207.
Freud, S. 1950a (trans. 1954e) *The Origins of Psychoanalysis. Letters to Wilhelm Fliess* (1887–1902). London: Imago Publ. Co.
Frijda, N.H., & Barendregt, J.T. 1981 Cognitive aspects of anxiety. Paper presented at the symposium "Origin, Prevalence & Treatment of Anxiety", Amsterdam.
Frijda, N.H. 1982 Barendregt over angst en depersonalisatie. Voordracht voor het Psychologen Congres, Amsterdam.
Gärling, T. 1969a/1969b Studies in visual perception of architectural spaces and rooms: I. Judgment scales of open and enclosed spaces.; II. Judgment of open and enclosed spaces by category rating and magnitude estimation. *Scand. J. Psychol.*, 18, 250–256 (I); 18, pp. 257–268 (II).

Gärling, T. 1970a/1970b Studies in visual perception of architectural spaces and rooms. III. A relation between judged depth and size of space; IV. The relation between judged depth to judged size of space under different viewing conditions. *Scand. J. Psychol*, 11, 124–131 (III); 11, 133–145 (IV).

Gibson, E.J., & Walk, R.D. 1960 The "visual cliff." *Scientific American*, 202, 64–71.

Gibson, J.J. 1950a *The Perception of the Visual World*. Boston: Houghton Mifflin Company.

Gibson, J.J. 1958 Visually controlled locomotion and visual orientation in animals. *Brit. J. Psychol*, 49, 182–194 (b).

Gibson, J.J. 1963 The useful dimensions of sensitivity. *American Psychologist*, 18, 1–15.

Gibson, J.J. 1966 *The Senses Considered As Perceptual Systems*. Boston: Houghton Mifflin Company.

Gibson, J.J. 1970 The theory of information pickup. In R.N. Haber (ed), *Contemporary Theory and Research in Visual Perception*. New York: Holt.

Gibson, J.J. 1982 Notes on Affordances. In E. Reed & R. Jones (eds), *Reasons for Realism*. New Jersey: Erlbaum Associates, 401–418 (1975 unpubl.).

Gibson, J.J. 1975 (a) Events are perceivable but time is not. In J.T. Fraser & N. Lawrence (eds), *The Study of Time*. New York: Springer-Verlag.

Gibson, J.J. 1979 (a) *The Ecological Approach to Visual Perception*. Boston: Houghton Mifflin Company.

Gregory, R.L. 1972 Cognitive contours. *Nature*, 238, 51–52.

Gregory, R.L. 1973 The Confounded Eye. In R.L. Gregory & E.H. Gombrich (eds), *Illusions in Nature and Art*. London: Duckworth.

Gregory, R.L. 1974 *Concepts and Mechanisms of Perception*. London: Duckworth.

Gregory, R.L. 1974 Perceptions as hypotheses. In S.C. Brown (ed), *Philosophy of Psychology*. London: MacMillan Press.

Gregory, R.L. 1981 *Mind in Science*. Cambridge/London: Cambr. Univ. Press.

Groddeck, G. 1923 *Das Buch vom Es*. Vienna: Int. Psychoanal. Verlag GmbH.

Guilford, J.P. 1954 *Psychometric Methods*. New York: McGraw-Hill. 2nd. ed.

Guirand, F. 1963/1935 *Greek Mythology*. London: Paul Hamlyn Ltd., (transl., Ames).

Haasen, P.P. van, 1972 *Van vaag naar helder, of toch niet zo helder*? Master's thesis, University of Amsterdam.

Hamlyn, D.W. 1983 *Perception, Learning and the Self. Essays in the Philosophy of Psychology*. London: Routledge & Kegan Paul.

Hansen, J. 1978 *De invloed van variatie in de collatieve variabele "complexiteitonzekerheid" op het perceptuele en emotionele gedrag van fobische en normale personen*. Master's thesis, University of Amsterdam.

Harris, C.S. 1963a Adaptation to displaced vision: Visual, motor, or proprioceptive change? *Science*, 140, 812–813.

Harris, C.S. 1963b *Adaptation to displaced vision: A proprioceptive change*. Doctoral dissertation, Harvard University.

Harris, C.S. 1980 Insight or Out of Sight?: Two examples of perceptual plasticity in the human adult. In C.S. Harris (ed), *Visual Coding and Adaptability*. Hillsdale, N.J.: Lawrence Erlbaum Assoc.

Hayward, S.C., & Franklin, S.S. 1974 Perceived openness-enclosure of architectural spaces. *Environment and Behavior*, 6, 37–52.

Heerden, J.H. van, 1982 *De zorgelijke staat van het onbewuste*. Doctoral dissertation. Amsterdam: Boom Meppel.

Held, R., & Bauer, J.A. 1974 Development of sensorially guided reaching in infant monkeys. *Brain Research*, 71, 265–271.

Helmholtz, H.L.F. von, 1965 (1866) On Perception and the Unconscious Conclusion. In R.J. Hernstein & E.G. Boring (eds), *A Source Book in the History of Psychology*, Cambridge, Massachusetts: Harvard University Press, 189–193.

Helmholtz, H.L.F. von 1962/1965 (1866–70) *Treatise on physiological optics*. Vol. 3, New York: Dover.

Helson, H. 1964 *Adaptation-level Theory. An Experimental and Systematic Approach to Behavior*. New York/London: Harper & Row.

Hesselgren, S. 1971 *Experimental Studies on Architectural Perception*. Stockholm: Nat. Swed. Inst. Build. Res., 104 pp.

Hirsch, H., & Spinelli, D.N. 1970 Distribution of receptive field orientation: Modification contingent on conditions of visual experiences. *Science*, 168, 869–871.

Hollingworth, H.L. 1910 The central tendency of judgment. *J. Philos. Psychol. & Sci. Meth.*, 7, 461–469.

Hume, D. 1739 *A Treatise of Human Nature: being an Attempt to introduce the experimental Method of Reasoning into Moral Subjects*. vol.I. London; *Philosophical Essays Concerning Human Understanding*, 2nd. ed., London, 1751 (No. 69).

Jackson, J. Hughlings 1965 (1884) On Dissolution of the Nervous System. In R.J. Herrnstein & E.G. Boring (eds), *A Source Book in the History of Psychology*, Cambridge, Mass.: Harvard University Press, pp. 233–236.

Jackson, J. Hughlings 1931 (1894) The Factors of Insanities. Reprinted in *Selected Writings of John Hughlings Jackson*, 2: 4115n. London: Hodder & Stoughton [1932].

James, W. 1950 (1890) *The Principles of Psychology*. Vols I & II. New York: Dover Publications, Inc.

Johansson, G., & Börjesson. E. 1989 Toward a New Theory of Vision. Studies in Wide-Angle Space Perception. In: *Ecological Psychology*, 1, 4, 301–331.

Jones, E. 1956 *Sigmund Freud, Life and Work, Vol. I*. London: The Hogarth Press.

Julesz, B. 1971 *Foundations of Cyclopean Perception*. Chicago, Il.: The University of Chicago Press.

Kanizsa, G. 1974 (1954) Contours without gradients or cognitive contours. *Italian J. Psychology*, 1, 93–112

Kaplan, B.(ed). 1964 *The Inner World of Mental Illness*. New York/London: Harper & Row.

Keats, J. 1985 (1817/1820) *The Complete Poems*. Harmondsworth, Middlesex: Penguin Books, Ltd.

Kelly, G.A. 1955 *The Psychology of Personal Constructs*. Vol. I (A theory of personality). New York: Norton.

Kernberg, O. 1966 Structural derivatives of object relationships. *Int. J. Psycho-Analysis*, 47, 236–253.

Kierkegaard, S. 1963 (1849) *Over de vertwijfeling. De ziekte tot de dood*(uit het Deens vertaald door H.A. van Munster en A.P. Klaver), Utrecht: Het Spectrum.

Klausner, S.Z. (ed). 1965 *The Quest for Self-control*. Classical Philosophies and Scientific Research. New York: The Free Press.

Klover, H. 1966 (1926) *Mescal and Mechanisms of Hallucinations*. Chicago: The University of Chicago Press.

Knoppers, M. 1976 Over definities, duinen en drijfzand. *Bulletin Persoonlijkheidsleer*, 4, 56–60.

Kohler, I. 1964 The formation and transformation of the perceptual world. (Translated by H. Fiss), *Psychological Issues*, 3, 4, 1–173.

Kok, R. & Lowich-Russell, V. 1980 *Waarnemings-aspecten van enkele fobici*. Master's thesis, University of Amsterdam.

Krogten, I.A.M.H. van & Schaper, W.W.F. 1976 Herenleed. *Bulletin Persoonlijkheidsleer*. 4, 93–102.

Lee, D.N., & Lishman, J.R. 1975 Visual proprioceptive control of stance. *J. Human Movement Studies*, I, 87–95.

Lee, D.N., & Lishman, J.R. 1977 Visual control of locomotion. *Scandinavian J. Psychology*, 18, 224–30.

Leeuw, P. de, 1977 *De invloed van structurele eigenschappen van stimulus situaties (m.n.variaties in de collatieve variabele "complexiteitonzekerheid") op het perceptuele en emotionele gedrag van fobische personen.* Master's thesis, University of Amsterdam.

Lohmann, W. 1984 *Aspecten van de waarneming en beleving van enkele fobici nader bekeken.* Master's thesis, University of Amsterdam.

Mace, W.M. 1977 James J. Gibson's strategy for perceiving: Ask not what's inside your head, but what your head's inside of. In R. Shaw & J. Bransford (eds), *Perceiving, Acting and Knowing. Toward an Ecological Psychology.* I Sect A,2. Hillsdale, New Jersey: Lawrence Erlbaum Associates, Inc.

Mach, E. 1897 Beiträge zur Analyse der Empfindungen, Jena, 1886. Translated from the German by C.M. Williams as *Contributions to the Analysis of the Sensations.* Chicago., 1897. By permission of Gustav Fischer Verlag, Jena (No. 110).

Mahler, M.S. 1968b On Human Symbiosis and the Vicissitudes of Individuation, *Infantile Psychosis, Vol .I.* New York: International Universities Press.

Mahler, M.S., Pine, F., & Bergman, A. 1975 *The Psychological Birth of the Infant Symbiosis and Individuation.* New York: Basic Books, Inc.

Marcel, A.J. 1983 Conscious and Unconscious Perception: An Approach to the Relations between Phenomenal Experience and Perceptual Process. *Cognitive Psychology*, 15, 238–300.

Marks, I.M. 1970 The Agoraphobic Syndrome (Phobic Anxiety State), *Archives Gen. Psychiatry*, 23.

Marks, I.M. 1978 *Living with Fear. Understanding and Coping with Anxiety.* New York: McGraw-Hill.

Marr, D. 1976 Early processing of visual information. *Philosophical Transactions of the Royal Society of London, Series B*, 275, 483–524;

Marr, D. 1982 *Vision: A Computational Investigation into the Human Representation and Processing of Visual Information.* San Francisco: W.H. Freeman and Company.

Masterson, J., & Rinsley, D.B. 1980 The Borderline Syndrome: Role of the mother. In R.F. Lax, S. Bach & J.A. Burland (eds), *Rapproachement. The Critical Subphase of Separation-Individuation*, New York: Jason Aronson.

Matte-Blanco, I. 1975 *The Unconscious as Infinite Sets. An Essay in Bi-logic.* London: Duckworth.

Matte-Blanco, I. 1988 *Thinking, Feeling, and Being.* Clinical reflections on the fundamental antinomy of human beings and world. London/New York: Routledge.

McCulloch, W.S. 1965 *Embodiments of Mind.* Cambridge, Mass: Cambridge MIT Press.

McGurk, H. 1974 Visual perception in young infants. In B. Foss (ed), *New Perspectives in Child Development.* London: Penguin Books.

McNab, B.I.E. 1981 The enemy without and within. A review and evaluation of some perception research on the effects of environmental stimulation on the behaviour of phobic patients. *Bulletin Persoonlijkheidsleer*, University of Amsterdam, 10, 1.

McNab, B.I.E. 1984 Van binnen ondermijnd, van buiten belaagd: Het perceptuele dilemma in de fobie. *Gedragstherapie*, 17, 1, Utrecht.

McNab, B.I.E. 1989 Hermeneut onder de methodologen, methodoloog onder de hermeneuten. Over leven en werk van Johan Barendregt. In: *Psychologie & Maatschappij*, Jaargang 13, 3, 235–252. September Uitgever: SUN, Nijmegen.

McNab, B.I.E., Batstra, W., & Vrouwe, E. 1975 *On the Perception of Tunnels by Tunnelphobic Subjects.* Internal report, University of Amsterdam.

McNab, B.I.E., Nieuwenhuijse, B., Jansweyer, B., & Kuyper, A. 1978 Height/distance ratio as a predictor of perceived openness-enclosure of space and emotional responses in normal and phobic subjects. *Ned. T. voor de Psychologie*, Van Loghum Slaterus, 33/6.

Melges, F.T. 1982 *Time and the Inner Future. A Temporal Approach to Psychiatric Disorders.* New York: John Wiley & Sons, Inc.

Michaels, C.E. & Carello, C. 1981 *Direct Perception*. Englewood Cliffs, New Jersey: Prentice-Hall, Inc.

Michon, J. 1967 *Timing in Temporal Tracking*. Institute for Perception RVO TNO, Soesterberg, The Netherlands.

Michotte, A. 1963 *The Perception of Causality*. London: Methuen & Co. Ltd.,

Miller, G.A. Sensitivity to changes in the intensity of white noise and its relation to masking and loudness. *J. Acoust. Soc. Amer.*, 19, 609–619.

Misumi, J. 1951 Experimental studies on the development of visual size constancy in early infancy. *Bulletin of the Fac. Literature, Kyusha University*, 1, 91–116.

Musil, R. 1953 *Der Man ohne Eigenschaften (1930–33)*. First published in Great Britain by Secher & Warburg Ltd., transl. as "The Man without Qualities".

Needleman, J. 1975 *Being-in-the-World. Selected Papers of Ludwig Binswanger*. (Translation and critical introduction to his existential psychoanalysis by J. Needleman.) New York: Basic Books Publ.,

Neisser, U. 1967 *Cognitive Psychology*. New York: Appleton-Century-Crofts.

Neisser, U. 1976 *Cognition and Reality*. San Francisco: W.H. Freeman and Company.

Nisbett, R.E., & DeCamp Wilson, T. 1977 Telling more than we can know: Verbal reports on mental processes. *Psychological Review*, 84, 3, 231–259.

Noyes, R., & Kletti, R. 1977 Depersonalization in response to life-threatening danger. *Comprehensive Psychiatry*, 18, 375–384.

Ornstein, R.E. 1969 *On the Experience of Time*. New York: Penguin Books.

Piaget, J. 1954 *The Construction of Reality in the Child*. (transl. by M. Cook), New York: Basic Books.

Piaget, J., & Inhelder, B. 1956 *The Child's Conception of Space*. (transl. by F.J. Langdon & J.L. Lunzer), New York: Humanities Press.

Piaget, J., & Inhelder, B. 1968 *The Psychology of the Child*. London: Routledge and Kegan Paul.

Piaget, J. 1969 *The Mechanisms of Perception*. (transl. by G.N. Seagrim), London: Routledge & Kegan Paul.

Piaget, J., In B. Inhelder, R. Garcia & J.J. Vonèche (eds) 1977 *Epistémologie génétique et équilibration (colloque de juillet, 1976)*. Neuchâtel/Paris: Delachaux & Niestlé.

Piët, S. 1986 *Het Loon van de Angst*. Doctoral dissertation, University of Amsterdam.

Powers, W.T. 1973 *Behavior: The Control of Perception*. Chicago: Aldine Publ. Co.,

Pribram, K.H. 1977 Some comments on the nature of the perceived universe. In R. Shaw & J. Bransford (eds), *Perceiving, Acting and Knowing. Towards an Ecological Psychology*. Hillsdale, New Jersey: Lawrence Erlbaum Associates, Inc.

Pribram, K.H. 1991 *Brain and Perception. Holonomy and Structure in Figural Processing*. Hillsdale, New Jersey: Lawrence Erlbaum Associates, Inc.

Pronko, N.H., Ebert, R. & Greenberg, R. 1966 A critical review of Theories of Perception. In A.H. Kidd & J.L. Rivoire (eds), *Perceptual Development in Children*. New York: International Universities Press.

Reed, E.S., & Jones, R.K. 1982 *Reasons for Realism. Selected Essays of J.J. Gibson*. New Jersey: Lawrence Erlbaum Associates Inc.

Reynolds, H. 1966 *Factors affecting the accuracy of visual tracking of a moving object when it has disappeared from sight* (Thesis). Cornell University Library.

Rilke, R.M. 1978. *The Notebook of Malte Laurids Brigge*. (transl. by J. Linton), London: The Hogarth Press.

Roazen, P. 1969 *Brother Animal: The Story of Freud and Tausk*. New York: Alfred A. Knopf.

Roberts, W.W. 1960 Normal and Abnormal Depersonalization. *J. Mental Science*, 106, 478–493.

Rock, I. 1983 *The Logic of Perception*. Cambridge, MA: MIT Press.

Rosen, G. 1968 *Madness in Society*. Chicago: University of Chicago Press.
Ross, H.E. 1974 *Behaviour and Perception in Strange Environments*. London: Allen & Unwin Ltd.
Russell, B. 1949/1974 *History of Western Philosophy*. London: Allen & Unwin Ltd.,
Sartre, J.P. 1943 *L'Etre et le Neant: essai d'ontologie phénoménologique*. Paris: Gallimard.
Schaper, W.W.F. 1974 Een relatietherapie-vorm voor fobici. *De Psycholoog*, IX. Amsterdam: Nederlands Instituut voor Psychologen (NIP).
Schiff, W. 1965 Perception of impending collision: A study of visually directed avoidant behavior. *Psychol. Monog.*, 79, 604.
Schiff, W., Caviness. J. & Gibson, J.J. 1962 Persistent fear responses in rhesus monkeys to the optical stimulus of "looming." *Science*, 136, 982–3.
Schneirla, T.C. 1959 An evolutionary and developmental theory of biphasic processes underlying approach and withdrawal. In M.R. Jones (ed), 1958 *Nebraska Symposium on Motivation*. Lincoln, University. of Nebraska Press, 1–135.
Schneirla, T.C. 1965 Aspects of stimulation and organization in approach/withdrawal processes underlying vertebrate development. In Lehrman, R.A. Hinde, & R. Shaw (eds), *Advances in the Study of Behavior*. London/New York: MacMillan, 2–75.
Seligman, M.E.P. 1971 Phobias and preparedness. *Behav. Ther.*, 2, 307–320.
Siegel, R.K. 1977 Hallucinations. In R.L. Atkinson & R.C. Atkinson (eds), *Mind and Behavior. Scientific American*, 125–132. San Francisco: W.H.Freeman and Company.
Sigman, E., & Rock, I. 1974 Stroboscopic movement based on perceptual intelligence. *Perception*, 3, 9–28.
Silverman, J. 1975 On the sensory bases of transcendental states of consciousness. In S.R. Dean (ed), *Psychiatry and Mysticism*, Chicago: Nelson-Hall, 365–398.
Spielberger, C.D. (ed.) 1966 *Anxiety and Behavior*. New York/London: Academic Press.
Spreiregen, P.D. 1965 *Urban Design: The Architecture of Towns and Cities*. New York: McGraw-Hill.
Strachey, J. 1976 Note on page 751 of IV of the Freud Standard Edition.
Stratton, G.M. 1965 Vision without inversion of the retinal image, *Psychological Review*, 4, 341–360, 463–481 (1897). Also in R.J. Herrnstein & E.G. Boring (eds), *A Source Book on the History of Psychology*, Cambridge, Mass: Harvard University Press.
Sulloway, F.J. 1980 *Freud, Biologist of the Mind. Beyond the Psychoanalytic Legend*. London: Fontana Paperbacks.
Thurstone, L.L 1959 *The Measurement of Values*. Chicago: University of Chicago Press.
Tibbetts, P. (ed). 1969 *Perception: Selected Readings in Science and Phenomenology*. Chicago: Quadrangle Press.
Tibbetts, P. 1972 Perceptual Theory and Epistemological Dualism: Some examples from experimental psychology. *The Psychological Record*, 22, 410–411.
Turvey, M.T. 1977 Preliminaries to a Theory of action with reference to Vision. In R. Shaw & J. Bransford (eds), *Perceiving, Acting and Knowing. Toward an Ecological Psychology*. Hillsdale, New Jersey: Lawrence Erlbaum Associates, Inc.,
Turvey, M.T., Shaw, R.E., Reed, E.S., & Mace, W.M. 1981 Ecological laws of perceiving and acting: In reply to Fodor and Pylyshyn (1981). *Cognition*, 9, 237–304.
Vernon, M.D. 1952 *A Further Study of Visual Perception*. Cambridge: Cambridge University Press
Vuyk, R. 1981 *Overview and Critique of Piaget's Genetic Epistemology* (1965–1980), Vols. I & II. London: Academic Press.Ltd.,
Weber, E.H. 1846/1849 Der Tastsinn und das gemeingefühl. In Wagner, R. (ed), *Handwörterbuch der Physiologie, III*. Braunschweig: Vieweg (No. 10).
Westphal, C. 1871/1872 Die Agoraphobie: eine neuropathische Erscheinung, *Archiv für Psychiatrie und Nervenkrankheiten*, Berlin, 3, 138–161.

Winer, B.J. 1962/1970 *Statistical Principles in Experimental Design*. New York: McGraw-Hill.

Winnicott, D.W. 1960 Ego distortion in terms of True and False Self. In: *The Maturational Processes and the Facilitating Environment*. London: The Hogarth Press and the Institute of Psycho-Analysis.

Winnicott, D.W. 1971/1982 *Playing and Reality*. London: Tavistock Publ. and Penguin Education Books.

Witkin, H.A. 1965 Psychological differentiation and forms of pathology. *J. Abnormal Psychology*, 70, 5, 317–336.

Wittgenstein, L. 1969 (1921) *Tractatus Logico-Philosophicus* (English translation by D.F. Pears and B.F. McGuiness), London: Routledge & Kegan Paul.

Wohlwill, J.F. 1966 The physical environment: A problem for a psychology of stimulation. In R.W. Kates and J.F. Wohlwill (eds), *Man's Response to the Physical Environment. Journal of Social Issues*, 22, 29–38.

Wohlwill, J.F. 1968 Amount of stimulus exploration and preference as differential functions of stimulus complexity. *Perception & Psychophysics* Vol. 4 (5), 307–312.

Wohlwill, J.F. 1970 The Emerging Discipline of Environmental Psychology. *American Psychologist*, 303–312.

Wolpe, J. 1966 In C.D. Spielberger, *Anxiety and Behavior*. New York: Academic Press, p. 182.

Woodworth, R.S. 1947 Reinforcement of perception. *Amer. J. Psychol.*, 60, 119–124.

Wurmser, L., & McDaniel, E. 1978 Phobic Neuroses. In G. Balis, L. Wurmser, E. McDaniel, & R.E. Grenell (eds), *Clinical Psychopathology. Psychiatric Foundations of Medicine*. Boston: Butterworth Publ. Inc., p. 252.

Zuuren, F.J. van, 1976 Slachtoffers van de openbare orde – een culturele benadering van de (agora)fobie. *Bulletin Persoonlijkheidsleer*, 4, 4, 103–137, University of Amsterdam.

Zuuren, F.J. van, 1982 *Fobie, situatie en identiteit. Een studie over de situatie-vermijding en identiteitsproblematiek van twee soorten fobici*. Doctoral dissertation Lisse: Swets & Zeitlinger, B.V.

Appendices

Appendix A: Intercorrelations between Constructcomponents for the Four Tunnelphobic Patients in Study I

Table 5.1e. Intercorrelations between constructcomponents for S 1 (claustrophobic patient in tunnels, elevators, etcetera)

Constructcomponent I															
C1 displeasing	1.00														
C2 pressure from above	.90	1.00													
C3 exit far off	.75	.83	1.00												
C4 difficult to oversee	.76	.72	.75	1.00											
C5 unfamiliar	.60	.72	.95	.68	1.00										
C6 long tunnel	.84	.91	.78	.68	.68	1.00									
C7 funneling	.79	.90	.65	.56	.53	.89	1.00								
C8 exit not visible	.46	.57	.85	.76	.91	.53	–	1.00							
C9 low ceiling	.75	.90	.89	.69	.82	.85	.78	.68	1.00						
C10 narrow opening	.75	.76	.56	.53	.–	.87	.84	.–	.67	1.00					
C11 dark	.78	.74	.76	.75	.62	.70	.58	.53	.60	.66	1.00				
C15 dismal	.84	.79	.68	.77	.59	.88	.79	–	.66	.88	.74	1.00			
C13 bend in tunnel	.41	–	–	–	–	–	–	.51	–	–	–	–	1.00		
C14 seems dead end	.24	–	.58	.54	.64	–	–	.72	–	–	–	–	–	1.00	
C20 traffic	.05	–	–	–	–	–	–	–	–	–	–	–	–	–	1.00

Constructcomponent II			
C14 seems dead end	1.00		
C16 don't know where you are	.62	1.00	
C17 narrow tunnel	–	.65	1.00

N.B. Except on "displeasingness", correlations r < .50 are not shown. Only constructs of component II with a correlation r ⩾ .50 are shown. The only constructs of component III that are highly intercorrelated (r = .72) are "exit not visible" and "seems a dead end" (underlined).

Table 5.1f. Intercorrelations between constructcomponents for S 2 (agoraphobic patient with a fear of being looked at)

Constructcomponent I																	
C1 displeasing	1.00																
C2 traffic	−.10	1.00															
C3 strange	.50	−.67	1.00														
C4 long tunnel	−.32	.66	−.65	1.00													
C5 old tunnel	.54	−.58	–	–	1.00												
C6 uncompleted	.30	−.57	.51	–	.62	1.00											
C7 ugly	.61	–	–	–	.82	–	1.00										
C8 traffic tunnel	−.28	.55	–	73	–	–	–	1.00									
C9 bend in tunnel	−.16	–	–	–	−.53	–	−.54	–	1.00								
C10 smooth walls	−.57	–	–	–	−.70	−.72	−.54	–	–	1.00							
C11 a real tunnel	−.12	–	–	–	–	–	–	.67	–	–	1.00						
C12 difficult to oversee	.66	–	.62	–	–	–	.61	–	–	–	–	1.00					
C13 no people	26	−.57	.53	–	–	.72	–	–	–	−.60	–	–	1.00				
C14 unsafe	.66	–	.60	–	–	–	.52	–	–	−.59	–	.87	.59	1.00			
C15 exit far off	−.27	–	–	.54	–	–	–	.71	–	–	–	–	–	–			
C16 other people inaccessible	−.55	–	–	–	.55	−.54	–	–	–	.77	–	−.70	−.77	−.79	1.00		
C17 dark	.59	–	–	–	–	–	–	–	–	−.52	–	.59	–	57	–	1.00	

Constructcomponent III					
C8 traffic tunnel	1.00				
C11 real tunnel	.55	1.00			
C18 narrow tunnel	–	–	1.00		
C20 low ceiling	–	–	.65	1.00	
C22 seems dead end	–	–	–	–	1.00

N.B. Except for "displeasingness", r-values < .50 are not shown. The underlined r-values show which constructs on the second component are highly intercorrelated. The constructs on the third component which are highly intercorrelated are shown below.

Table 5.1g. Intercorrelations between constructcomponents for S 3 (agoraphobic-social phobic-claustrophobic patient, with a fear of being far from home)

Constructcomponent I														
C1 displeasing	1.00													
C2 dark	.86	1.00												
C3 sombre	.91	.94	1.00											
C4 low ceiling	.29	–	–	1.00										
C5 bend in tunnel	−.42	−.54	−.51	–	1.00									
C6 narrow tunnel	.44	–	–	.71	–	1.00								
C7 traffic tunnel	−.06	–	–	–	–	–	1.00							
C8 strange	.81	78	.77	–	–	–	–	1.00						
C9 other people inaccessible	−.83	−.77	−.84	–	–	−.54	–	−.55	1.00					
C10 unsafe	.67	.70	.69	.52	–	–	–	.78	−.53	1.00				
C11 exit far off	−.11	–	–	–	–	–	.67	–	–	–	1.00			
C12 long tunnel	−.01	–	–	−.57	–	–	.75	–	–	–	.63	1.00		
C13 no people	.71	.54	.60	–	–	.50	–	–	−.74	–	–	–	1.00	
C14 difficult to oversee	.69	.73	.63	–	–	–	–	–	−.72	.50	–	–	.61	1.00

N.B. The underlined r-values show which constructs on the second component are significantly correlated. None of the constructs on the third component are significantly correlated.

Table 5.1h. Intercorrelations between constructcomponents for S 4 (travel phobic-and tunnel phobic patient, with a fear of being far from home)

Constructcomponent I

C1 displeasing	1.00												
C2 cars	.64	1.00											
C3 traffic tunnel	.58	.90	1.00										
C4 long tunnel	.77	.87	.79	1.00									
C5 a real tunnel	.71	.80	73	.97	.100								
C6 exit far off	.58	–	.57	.66	.64	1.00							
C7 suffocating	.85	.66	.59	.80	.76	.63	1.00						
C8 exit not visible	.30	–	.52	–	.68	.68	–	1.00					
C9 lonely	.73	–	–	–	–	–	.74	–	1.00				
C10 difficult to oversee	.65	–	–	–	–	–	.50	–	.65	1.00			
C11 no possibility to turn away	.30	–	–	.57	.57	–	.54	–	–	–	1.00		
C12 sombre	.75	–	–	–	–	.65	.65	–	.58	.61	–	1.00	
C13 narrow opening	.69	–	–	–	–	.54	.69	–	.71	.70	–	.58	1.00

Constructcomponent II

C1 displeasing	1.00										
C2 cars	.64	1.00									
C3 traffic tunnel	.58	–	1.00								
C9 lonely	.73	–	–	1.00							
C10 difficult to oversee	.65	–	–	.65	1.00						
C13 narrow opening	.69	–	–	.71	.70	1.00					
C14 don't know were you are	.43	–	–	–	–	.51	1.00				
C15 no people	–.03	–	.63	–	–	–	–	1.00			
C18 narrow	.36	–	–	–	–	.63	.65	.58	1.00		
C19 dark	.37	–	–	–	.53	–	–	–	–	1.00	
C20 quiet	.11	–	–	–	–	.50	–	.66	51	–	1.00

Constructcomponent III

C6 exit far off	1.00			
C8 exit not visible	.58	1.00		
C16 end of tunnel	–	–.61	1.00	
C20 quiet	–	–	–	1.00

N.B. Except on "displeasingness" r-values < .50 are not shown.

Appendix B: Means and standard deviations for the different variables in studies II–V; and mean z-scores for the subgroups manifesting different strategies

Table 6.1a (depth estimation – normals) and **Table 6.1b** (perceived enclosure – phobics). Means and s.ds on the variables depth estimation and perceived enclosure of architectural spaces as a function of H/D and B/D ratios; and mean z-scores for the different subgroups, manifesting different strategies [Study III]

Depth estimation (Normals; n = 33)					Perceived enclosure (Phobics; n = 32)					
	H/D ratio					H/D ratio				
	.25	.50	.75	1.00		.25	.50	.75	1.00	
	(15)	(30)*	(45)	(60)						
Means	39.36	41.37	44.61	47.81		3.23	3.67	4.00	4.12	
s.d.	13.48	13.88	22.12	21.82		1.47	1.17	1.12	1.33	
Mean z-scores for the subgroups:										
N1(n = 18)	−.61	−.57	−.43	−.56	P1(n = 4)	−.91	−.73	−.76	−.82	as a
N2(n = 6)	.57	.71	−.07	−.40	P2(n = 3)	1.31	.63	−.31	−.82	function
N3(n = 4)	−.31	.47	.46	.96	P3(n = 6)	−.47	−.28	.25	.58	of B/D
N4(n = 5)	1.75	.82	1.26	1.71	P4(n = 3)	.86	1.06	.81	.76	ratio: 1.0
Mean z-scores for the subgroups:										
N5(n = 1)	2.27	1.34	4.28	1.28	P5(n = 5)	−.13	−.67	−1.02	−.88	as a
					P6(n = 5)	−.90	−.23	.27	.41	function
					P7(n = 6)	1.03	.79	.63	.41**	of B/D
					P8(n = 1)	−2.08	−2.91	−3.03	−3.67	ratio:.50

* = standard stimulus in depth estimationtask   ** see text for explanation

Table 6.1c Means and s.ds on the variable perceived complexity in abstract stimuli, as a function of six classes of complexity and two levels of complexity (Simple and Complex); and mean z-scores for the different subgroups (phobic patients) [Study IV]

Collative variables		I	II	III	IV	V	VI	
Means	S	1.53	2.24	1.54	1.86	1.84	1.91	S = simple stimulus
(n = 24)	C	1.61	3.54	3.60	5.10	3.48	3.84	C = complex stimulus
s.d.	S	.79	1.73	1.32	.91	1.10	1.32	
s.d.	C	.87	1.95	1.66	1.61	1.80	1.64	
Mean z-scores for subgroups:								
P1 (n = 16)	S	−.46	−.54	−.41	−.15	−.28	−.01	
	C	−.46	−.39	−.16	−.03	−.08	−.16	
P2 (n = 5)	S	.76	.70	.20	.99	.46	−.37	
	C	.53	1.16	−.03	−.02	−.03	.17	
P3 (n = 2)	S	.59	2.26	1.49	−.91	−.64	−.72	
	C	1.60	−.79	.82	−.59	.22	−1.41	
P4 (n = 1)	S	1.86	.43	2.62	−.91	3.04	3.72	
	C	1.60	1.77	.82	1.27	.78	1.92	

Table 6.1d Means and s.ds on the variable perceived complexity in street situations, as a function of five levels of complexity for normal subjects and phobic patients; and mean z-scores for the different subgroups [Study V]

Subjects	Complexity levels I	II	III	IV	V					
Means						s.d.				
N1 (n = 30)	2.32	2.35	2.61	3.57	4.90	.79	.79	.74	.90	1.12
N2 (n = 20)	2.21	1.90	2.72	3.86	5.09	.75	.67	.92	1.00	.83
(combined): (n = 50)	2.27	2.17	2.65	3.69	4.98	.78	.74	.82	.98	1.01
Phobics (n = 12)	1.87	2.23	2.89	4.21	5.31	.85	1.28	1.89	1.78	1.57
Mean z-scores for subgroups:										
N1 (n = 22)	.61	.74	.37	.11	.01		N = normals			
N2 (n = 17)	−.84	−.54	−.70	−.74	−.33		P = phobics			
N3 (n = 9)	−.54	−.68	−.09	.68	.60					
N4 (n = 2)	2.43	1.19	.63	−.64	−1.46					
P1 (n = 3)	−.40	−.32	.15	.85	1.22					
P2 (n = 4)	−1.17	−1.54	−1.47	−1.21	−1.52					
P3 (n = 3)	−.87	2.27	2.59	2.02	1.49					
P4 (n = 2)	1.15	.66	.56	1.69	1.80					

Table 6.1e Mean z-scores for tunnel phobics and other phobics, and normal subjects with respect to the experiential variables "funneling effect", "busyness or crowdedness", and "darkness, dismalness or sombreness" in (car-, bicycle-, and pedestrian-)tunnels, corridors and street lanes [Study II]

Source	Funneling effect 1	2	(S)	4	Busyness/crowdedness 1	2	(S)	4	Darkness/dismalness etc. 1	2	3	4
Cartunnels:												
N1 (n = 3)	2.06	1.52	.05	(n = 4)	2.77	2.29	−1.52	(n = 4)	.27	.18	1.95	1.15
N2 (n = 2)	−.14	.05	−.65	(n = 1)	−.91	1.69	−2.64	(n = 1)	−.11	−1.10	−1.10	.88
P1 (n = 10)	2.66	2.11	.04	(n = 9)	2.00	1.66	−1.52	(n = 10)	−.08	1.16	2.00	.59
Bicycle/pedestriantunnels:												
N1 (n = 3)	2.13	1.02	−.88	(n = 4)	2.59	2.17	−.24	(n = 4)	.16	1.89	.40	.69
N2 (n = 2)	−1.05	−.66	−1.61	(n = 1)	−2.76	−2.55	1.36	(n = 1)	1.98	2.22	2.64	3.30
P1 (n = 9)	1.82	1.38	−1.13	(n = 3)	1.12	2.32	1.95	(n = 9)	1.35	1.20	.01	.69
P2 (n = 1)	−1.90	−2.31	−.09	(n = 6)	2.69	1.31	−.98	(n = 1)	−1.11	−1.81	2.64	−.37
			P3	(n = 1)	0.00	−.54	−.57					
Corridors:												
N1 (n = 4)	.94	.51	−.72	(n = 5)	2.79	1.27	−2.74	(n = 3)	2.50	1.34	1.66	.40
N2 (n = 1)	−1.11	−.29	−.90									
P1 (n = 10)	2.25	1.52	−.56	(n = 6)	2.91	1.27	−2.46	(n = 9)	2.65	1.35	1.94	.68
			P2	(n = 3)	−.16	.01	−1.51	(n = 1)	−.99	−.94	−1.87	.90
			P3	(n = 1)	−3.30	−.54	−1.65					
Street lanes:												
N1 (n = 3)	2.36	2.75	−1.36	(n = 5)	2.13	2.08	−1.47	(n = 5)	2.45	1.63	.73	.09
N2 (n = 2)	.04	1.42	−.59									
P1 (n = 8)	1.65	1.52	−.99	(n = 9)	3.23	2.56	−1.09	(n = 2)	−2.00	−2.25	−1.76	2.12
P2 (n = 2)	0.00	.59	−.05	(n = 1)	0.08	−.23	−1.57	(n = 8)	3.03	2.34	.54	.38

(S) = position standard stimulus. No further analyses of variance were carried out on these groups, but these few deviating subjects are used as a further illustration. We know from Chapter V, that normals and phobics did not differ on perceived complexity, responding in similar ways to all levels of stimulation.

Appendix C: Table 7.1 items of the questionnaire Perceptual disorientation, derealization and depersonalization (derived from Cappon et al., 1961)

Item number:* [Perceptual disorientation]

Have you ever had the awareness that:

13. The space around you seems to become smaller, while you know that in fact it has not changed?
14. The space around you seems to become larger, while you know that in fact it has not changed?
19. Time seems to pass much faster, while you know that in fact it has not changed?
20. Time seems to pass much slower, while you know that in fact it has not changed?
15. Your body, or some part of it, seems to become smaller, while you know that in fact it has not changed?
16. Your body, or some part of it, seems to become larger, while you know that in fact it has not changed;
21. Your body, or some part of it, seems to become lighter, while you know that in fact it has not changed?
22. Your body, or some part of it, seems to become heavier, while you know that in fact it has not changed?
23. Your body, or some part of it, seems to be moving in space (e.g., whirling), while you know this is not actually so?
25. Your body or some part of it, seems to change its position or place in space, while you know this is not actually so?
17. Objects or people around you seem to become smaller, while you know this is not actually so?
18. Objects or people around you seem to become larger, while you know this is not actually so?
24. Objects or people around you seem to be moving in space (e.g., whirling), while you know this is not actually so?
26. Objects or people around you seem to change their position or place in space, while you know this is not actually so?

[Derealization]

1. Space seems to be infinite?
2. Space seems to be collapsed (*ineengeschrompeldlijkt)*?
5. Time seems to be infinite or nonexistent?
4. Objects or people around you seem to disappear into space or melt into space?
9. Objects or people around you seem to be floating in a strange or unreal way, and are coming up close (*opjeafkomen*)?
12. You are in an unreal world in which objects or people around you seem strange and unreal?
27. The colour or brightness of objects in your surroundings seem to become stronger than is usually the case?
28. The colour or brightness of objects in your surroundings seems to become weaker than is usually the case?
29. Sounds of people, animals, or objects seem duller, more muffled or farther away than is usually the case?
30. Sounds of people, animals, or objects seem harsher, more penetrating, or nearer than is usually the case?
31. Objects seem to feel warmer and look more vivid than is usually the case?
32. Objects seem to feel chilly and look more lifeless than is usually the case?
34. You have little or no control over people or objects in your surroundings?

[Depersonalization]

Item number:* [Perceptual disorientation]	
3.	Your body, or some part of it, disappears or melts into space;
6.	Your body, or some part of it, becomes weightless?
7.	Your body, or some part of it, sinks into the earth or space?
8.	Your body, or some part of it, floats in a strange or unreal way?
10.	You are outside your body, or apart from it?
11.	You feel as if you were someone else?
13.	You are losing control over yourself or in danger of doing so?

* The item numbers denote the order in which the item appeared on the questionnaire.

Name Index

Subject Index